Journal of Chromatography Library — Volume 1

CHROMATOGRAPHY OF ANTIBIOTICS

JOURNAL OF CHROMATOGRAPHY LIBRARY

Volume 1   Chromatography of Antibiotics
           by G.H. Wagman and M.J. Weinstein

Journal of Chromatography Library — Volume 1

CHROMATOGRAPHY OF ANTIBIOTICS

Gerald H. Wagman, Manager
Antibiotics Research Department, Schering Corporation, Bloomfield, New Jersey

Marvin J. Weinstein, Director
Microbiology Research Division, Schering Corporation, Bloomfield, New Jersey

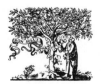

ELSEVIER SCIENTIFIC PUBLISHING COMPANY
AMSTERDAM — LONDON — NEW YORK 1973

ELSEVIER SCIENTIFIC PUBLISHING COMPANY
335 Jan van Galenstraat
P.O. Box 1270, Amsterdam, The Netherlands

AMERICAN ELSEVIER PUBLISHING COMPANY, INC.
52 Vanderbilt Avenue
New York, New York 10017

Library of Congress Card Number: 72-97439

ISBN: 0-444-41106-2

Printed in The Netherlands

ACKNOWLEDGEMENTS

We wish to express our appreciation for the valuable assistance given to us by the Library Staff of the Schering Research Laboratories, in particular to Mrs. Corinne McGee for literature searches and to Dr. Elizabeth Shecket for some of the translations. Also, we thank Mrs. Alyson Cooper for transcription of data and we especially acknowledge the work of Mrs. Patricia Bzdek whose tireless efforts in typing the entire manuscript helped make this book possible. Special thanks are extended to Dr. Preston L. Perlman, Vice President Laboratory Research and the late Dr. Augustus Gibson, Vice President for Research and Development, for their kind consideration of this project.

The authors remember . . . . .

A little over twenty years ago, in the late 1940's and early 1950's the authors were engaged in antibiotic screening and other microbiological research projects; we remember well the introduction and development of the new analytical tool, paper chromatography. It was finding its place in the analysis of various biologically interesting substances such as alkaloids, steroids, vitamins, amino acids and finally antibiotics.

Researchers struggled with this new technique in antibiotic screening which moved the arena of discovery from the hallowed halls of the organic chemist closer to the corner laboratory of the microbiologist. With this new weapon, properly employed, it became possible to demonstrate differences among substances but not necessarily similarities. This is the goal of any screening program: one searches for novelty, not for sameness. The labors of the chemist could now be conserved for final chemical identification and physical characterization. The microbiologist was now able to declare with a good deal more confidence what the observed activities were not.

The use of paper, and later, thin layer chromatography, permitted antibiotic screening to make genuine advances. As increasing numbers of new antibiotics tumbled from the fermentation broths, identification of authentic discoveries became increasingly more difficult. The search, however, is far from being over, and for the imaginative and perservering researcher, there are still useful agents to be found.

It is for the diligent screener that this book has been prepared. It is an antibioticist's *vade mecum*. We have found this data compilation on the chromatography of antibiotics most useful for our purposes and hope it will be found applicable and time saving for others.

This book is primarily for use as a consolidated reference for the specific chromatographic identification of antibiotics. As an operating manual, one might ask if this is a propitious time to introduce such a book. Hasn't the antibiotic discovery era come and gone? We think not. In spite of the frequent funereal pronouncements that the discovery of new antibiotics is in a moribund state, new entities are regularly brought to life. From our laboratory, during the past 10 years, the discovery of gentamicin, halomicin, everninomicin, megalomicin, rosamicin and sisomicin have been reported up to the time of this writing.

There was a hiatus in the discovery of clinically useful antibiotics from the middle 1950's, when kanamycin was discovered, until the Third Interscience Conference on Antimicrobial Agents and Chemotherapy, in 1963, when both lincomycin and gentamicin were announced. The utility of the new aminoglycoside, gentamicin, was unique with its wide spectrum of gram-negative activity, including *Pseudomonas* organisms, as well as activity against gram-positive bacteria, and most important, limited but definable and minimal toxicity. This initiated a re-evaluation of basic, resin extractable antibiotics which had been shelved in various screening program refrigerators. In the last few years a plethora of aminoglycoside antibiotics have been reported; tobramycin, kanendomycin, dideoxy-kanamycin B, ambutyrosine, negamycin, sisomicin and BBK-8, to name several.

This renaissance was by no means limited to aminoglycoside antibiotics. Indeed new polypeptides, ansamycins, macrolides and other novel chemical types have been discovered in recent years.

We believe that antibiotics are alive and well and will continue to be found. We offer this book as a guide to the investigator who takes up this hunt.

Bloomfield, N.J.
February, 1973

Gerald H. Wagman
Marvin J. Weinstein

TABLE OF CONTENTS

Chromatographic Classification of Antibiotics 1

Detection of Antibiotics on Chromatograms 7

Comments on the Use of this Index 13

Abbreviations 14

Index — Chromatography of Antibiotics 17

Index by Compound 225

CHROMATOGRAPHIC CLASSIFICATION OF ANTIBIOTICS

Over the years many investigators have devised numerous procedures for classification and identification of antibiotics by use of chromatographic techniques. In earlier years, these various chromatographic systems were quite usuable because of the relatively small number of antibiotics compared to the present. With the thousands of antibiotics currently known, systematic chromatographic classification of this large number of compounds is extremely difficult. It is possible to group many of these substances, but in order to identify very closely related antibiotics in a particular group the use of many additional chromatographic systems may be required. This book is not written as a means of systematic chromatography but hopefully as an aid in identifying very similar compounds by use of specific chromatographic techniques. A number of methods proposed for classification of antibiotics into groups and within groups will be reviewed for use in the preliminary or presumptive identification of some of these compounds. More definitive identification should be possible by selective use of the index comprising the body of the book.

In 1959 Miyazaki *et al.*[1] described a method of grouping antibiotics according to their salting out chromatograms. The antibiotics were examined by means of ascending paper chromatography. As solvents, distilled water and increasing concentrations of ammonium chloride (0.5 to 20% and saturated solution) were used. Location of the antibiotic zones were determined by bioautographic methods. Using this technique the antibiotics were divided into four major groups. In group A the R_f values were not correlated with the concentration of the ammonium chloride solution, identical values being found at all concentrations and in distilled water. Group B consisted of the antibiotics which had an R_f value of 0 in distilled water and increasing R_f values with increasing concentrations of ammonium chloride. Group C displayed the highest R_f value in distilled water and lowered values with increasing concentration of the ammonium chloride solution. Group D consisted of antibiotics which did not display any movement whatever in the solvent from the starting point. This systematic method was extended by Uri[2] who added two additional groups. Group E consisted of antibiotics which had an R_f value of 0 in distilled water and an initial increase with rising concentrations of ammonium chloride with the maximum (R_f approximately 1) in 5% salt solution. Beyond this a decrease occurred. This type of paper chromatogram was typical for the macrolides such as oleandomycin, erythromycin, and carbomycin. Within the macrolide group further differentiation was possible. An additional grouping, F, was made, which at that time consisted of only one antibiotic, desertomycin. By connecting the R_f values using a variety of concentrations of ammonium chloride solution paraboloid curves were obtained which were different for different antibiotics.

Paris and Theallet[3] were able to separate 23 antibiotics which were described in the French Pharmacopia into seven groups utilizing paper and TLC as well as electrophoresis. The groups were as follows: (1) penicillin and derivatives, (2) heterocyclic compounds containing amino groups such as the aminoglycosides, (3) macrolides, (4) tetracyclines, (5) chloramphenicol and viomycin, (6) polypeptides, and (7) polyenes.

Blinov and co-workers[4] in 1969 were able to separate over 300 antibacterial preparations into five groups according to a chromatographic scheme.

Probably the greatest single influence in the systematic analysis of antibiotics was that of Betina[5] who, in 1964, attempted to establish a systematic chromatographic separation of 62 known antibiotics. These were distributed into five classes and further into 14 sub-classes according to their R_f values in four principle solvent systems. Betina felt that antibiotics are a very heterogeneous group of biologically active compounds which cause great difficulty in working out systematic chromatographic analysis. Therefore he developed the analysis along the lines previously noted. By using what are referred to as "summarized chromatograms" it was possible to graph the R_f's of each antibiotic in a number of solvent systems. This results in a kind of curve or plot for an unknown which can be compared to plots of known antibiotics belonging to appropriate classes and sub-classes.

Betina further analyzed antibiotics by means of "pH-chromatography". By the use of this chromatographic method the ionic character of unknown antibiotics and also the general possibilities of their isolation can be determined. A series of strips of chromatographic papers impregnated with buffers in the range of pH 2–10 is used for each antibiotic. For the development of the chromatograms, an appropriate water-saturated organic solvent is used as the mobile phase. Salting out chromatography as described previously was also utilized to further characterize the antibiotics.

Using techniques previously described, Barath and co-workers[6] classified the antibiotics from crude concentrates of fermentation media and from the mycelia of 50 strains of soil fungi. Utilizing the systematic paper chromatographic methods with bioautographic techniques against *Bacillus subtilis*, *Escherichia coli*, *Saccharomyces cerevisiae* and *Candida pseudotropicalis*, the antibiotics were grouped into a series of classes which permitted the authors to choose strains that produced antibiotics with specific activities.

Utilization of hydrolysis–gas chromatography for differentiation and characterization of antibiotics was described by Brodasky[7]. In most cases, this information, together with conventional chromatography and infra-red and ultraviolet spectra, was sufficient to establish identity or dissimilarity. Both high and low temperature pyrolysis were described. The general lability of antibiotics makes them suitable compounds for pyrolysis studies. A number of examples of differentiation of antibiotics in both temperature ranges were given.

For screening of new antibiotics, Maeda *et al*.[8] have applied the use of high voltage paper electrophoresis for separation and identification of these substances. The relative mobilities of 92 antibiotics in two groups are listed according to their extraction properties. Antibiotics in Group 1 are those which are able to be extracted by solvent techniques. Most antibiotics assigned to Group 2 are adsorbed on weak cation exchange resins such as Amberlite® IRC 50 or strong cation exchange resins such as Amberlite ® IR 120.

The behavior of 16 antibiotics were examined by Dobrecky and co-workers[9] by means of thin layer chromatography using Silica Gel G, Aluminum Oxide G, and Cellulose MN300. A number of solvents were used. Antibiotic zones were detected by spraying with ninhydrin, sulfuric acid or by UV.

An extension of the classification of antibiotics by thin layer chromatography was proposed by Aszalos and co-workers[10]. The authors present what is called "instant thin layer chromatography (ITLC)" which attempts to rapidly assess the probability that an antibiotic in question is an already known one. The authors used 84 antibiotics in this study. They state that the method will not identify an individual antibiotic in a crude mixture but it will narrow the choice of identities to a small number. Thereafter, additional chemical, physical and microbiological testing are required to distinguish the individual antibiotics. The prime criteria employed by the authors in their method of classification was the occurrence of movement of an antibiotic in a specific solvent system. Analysis of the antibiotics tested utilizing 3 primary solvent systems produced a scheme containing four primary groups. Application of 11 additional solvent systems to the members of the four primary groups yielded 15 sub-groups. The authors state that differentiation of antibiotics based on the characteristics of the ITLC system is more reliable than is differentiation based on potentially misleading differences in R_f values. The only use made of R_f values in this scheme is to demonstrate the movement of the antibiotic.

Sephadex has been used in thin layer chromatography for the identification of antibiotics by Zuidweg et al.[11] With this medium a buffer solution was used instead of organic solvents. A combination of Sephadex TLC and bioautography was applied to qualitative analysis of mixtures of particular antibiotics. The authors stated that the advantage of the combination of Sephadex TLC and the bioautography is the elimination of false inhibition zones due to incomplete removal of inorganic solvents which sometimes occurs with conventional chromatographic methods. Descending chromatography was used and the layers were prepared by mixing Sephadex G-15 (40–120 μg) with 0.025 M phosphate buffer at pH 6.0 containing 0.5 M sodium chloride. The suspension was spread in a layer of 0.5 mm thickness and plates allowed to dry at room temperature for about 1 hour and then transferred to a moist chamber where they were kept in a horizontal position for at least 24 hours. Plates were run in sandwich arrangements using descending chromatography for about 60–90 minutes. After development the Sephadex chromatographic plates were pressed on seeded agar layers covered with a sheet of lens tissue paper and allowed to remain in contact for 30 minutes, the lens paper removed, and the agar plate incubated at the optimal growth temperature of the test organism. The organisms used were *Bacillus subtilis*, *Staphylococcus aureus* and *Saccharomyces cerevisiae*. Utilizing this technique 17 antibiotics were successfully separated.

Thin layer chromatography using Kieselgel G (Merck) was utilized by Schmitt and Mathis[12] for separation of 42 antibiotics. Utilizing three selective solvent systems, the authors were able to distribute these antibiotics into four groups. The antibiotics of closely related chemical composition generally fell in the same chromatographic group; for example, macrolides in group two, tetracyclines in group three and aminoglycosides in group four. A number of miscellaneous antibiotics fell into the first group. These included cephalosporins, penicillins, chloramphenicol, rifamycin, etc. The antibiotics were detected after development by two reagents containing paradimethylamino-benzaldehyde.

A number of systems have been proposed for classification of specifically related antibiotics as opposed to the previously discussed schemes for classification of a variety of antibiotic types. Yakima[13] was one of several investigators to propose a system for the classification of antifungal antibiotics. The author used summarized papergrams with six different solvent systems and compared the studies of this classification with results obtained by electrophoretograms, diffusion curves, antifungal spectrum and identification by ultraviolet absorption spectrum. Twenty four antifungal antibiotics were tested and were classified into 11 groups. It was difficult to differentiate closely related substances such as actidione and formicidin. However, it was concluded that the patterns obtained would be useful not only for the identification of antifungal agents produced in agar or broth but also for the selection of solvents employed in purification procedures. Using electrophoresis, diffusion curves and antifungal spectrum, correlations such as were found by solvent extractabilities or solvent solubilities were unable to be differentiated. Utilizing the summarized papergram system, the author could classify 17 antifungal substances produced by streptomyces into seven groups, four substances produced by fungi into two groups, and three substances produced by bacteria into two groups.

At approximately the same time Ammann and Gottlieb[14] worked out a paper chromatographic technique for the separation of antifungal antibiotics on the basis of their R_f values in five solvent systems. Rather than utilizing the summarized papergram method, the authors described R_f values of 15 antifungal antibiotics, six of which also showed antibacterial activity, by utilizing a flow chart for the separation of the agents on the basis of the chromatographic data.

In 1956, paper chromatography followed by bioautography was shown to be useful for differentiating antibiotics produced by the *Bacillus* species in a screen program by Snell and co-workers[15]. Most of the antibiotics active against gram positive bacteria and several polypeptide antibiotics produced by other microorganisms have been separated. A solvent mixture of *t*-butanol, acetic acid and water proved to be most satisfactory ry for giving a good initial spread of the entire group of antibiotics tested. After determination of the rate of movement in the first solvent, a series of additional solvent systems were used for specific areas of mobility in order to eventually separate the antibiotics. One of the major difficulties in this system is the fact that most of the organisms produced a multiplicity of antibiotics and the production of only one antibiotic appeared to be the exception rather than the rule. Thus, if a major spot was readily observed, it was more easy to key the particular antibiotic.

Blinov and co-workers[16] worked out a scheme for classification of antibiotics having indicator properties by means of paper chromatography. They applied a paper chromatographic method to a study of over 20 preparations of indicator antibiotics (blue in an alkaline medium and red in an acid medium). These authors showed that the antibiotics under study contained not less than 15 different compounds which were divided into five groups. The largest group, the mycetin—violarin group was partitioned into approximately 10 different components. A classification scheme was suggested for these antibiotics which enables rapid comparison of the isolated antibiotic with at least 15 different compounds of this group.

Thin layer chromatography was utilized by Ikekawa *et al.*[17] for resolving approximately 50 antibiotics utilizing seven different solvent systems. The method used Silica Gel G TLC plates and detection of the spots with 10% potassium permanganate and 0.2% bromophenyl blue solution or by color reactions characteristic to the particular antibiotic under test. Of particular interest are several solvent systems for separation of certain groups of antibiotics. Chromatography using ethanol:conc. ammonium hydroxide:water (8:1:1) was useful for the macrolide antibiotics as a group. Propanol:pyridine:acetic acid:water (15:10:3:12) was useful for differentiating the water soluble basic antibiotics. Differentiation of peptide antibiotics was accomplished with butanol:acetic acid:water (3:1:1) and ethanol:conc. ammonium hydroxide:water (8:1:1) was useful for identification of the polyene antibiotics. The solvent system selected by the thin layer chromatography can be applied to column chromatography for preparative separations.

Using the solvent system propanol:pyridine:acetic acid:water (15:10:3:12) on cellulose powder thin layer plates gave excellent separations of the water-soluble antibiotics according to Ito *et al.*[18] Ninhydrin reagents or oxidized nitroprusside reagent were used as the identification system. Based on R_f and color, 20 basic antibiotics were separated. For six closely related compounds in terms of R_f, the solvent system consisting of water-saturated butanol plus 2% p-toluenesulfonic acid was successful in differentiation.

A number of schemes for identification of antibiotics of the macrolide group have been composed. Sokolski and co-workers[19] were able to chromatograph some of the macrolide antibiotics by using Whatman No. 1 paper and 11 different solvent systems. Igloy et al.[20] felt that the solvent systems proposed were not completely satisfactory for separation of closely related macrolides. In their experiments they endeavored to formulate solvent systems which allowed for maximum separation of the macrolide antibiotics from other antibiotics together with maximum separation of individual members within this group, and furthermore allowed the reproducible estimation of samples of low biological activity. The principal of the separation method is based on the structural specificity of macrolide antibiotics and utilizes Schleicher—Schüll 2043/b paper strips with four solvent systems. Chromatograms were bioautographed against B. subtilis. The solvent systems in each case contained a polar and a non-polar solvent; the water content of the mixtures were standardized by shaking with 1/10 volume of a 30% aqueous sodium chloride solution. The adjustment of the pH of the paper was carried out by impregnating it with M/phosphate buffers of pH 4.7, 6.0, 7.0 and 8.0 respectively. The most effective solvent mixtures were composed of an alcohol and a non-polar solvent saturated with a concentrated solution of sodium chloride, and buffered to various pH values with mixtures of organic acids and bases. The solvents tested were shown to be suitable for the identification of these antibiotics in fermentation broths of the producing organisms. More recently, Silica Gel G thin layer plates were utilized by Ochab and Borowiecka[21] for separation of the macrolide group, which these authors state were difficult to identify on paper. Out of 17 solvent systems investigated, four were found to be the most useful. After development, plates were dried at room temperature for 1 hour at $100-110°$ for about 20 minutes and sprayed with a 0.05% solution of xanthydrol in glacial acetic acid with 2 ml of concentrated HCl, and finally with a 10% solution of phosphomolybdic acid in ethanol. After heating, various colors dependent on the macrolide tested were formed. With the four solvent systems used, by noting the R_f and the color it was possible to separate five of the more common macrolide antibiotics.

One of the latter authors (Borowiecka)[21] devised a thin layer technique for chromatography of glycosidic antibiotics. Group separation was obtained with all solvent systems tested with a thin layer composed of Kieselgel G plus Kieselguhr G (1:2). Similarly, Roets and Vanderhaeghe[22] utilized different color reactions and chromatographic systems on paper or Silica Gel thin layer plates for the identification of 14 aminoglycoside and peptide antibiotics.

Cephalosporin C and its semi-synthetic derivatives have been separated and identified by thin layer chromatography using Silica Gel G layers by Buri[23]. Using heat activated plates and a solvent consisting of isopropanol:methanol:pH 5 buffer (30:105:15) and spraying the developed, dried plates with an iodine-starch detection system it was possible to separate the cephalosporins and their derivatives.

Thin layer chromatography of compounds with chelating ability, particularly a variety of tetracyclines and their derivatives, was carried out by Nishimoto and co-workers[24]. Silica Gel thin layer plates pretreated with disodium-EDTA were utilized with excellent results. Changes in the behavior of tetracycline and oxytetracycline with pH and temperature were studied and the effects of citric acid, boric acid and Ca^{++} on these compounds were determined.

It is not possible to go into details of all of the aforementioned chromatographic methods for differentiating various antibiotics because of the enormous amount of data in some of the publications reviewed here. It is suggested that direct examination of the publications mentioned should be made in order to better evaluate the system or systems most useful for particular separations. It is hoped that this book will be useful in aiding in the positive identification of these antibiotics or antibiotic complexes separated by preliminary systematic chromatography.

REFERENCES

1 J. Miyazaki, K. Omachi and T. Kamata, *J. Antibiotics*, 6 (1953) 6.
2 J. Uri, *Nature*, 183 (1959) 1188–1189.
3 R. Paris and J.-P. Theallet, *Ann. Pharm. Franc.*, 20 (1962) 436–442.
4 N.O. Blinov, E.P. Oparysheva, Yu.M. Khokhlova, A.V. Lesnikova, K.M. Khryashcheva and A.S. Khokhlov, *Antibiotiki*, 14 (1969) 275–287.
5 V. Betina, *J. Chromatog.*, 15 (1964) 379–392.
6 Z. Barath, V. Betina and P. Nemec, *J. Antibiotics*, 17 (1964) 144–147.
7 T.F. Brodasky, *J. Gas Chromatog.*, 5 (1967) 311–318.
8 K. Maeda, A. Yagi, H. Naganawa, S. Kondo and H. Umezawa, *J. Antibiotics*, 22 (1969) 635–636.
9 J. Dobrecky, E.A. Vazquez and R. Amper, *SAFYBI*, 8 (1968) 204–208; *Chem. Abstr.*, 71 (1969) 42362r.
10 A. Aszalos, S. Davis and D. Frost, *J. Chromatog.*, 37 (1968) 487–498.
11 M.H.J. Zuidweg, J.G. Oostendorp and C.J.K. Bos, *J. Chromatog.*, 42 (1969) 552–554.
12 J.-P. Schmitt and C. Mathis, *Ann. Pharm. Franc.*, 26 (1970) 205–210.
13 T. Yajima, *J. Antibiotics*, 8 (1955) 189–195.
14 A. Ammann and D. Gottlieb, *Appl. Microbiol.*, 3 (1955) 181–186.
15 N. Snell, K. Ijichi and J.C. Lewis, *Appl. Microbiol.*, 4 (1956) 13–17.
16 N.O. Blinov, G.Z. Yakubov, C.A. Betlugina and Yu.M. Khokhlova, *Mikrobiologiya*, 30 (1961) 642–650.
17 T. Ikekawa, F. Iwami, E. Akita and H. Umezawa, *J. Antibiotics*, 16 (1963) 56–57.
18 Y. Ito, M. Namba, N. Nagahama, T. Yamaguchi and T. Okuda, *J. Antibiotics*, 17 (1964) 218–219.
19 W.T. Sokolski, S. Ullmann, H. Koffler and P.A. Tetrault, *Antibiot. and Chemotherap.*, 4 (1954) 1057–1060.
20 M. Iglóy, A. Mizsei and I. Horvath, *J. Chromatog.*, 20 (1965) 295–298.
21 S. Ochab and B. Borowiecka, *Dissert. Pharm. Pharmacol.*, 20 (1968) 449–451.
22 B. Borowiecka, *Dissert. Pharm. Pharmacol.*, 22 (1970) 345–350.
23 E. Roets and H. Vanderhaeghe, *Pharm. Tijdschr. Belg.*, 44 (1967) 57–64; *Chem. Abstr.*, 67 (1967) 67633k.
24 P. Buri, *Pharm. Acta Helv.*, 42 (1967) 344–349.
25 Y. Nishimoto, E. Tsuchida and S. Toyoshima, *Yakugaku Zasshi*, 87 (1967) 516–523; *Chem. Abstr.*, 67 (1967) 67635n.

DETECTION OF ANTIBIOTICS ON CHROMATOGRAMS

Numerous methods are used for the detection of antimicrobial agents on chromatograms and these are divided into several categories; chemical detection by use of suitable reagents, bioautographic detection of biologically active components, the use of ultraviolet light for the detection of fluorescent or absorbing spots, and the use of radioisotopic scanning for radioactive antibiotics produced by the addition of tracers to the various media in which the antibiotics were produced, or by other means. Methods for visualization by chemical means or by ultraviolet light will not be discussed in any great detail because these techniques have been known and used for many years in the detection of numerous substances on chromatograms. Several of the more general and useful techniques for the detection of antibiotics will be discussed. Specific chemical methods are given for particular antibiotics listed in the index. Likewise, radioisotopic detection is described under the designated antibiotic to which it applies. General methodology will be mentioned. Because of its extreme importance to the detection of antibiotics on both paper and thin layer plates, various bioautographic techniques will be explored in some detail.

Bioautography of developed chromatograms is carried out by similar methods in most laboratories. The authors use Pyrex baking dishes approximately 8.5 inches wide by 13.5 inches long by 1.75 inches deep ($21.6 \times 34.3 \times 4.4$ centimeters) with stainless steel covers. Similar types of flat dishes constructed of plate glass or plastic have also been used by numerous investigators.

A large variety of microorganisms including bacteria, fungi, and viruses have been used to detect various antibiotics under test. Typically, a 200 ml portion of a base layer agar is poured into a baking dish resting on a level surface and allowed to harden. To 100 ml of agar is added 1.0 ml of the working inoculum, mixed well, and poured on top of the base layer.

Occasionally, air bubbles form on the surface of the agar; if so, a Bunsen Burner flame can be passed rapidly over the agar to break them down. The plates are then allowed to harden. Or, a detergent can be incorporated in the medium.

A number of useful agar media can be found in two excellent books: Analytical Microbiology by Kavanaugh[1], or in Assay Methods of Antibiotics by Grove and Randall[2].

Paper chromatograms are placed in contact with the agar and allowed to remain so for a period of from several minutes to several hours depending on the organism that is used and the diffusibility of the antibiotic that has been chromatographed. In analytical techniques where paper strips are used to determine unknown quantities of antibiotics in samples for assay, the strips are placed evenly spaced on the seed layer of the agar, carefully laying them on the surface beginning at the origin. Generally, alternate standards and unknowns are plated if possible with no two like standards on a plate, such as described by Wagman et al[3]. In a number of techniques, in order to enhance zone sizes, the strips are allowed to diffuse at 20°C for 1 hour before being placed in a 37°C incubator. In all methods that are generally utilized for bioautography of the chromatograms, the plates are incubated for approximately 18 hours (overnight) and the zones of inhibition on the grown plates are ready for observation or measurement.

Bioautographic methodology can also be used for characterization of antiviral agents.

Herrmann and Rosselet[4] have described an adaptation of the Dulbecco virus-plaque technique[5] for this purpose. Paper chromatograms were sterilized by means of ethylene oxide after drying and were placed for 5 minutes on agar overlays of virus infected cultures. After removal of papers, baking dishes were sealed with Saran Wrap (Dow Chemical Co.), then incubated for 4 days at 36°C. The cell sheet was then stained with a second agar overlay containing indonitrotetrazolium chloride and within a few hours plaques were readily observed. It was found that zone sizes varied, dependent on the time after virus infection that the paper was applied to the agar. The longer the time period after infection, the smaller the zones were that were formed. When very sensitive tests are needed, the authors recommended applying the paper very soon after virus infection of overlay cultures. When sensitivity is not important but a more accurate determination of the area of antiviral activity is required, then application of the paper can be delayed.

Bioautography of thin layer chromatograms is used routinely for the detection of antimicrobial substances, but is somewhat more difficult to handle because of the inflexibility of a glass backed plate which does not always permit the layer to conform to the agar. This lack of contact between the entire surface and the agar can result in poorly defined or missing spots.

To avoid the adherence of the adsorbent to the agar surface a number of methods have been used. Probably the most common technique is that described by Meyers and Smith[6] who inserted a sheet of filter paper between the plate and the agar surface. Initially, the Meyers and Smith technique consisted of incubating the developed chromatographic plates for 16 hours at 4°C to allow diffusion of the antibiotic into the agar. The chromatographic plate and filter paper were removed and the seeded agar examined after an additional overnight incubation at 37°C. In order to avoid two overnight incubation periods the latter authors substituted *Streptococcus lactis*, facultative in respect to oxygen, as a replacement for *Staphylococcus aureus*. Using this culture it proved possible to obtain results after overnight incubation at 37°C with the chromatographic plates and filter paper laying on the agar surface. Growth of this organism occurred only under the area covered by the glass plate.

In our laboratories, however, we have modified this procedure to incubate the glass plate on the agar with a strip of Whatman No. 1 filter paper between the plate and the agar for periods ranging from several minutes to 1 hour. The paper and glass plate are both removed and the seeded agar incubated as is normal for paper chromatograms. We have had satisfactory results with a variety of microorganisms seeded in the agar using this technique; however, the zone sizes and diffusion rates are dependent upon the amount of material spotted on the chromatographic plate and the thickness and type of layer.

As a modification of the Meyers and Smith method, Meyers and Erikson[7] have altered the technique by incorporating 0.1% potassium nitrate into both the basal and seed agar layers described in the previous paper and have found that good growth of the organism occurred under the glass plate. The theory of this technique is that an organism would grow under these conditions if given a compound capable of replacing oxygen as an oxident in terminal respiration. Under the conditions described, the test organism was as sensitive to a variety of antibiotics as it was when paper chromatograms of the same antibiotics were tested.

Another technique for increasing visualization of the zones of inhibition is to incorporate tetrazolium dye in the agar overlay, or to add a solution of tetrazolium to the grown organism after incubation and let the agar stand for a length of time. Either method results in a reddish area of growth against a clear zone of inhibition. In general, addition of 1.0 ml of a 2% aqueous (w/v) solution of 2,3,5-triphenyl-2H-tetrazolium chloride per 100 ml of seed layer is satisfactory.

In order to enhance the visualization of the zones of inhibition, Begue and Kline[8] have tested a large variety of tetrazolium salts which are commercially available in order to determine the optimum conditions for color formation with these various compounds. Their conclusion was that not all tetrazolium salts will produce desired results and each investigator may have to find the best agent experimentally for his own system. Of the salts which were tested, the one which was generally most satisfactory was para-iodonitro-tetrazolium violet. This was sprayed as an aqueous solution at a concentration of 2 mg per ml after incubation and bioautograms allowed to react for approximately 30 minutes for *Bacillus subtilis* or *Sarcina lutea* and up to 2 hours as in the case of *Pseudomonas syringae*.

An interesting method used to plate thin layer chromatograms is described by Narasimhachari and Ramachandran[9] who used the method of taking a micro thin layer of the developed, dry thin layer chromatogram by pressing a transparent cellulose adhesive tape such as "Scotch" tape of suitable width on the thin layer plate. The Scotch tape is then carefully removed from the plate and gently tapped on the nonadhesive side to remove any loose adsorbent material. It is then stretched on a nutrient agar plate freshly seeded with a suitable test organism. It is important that the tape is fully stretched without any folds. The latter authors recommend testing to determine whether the tape or the solvent free adsorbent has any effect on the test organism. This is done by pressing a similar length of tape on the thin layer medium at a place where no compound was applied and then contacted on the seeded plate as a control strip. They found that neither the tape nor any of the adsorbent material had an inhibitory action on the test organisms used in their studies.

Several methods have been devised by Hamilton and Cook[10] while using the phyto-pathogenic organism *Xanthomonas pruni* which did not reduce tetrazolium dyes, is an obligate aerobe, and its normal growth is very slow. *X. pruni* hydrolyzes gelatin and starch and produces acid from several sugars. These characteristics can be made indirect indicators of growth. Gelatin hydrolysis as an indicator of microbial growth was determined by incorporating 0.4% gelatin into the nutrient agar. After the incubation period, the agar was flooded with a solution of 10% mercuric sulfate in 2.5 M hydrochloric acid which causes the unhydrolyzed gelatin to form a white precipitate. The zones of inhibition are white and the growth areas have the normal slight turbidity of nutrient agar. They determined starch hydrolysis as an indicator of microbial growth by incorporating 0.2% soluble starch into the nutrient agar. After incubation the agar was flooded with a mixture of 1% iodine in 2% aqueous potassium iodide. The unhydrolyzed starch forms a blue complex with iodine resulting in blue zones of inhibition and faint yellow areas of growth. Acid production was detected by incorporating bromcresol purple (1 ml of a 1.6% solution in ethanol per liter of medium) into nutrient agar containing 1% glucose. The microorganism produced slight amounts of diffusible acids and the zones of inhibition were purple and the growth areas were yellow.

Another interesting technique was devised by Homans and Fuchs[11] who found that it was possible to directly spray a thin layer chromatogram with a spore suspension of a fungus contained in a glucose minimal medium and which gave most reliable results. After locating UV absorbing spots, the chromatograms were sprayed with a conidial suspension of a fungus in a medium prepared as follows. The stock solution contains (per liter of tap water), 7 grams KH_2PO_4, 3 g $Na_2HPO_4 \cdot 2H_2O$, 4 g potassium nitrate, 1 g $MgSO_4 \cdot 7H_2O$ and 1 g sodium chloride. This solution is autoclaved at 120°C for twenty minutes. Just before making the conidial suspension, 10 ml of a 30% aqueous solution of glucose is added per 60 ml of this solution. During spraying, care should be taken to avoid the plates becoming too wet. After spraying, the thin layer plates are incubated at a moist atmosphere for two to three days at 25°C. Inhibition zones indicate the presence of the original fungitoxic product, plus if present, conversion or decomposition products which are fungitoxic. The authors have applied this technique to a number of compounds using many fungi such as *Aspergillus niger*, *Ascochyta pisi*, *Botrytis cinerea*, *Colletotrichum lindemuthianum*, *Fusarium colmorum* and *Penicillium expansum*, for example.

Thin layer chromatograms have the disadvantage of adherence of the absorbent to the agar surface when carrying out bioautographic methods. This problem can be avoided as shown by Wagman and Bailey[12] by the use of a silicic acid–glass fiber sheet (ChromAR sheet 500, code 2182, Mallinckrodt Chemical Works, St. Louis, Mo., U.S.A.). This sheet is composed of approximately 70% silicic acid and 30% micro fiber glass and can be cut to the desired size with a pair of scissors or a paper cutter. Although the sheet does not have high tensile strength, if one is careful it is easily handled. This medium has been used in our laboratories for some length of time with excellent results.

The ChromAR sheet has several advantages over TLC plates: (1) it conforms entirely to the agar surface, making complete contact; (2) the adsorbent does not adhere to the agar, therefore no paper need be used to separate the sheet from the agar; (3) much lower levels of antibiotic often need to be spotted compared to TLC plates, apparently due to a more efficient transfer of material from sheet to agar; and (4) in a number of chromatographic solvent systems development was up to twice as rapid as with TLC plates.

Visualization of antibiotics on chromatograms by chemical means are essentially the same as for numerous other compounds which are routinely separated by chromatography. Probably the most common reagent is ninhydrin which is primary used for detection of amino acids. This reagent is extremely satisfactory for detecting aminoglycoside and polypeptide antibiotics, and a variety of other amino-containing compounds. Because various investigators have their own preferences in making up ninhydrin solutions, the methodology for preparing each of these sprays is discussed under the individual antibiotics in the Index. Another reagent not usually used in most chromatographic methods but which is useful in antibiotic detection, particularly for those antibiotics containing a guanidine group such as streptomycin and viomycin, is the Sakaguchi reagent. An excellent method for detection of Sakaguchi positive antibiotics is described by Szilagyi and Szabo[13] by use of n-bromosuccinimide. The chromatographic paper strips were dipped into a 0.01% solution of 1-naphthol in 5% methanolic sodium hydroxide, dried in air, and the spots developed by a cooled 0.5% solution of n-bromosuccinimide and stabilized by a 40% solution of urea. A red color develops in the presence of Sakaguchi positive compounds.

One very useful compound for location of spots on thin layer chromatograms is iodine vapor. This is most easily accomplished by placing some crystals of iodine in the bottom of a small glass chromatographic chamber, covering with a glass top, and simply standing the dried thin layer chromatogram in the jar. Upon exposure to the iodine vapor, brownish yellow spots corresponding to those antibiotics which are positive to the iodine, can be recognized. An alternative technique is to make a saturated solution of iodine in petroleum ether and either dip or spray the plate with this solution. Similar results to exposure to iodine vapor are found. Studies by Brown and Turner[14] have indicated that neither calcium sulfate (present as a binder in the silica gel) nor ultraviolet sensitizer affect the rate of iodination. Furthermore, results are unchanged when plates are dried at 80°C prior to iodination, to insure that no traces of organic solvent remain absorbed on the silica gel as a reaction medium. The only disadvantage to this technique is that the color fades rapidly as the plates are exposed to air. The degree of fading can be reduced somewhat by covering the chromatogram with glass.

Radioisotopic scanning for labelled antibiotics will not be discussed here. Several methods are noted under specific antibiotics in the Index. However, a technique for autoradiography of thin layer radiochromatograms utilizing Polaroid film have been developed by Tio and Sisenwine[15] which bears noting for permanent records of these TLC plates. The authors have constructed a light-tight casette for $4 \times 5''$ Polaroid type 57 or 58 film packets. The film holder with the front side of the packet (that is the side normally toward the lens) facing the radiochromatogram is inserted into the holder and the protective envelope is then withdrawn. Exposure times depend upon the activity of the material on the TLC plates. For details on construction it is suggested that the original paper be consulted. A typical radiochromatogram containing 10,000 d.p.m. of $[^{14}C]$ glycine and 1 million d.p.m. of $[^{3}H]$ valine was exposed to Polaroid type 57 film (black and white) for 96 hours. The same radiochromatogram, when exposed to Polaroid type 58 film gave a positive print after 240 hours which exhibited a very faint blue area due to the tritiated material and greenish white area due to ^{14}C. Greater activities of tritium or longer exposure time produced brighter areas. The whiteness of the ^{14}C also increased on longer exposure times. For type 57 film exposures were similar to those for autoradiographs on X-ray film using a wet process development. In particular, the ability to differentiate ^{14}C and ^{3}H makes this method useful in studies where doubly labelled antibiotics must be chromatographed and recorded.

One additional technique for removing chromatographic layers bears note. This method, described by Kuranz[16] is useful for removal of the active silica gel layer from Eastman Chromagram Sheet and for its subsequent replication. The author has found that by firmly pressing number 810 Magic Mending Tape (Minnesota Mining and Manufacturing Co., St. Paul, Minnesota, U.S.A.) over the chromatogram and subsequently removing it, the silica gel layer can be transferred almost intact from the supporting plastic adhesive layer of the tape. Since the thickness of the tape is in the order of 0.0027 inches the thickness of the chromatogram has been greatly reduced. This method is very useful for producing replicates of single chromatograms and it is very satisfactory for inclusion in notebooks or for other permanent record storage. The author further states that this process can be repeated several times to produce multiple, though obviously less distinct, copies.

Some additional techniques have been found useful in our laboratories for the chromatography of antibiotics and will be briefly described.

A useful method for increasing the detection sensitivity of paper strips during bioautography is to leave them in contact with the agar surface throughout the incubation period, thus increasing the diffusion of even trace quantities of antibiotics present and making such zones readily apparent. Another interesting method, particularly for aminoglycoside antibiotics, is to bioautograph paper chromatograms after first spraying with ninhydrin and developing the color; colored areas and zones of activity can be easily correlated, since in most instances enough active substances remain to give zones of inhibition on the seeded agar plates.

Many chemical methods used for detection of a variety of substances are also useful for location of antibiotics. For both paper and TLC numerous reagents described in Spot Tests in Organic Analysis by Feigl[17] can be utilized to detect antibiotics on chromatograms. One method useful for TLC spot detection that we have found particularly helpful is charring with sulfuric acid, i.e. concentrated sulfuric acid in methanol is sprayed onto a developed, preheated (110°C) thin layer plate. This results in dark zones against a white background and is a very sensitive detection agent for many antibiotics. Finally, chromatography of antibiotic hydrolysates followed by a ninhydrin spray is a useful "fingerprint" technique for comparison of similar substances, most particularly for identification of aminoglycosides.

For measurement of R_f's a very simple, reliable tool is a piece of elastic tape marked with ten equal calibrations and subdivisions (0 to 1.0). This can be mounted with the zero end held fast to a strip of metal and a movable clamp attached to the opposite end of the tape. The "0" is positioned at the origin and the "1.0" placed at the front. The R_f can then be read directly from the scale opposite the antibiotic zone.

A rapid, simple means of recording chromatographic data is the use of Polaroid equipment. Even an elementary camera on an inexpensive stand can be used for photographing chromatograms or bioautographic plates. These can be copied in color or black and white and used as permanent laboratory records and are available immediately after photography.

Other specific techniques for detection of particular antibiotics will be discussed under chromatography of the antibiotic in the Index.

REFERENCES

1 F. Kavanaugh, Editor, *Analytical Microbiology* (1963). Academic Press, New York.
2 D.C. Grove and W.A. Randall; *Assay Methods of Antibiotics. A Laboratory Manual* (1955). Medical Encyclopedia, Inc., New York.
3 G.H. Wagman, E.M. Oden and M.J. Weinstein, *Appl. Microbiol.*, 16 (1968) 624—627.
4 E.C. Herrmann and J.-P. Rosselet, *Proc. Soc. Expt. Biol. and Med.*, 104 (1960) 304—306.
5 R. Dulbecco, *Proc. Nat. Acad. Sci.*, 38 (1952) 747.
6 E. Meyers and D.A. Smith, *J. Chromatog.*, 14 (1964) 129—132.
7 E. Meyers and R.C. Erickson, *J. Chromatog.*, 26 (1967) 531—532.
8 W.J. Begue and R.M. Kline, *J. Chromatog.*, 64 (1972) 182—184.
9 N. Narasimhachari and S. Ramachandran, *J. Chromatog.*, 27 (1967) 494.
10 P.B. Hamilton and C.E. Cook, *J. Chromatog.*, 35 (1968) 295—296.
11 A.L. Homans and A. Fuchs, *J. Chromatog.*, 51 (1970) 327—329.
12 G.H. Wagman and J.V. Bailey, *J. Chromatog.*, 41 (1969) 263—264.
13 I. Szilagyi and I. Szabo, *Nature*, 181 (1958) 52—53.
14 W. Brown and A.B. Turner, *J. Chromatog.*, 26 (1967) 518—519.
15 C.O. Tio and S.F. Sisenwine, *J. Chromatog.*, 48 (1970) 555—557.
16 R. Kuranz, *J. Chromatog.*, 28 (1967) 446.
17 F. Feigl, *Spot Tests in Organic Analysis*, 7th edn. (1966). Elsevier Publishing Co., Amsterdam.

COMMENTS ON THE USE OF THIS INDEX

The index which follows is divided into two major sections; the first segment lists antibiotics in alphabetical order. The second segment lists numbered or letter/number combinations of antibiotics so designated in the literature. Antibiotics which have not been assigned names or numbers are listed under the organism from which they were derived. These organisms will be found in the generalized alphabetical sequence.

The chromatographic methods for those antibiotics listed are presented in the following order: paper chromatography (PC), thin layer chromatography (TLC), electrophoresis (ELPHO), counter current distribution (CCD), and gas chromatography (GSC, GLC). In numerous instances one or more of the items shown under each heading may have been left blank. This is because either no information regarding the particular feature was presented in the literature or it was not clearly defined. For example, in paper chromatography the type of paper used may not be given. In most instances, it can usually be assumed that a paper such as Whatman No. 1 will suffice and that other substitutes will also be satisfactory. R_f values on other papers may not be identical to those presented in the literature. However, it was felt that in most of these cases enough information could be gleaned to make the system or systems described of some use in the laboratory. In those techniques where detection methodology is not given, it can usually be assumed that a bioautographic method was used or can be used against a sensitive organism.

In many descriptions the R_f values are noted to be estimated. In general these were derived as accurately as possible from photographs, drawings, or graphic reproductions of mobilities as closely as could be determined. In order to enable comparisons to be made with other chromatographic systems described in the index, it was felt that this data would be more useful rather than to punctuate the text with numerous and varied types of illustrations.

Solvent proportions shown in the text are in all instances presumed to be ratios by volume unless otherwise noted.

A listing of abbreviations which are used in the index is found on the following pages.

ABBREVIATIONS

Most of the abbreviations follow those used in the Journal of Chromatography.

A	amperes
abs.	absolute; e.g. abs. alcohol
A.F.S.	amperes full scale
aq.	aqueous
atm	atmosphere
av.	average
b.p.	boiling point
C	Celsius, centigrade
ca.	about
calc.	calculated
CCD	counter-current distribution
Ci	Curie
C	Coulombs
cm	centimeter
conc.	concentrated
concn.	concentration (c or C in formulas)
const.	constant
corr.	corrected
c.p.m.	counts per minute
$E^{1\%}_{1\,cm}$	extinction coefficient (1% solution, 1 cm light path)
ECD	electron capture detector
ELPHO	electrophoresis
equiv., mequiv.	equivalent, milliequivalent
eV	electron volt
°F	degree Fahrenheit
FID	flame ionization detector
Fig., Figs.	figure, figures
f.s.d.	full-scale deflection
ft.	foot
g	gram
GC	gas chromatography
GLC	gas-liquid chromatography
GSC	gas-solid chromatography
h	hour(s)
I (or, μ)	ion strength
I.D.	inner diameter
in.	inch(es)
insol.	insoluble
IR	infrared

I.U.	international unit
K	distribution coefficient
k	kilo
kg	kilogram
l	liter(s)
lb.	pound
m	meta
M	mega (=$\times 10^6$)
m	milli- ($\times 10^{-3}$), metre(s)
μ	micro ($\times 10^{-6}$), micron (10^{-6} m = 10^{-4} cm)
M	molar (grammol./l)
max.	maximum
MeV	mega electron volt(s)
mg	milligram(s)
min	minute(s)
ml	milliliter(s)
mμ	millimicron (10^{-9} m = 10^{-7} cm – nm)
mol. wt.	molecular weight
m.p.	melting point
n	nano ($\times 10^{-9}$)
N	normal (solution)
n-	normal in organic chemical names, e.g. n-butylamine
ng	nanogram = mμg = 10^{-9} g
nm	nanometer (10^{-9} m = mμ)
No.	number
o-	ortho
O.D.	optical density, also outer diameter
p-	para
PC	paper chromatography
pH	hydrogen ion exponent
pK	K = equilibrium constant, cf. pH
p.p.m.	parts per million
ppt.	precipitate
p.s.i.	pounds per square inch
radioactivity	superior preceding the element, e.g. ^{32}P; (^{14}C) amino acids; ^{14}C-labelled
ref., refs.	reference, references
R_f	distance travelled by the zone/distance travelled by liquid front
R_m	log ($1/R_F$-1)
R_x	distance travelled by the zone/distance travelled by reference substance X
r.p.m.	revolutions per minute
s-	symmetrical, e.g. s-tetrachloroethane
satd.	saturated
satn.	saturation
S.D.	standard deviation

S.E.	standard error (deviation) of mean of series
sec	second(s)
sec.-	secondary, e.g. sec.-butylamine
soln.	solution
sp. gr.	specific gravity
t-	tertiary, e.g. t-butanol
TLC	thin-layer chromatography
t_r	retention time
UV	ultraviolet
V, mV	volt, millivolt
vol.	volume
vs.	versus, against
v/v	volume per volume
wt.	weight
w/v	weight in volume
w/w	weight per weight
>	greater than; faster than
<	less than; slower than

INDEX — CHROMATOGRAPHY OF ANTIBIOTICS

AABOMYCIN A
PC.
1. **Paper:**
    Solvent:
    A. Benzene.
    B. Chloroform.
    C. Ethyl acetate.
    D. Ethyl acetate:benzene (1:1).
    E. Chloroform:benzene (1:1).
    F. Benzene:ethyl acetate (1:2).
    Detection:
    Bioautography against *Piricularia oryzae*.
    R_f:

Solvent	R_f
A	0.00
B	0.00
C	0.80
D	0.10
E	0.00
F	0.23

Ref:
German, "Offenlegungsschrift" 1,961,746 (1970).

TLC.
1. **Medium:**
    A. Silica Gel G.
    B. Alumina.
    Solvent:
    A. Ethyl acetate.
    B. Benzene.
    C. Ethyl acetate:benzene (1:1).
    D. Ethyl acetate:benzene (2:1).
    E. Ethyl acetate:benzene (1:2).
    F. Chloroform.
    G. Ethyl ether.
    H. Methanol.
    I. Acetone.
    Detection:
    A. Bioautography against *Piricularia oryzae*.
    B. Concentrated sulfuric acid followed by heating.
    R_f:

Solvent	$R_f^\star$ Medium A	B
A	0.82	0.70
B	0.00	0.00
C	0.35	0.10
D	0.47	0.23
E	0.10	0.00
F	0.00	0.00
G	0.80	0.79
H	0.96	0.93
I	1.00	1.00

$\star R_f$ same for both detection methods.
Ref:
S. Aizawa, Y. Nakamura, S. Shirato, R. Taguchi, I. Yamaguchi and T. Misato, J. Antibiotics, 22 (1969) 457–462.

ELPHO.
1. **Medium:**
    Sephadex sheet.
    Buffer:
    A. Phosphate, pH 7.0.
    B. Phosphate, pH 10.5.
    Conditions:
    15 mA, 30 min.
    Detection:
    Bioautography against *Piricularia oryzae*.
    Mobility:
    Buffer (A), no movement; (B) moved slightly to anode.
    Ref:
    As TLC (1).

ABLASTMYCIN
PC.
1. **Paper:**
    Solvent:
    n-Propanol:pyridine:acetic acid:water (15:10:3:12), descending, 18 h.
    Detection:
    R_f:
    Spot moved 23 cm from origin.
    Ref:
    T. Hashimoto, M. Kito, T. Takeuchi, M. Hamada, K. Maeda, Y. Okami and H. Umezawa, J. Antibiotics, 21 (1967) 37.

ELPHO.
1. **Medium:**
    Whatman No. 3 MM Paper.
    Buffer:
    Formic acid:acetic acid:water (25:75:900).
    Conditions:
    3000 V, 100–150 mA for 30 min.
    Detection:
    Ninhydrin, UV absorption; biological activity.

Mobility:
Ref:
As PC (1).

ACRYLAMIDINE
PC.
1. **Paper:**
Toyo Filter Paper No. 51.
Solvent:
A. Wet butanol.
B. 20% Ammonium chloride.
C. 75% Phenol.
D. 50% Acetone.
E. Butanol:methanol:water (4:1:2) + 1.5% methyl orange.
F. Butanol:methanol:water (4:1:2).
G. Benzene:methanol (4:1).
H. Water.
Detection:
A. Iodine.
B. Nitroprusside reagent.
C. Potassium permanganate.
D. UV.
R_f:

Solvent	R_f
A	0.20 (est)
B	0.95 (est)
C	0.78 (est)
D	0.70 (est)
E	0.67 (est)
F	0.43
G	0.00 (est)
H	0.89 (est)

Ref:
K. Yagishita, R. Utahara, K. Maeda, M. Hamada and H. Umezawa, J. Antibiotics, 21 (1968) 444–450.

TLC.
1. **Medium:**
Eastman chromatogram Sheet 6061.
Solvent:
1-Butanol:glacial acetic acid:water (4:1:5).
Detection:
As PC (1).
R_f:
0.56.
Ref:
As PC (1).

ACTINOBOLIN
PC.
1. **Paper:**
Solvent:
n-Butanol:acetic acid:water (10:1:4); ascending.
Detection:
R_f:
0.12 to 0.19 (actinobolin acetate).
Ref:
T.H. Haskell, J. Ehrlich, R.F. Pittillo and L.E. Anderson, U.S. Pat. No. 3,043,830, July 10, 1962.

ACTINOLEUKIN
TLC.
1. **Medium:**
Silica Gel G.
Solvent:
Ethyl acetate:acetone (9:1).
Detection:
R_f:
0.11, 0.57, 0.74.
Ref:
S. Omura, Y. Lin, T. Yajima, S. Nakamura, N. Tanaka, H. Umezawa, S. Yokoyama, Y. Homma and M. Hamada, J. Antibiotics, 20 (1967) 241.

ACTINOMYCINS
PC.
1. **Paper:**
Solvent:
A. Ethyl acetate:n-butyl ether:2% aq. naphthalene-2-sulfonic acid (1:1:2).
B. Ethyl acetate:n-butyl ether:10% aq. sodium-o-cresotinate (1:3:4).
Detection:
R_f:

Actinomycin	R_D*	
	Solvent A	Solvent B
A	1.80, 2.16, 2.46	1.24, 1.71, 4.5
B	1.00, 1.80	(0.55)**, 0.76, 1.00, *1.24****, (1.71), (2.07)
C	*1.57*, 2.00	*1.59*, 2.52
D	1.00	(0.55), (0.76), *1.00*, 1.59

* R_D value is ratio of distance run by component compared with that of major component of actinomycin D.
** ( ) indicates minor component.
*** Italics indicates major component.

Ref:

R.A. Mancher, F.J. Gregory, L.C. Vining and S.A. Waksman, Antibiotics Annual 1954–1955, pp. 853–857.

2. **Paper:**

Solvent:

Ethyl acetate:n-butyl ether:2% aq. naphthalene-2-sulfonic acid (1:1:2). Acetone solution of actinomycins placed along entire starting line.

Detection:

A. Color.

B. Bioautography against *B. cereus* made resistant to naphthalene-2-sulfonic acid by gradient plate technique. Chromatograms plated on seeded agar for 3 min and incubated at 28°C for 24 h. Quantitative estimation done by densitometric scanning and measuring area enclosed by each plate.

R_f:

Indicates % of component at each R_D value, where R_D is as in PC (1).

Actinomycin A (Sample 1): 1.00 (54.1),
                                              1.80 (12.4),
                                              2.16 (0.7),
                                              2.46 (2.8).

Actinomycin A (Sample 2): 0.07 (9.5),
                                              1.00 (28.1),
                                              1.80 (59.3),
                                              2.16 (3.1).

Actinomycin B: 0.07 (12.5), 1.00 (27.6),
                       1.80 (59.9).

Actinomycin C: 1.00 (10.9), 1.57 (52.0),
                       2.00 (37.1).

Actinomycin D: 1.00 (100).

Ref:

F.J. Gregory, L.C. Vining and S.A. Waksman, Antibiotics and Chemotherapy, 5 (1955) 409–416.

3. **Paper:**

Schleicher and Schull 2043 bmgl.

Solvent:

A. n-Dibutyl ether:n-butanol (5:1)/2% aq.

soln. of β-naphthalene sulfonic acid sodium salt.

B. Isoamylacetate/5% aq. soln. of β-naphthalene sulfonic acid sodium salt.

Detection:

R_f:

	R_{C_2} *							
Solvent	C_0	C_1	C_1a	C_2	C_2a	C_3	C_3a	C_4
A	0.25	0.69	0.81	1.0	1.15	1.39	1.56	1.75
B	0.20	0.64	–	1.0	1.21	1.55	1.79	–

*R_{C_2}: Value is ratio of distance run by component compared with C_2.

Ref:

K.H. Zepf, Experientia 14 (1958) 207–208.

4. **Paper:**

Whatman No. 1 (Ascending or circular).

Solvent:

n-Dibutyl ether:ethyl acetate:2% naphthalene-β-sulfonic acid (3:1:4). Paper is dipped in aq. phase and blotted between sheets of filter paper.

Detection:

Color. Deep red color of naphthalene-β-sulfonic acid salt facilitated detection of zones. Identical separations achieved by either ascending or circular chromatography.

R_f:

	R_f				
Sample	0.02	0.30	0.47	0.54	0.60
Actinomycin A (produced in 1940)		xxx*		xx	
Actinomycin A (produced in 1953)	x	xx		xxx	
Actinomycin B	x	xx		xxx	
Actinomycin C		x	xx		xx
Actinomycin D		xxxx			

*x = relative intensity of zones.

Ref:

L.C. Vining and S.A. Waksman, Science, 120 (1954) 389–390.

5. **Paper:**

Solvent:

n-Butanol:pyridine:water (4:1:5, upper phase).

Detection:

R_f:

Actinomycin, 0.9; actinomycin monolactone, 0.75; actinomycin acid, 0.5.

Ref:

D. Perlman, A.B. Mauger and H. Weissbach, Antimicrobial Agents and Chemotherapy, 1966 (1967) 581–586.

6. **Paper:**

(Circular). Whatman No. 2, 15 cm diam.

Solvent:

Ethyl acetate:n-butyl ether:2% aq. naphthalene-2-sulfonic acid (1:3:4). Paper dipped in lower phase and blotted between sheets of clean filter paper. Samples applied to segments of circle near center of paper. Development time about 30 min.

Detection:

R_f:

Ref:

As PC (2).

7. **Paper:**

(Circular). Whatman No. 2.

Solvent:

A. Di-n-butyl ether:s-tetrachloroethane:10% aq. sodium-o-cresotinate (2:1:3).

B. Di-n-butyl ether:s-tetrachloroethane:10% aq. sodium-o-cresotinate (5:1:6).

C. Di-n-butyl ether:ethyl acetate:10% aq. sodium-o-cresotinate (2:1:3).

Detection:

UV light of 2570A; zones appear as dark absorbing areas against a fluorescent background.

R_f:

Solvent 1

Actinomycin Complex	$R_{D, IV}$* (% composition)					
	I	II	III	IV	V	VI**
	0.27	0.40	0.56	1.00	1.35	1.55–1.97
X	4.9	Trace	Trace	11.5	84.6	Trace
B	9.5	Trace	Trace	28.1	59.3	3.1
A	6.6	2.9	Trace	66.7	23.8	Trace
D	Trace	Trace	Trace	100	Trace	—

	$R_{D, IV}$*		
C	1.00 (C_1)	1.43 (C_2)	1.99 (C_3)
	10.3	48.3	41.4

Solvent 2

		Actinomycin Complex Group		
$R_{D, IV}$*		B	V_{VI}	C
I	0.20	x***		
II	0.39	x		
III	0.63	x		
IV	1.00	x		x (C_1)
V	1.20	x	x	
VI_a	1.77	Trace	x	x (C_2)
VI_b	2.20	Trace	x	
VI_c	2.66	Trace	x	x (C_3)
VI_d	2.90	Trace	x	
VI_e	3.27	Trace	x	

Solvent 3

Actinomycin	$R_{D, IV}$*
B_{VI_c}	2.13
C_3	2.90

*   Relative to D_{IV}.
** Values greater than 1.35 have been referred to collectively as component VI.
***Present.

Ref:

G.G. Rousos and L.C. Vining, J. Chem. Soc. (1956) 2469–2474.

8. **Paper:**

(Circular).

Solvent:

A. As PC (5).

B. Ethyl acetate:n-butyl ether:10% aq. sodium-o-cresotinate (1:3:4).

Detection:

R_f:

	R_D* Values	
Actinomycin	Solvent 1	Solvent 2
B zone I	0.00	0.00, 0.08, 0.25
B zone II	0.07	0.40
B zone III	1.00	0.76
B zone IV	1.00	1.00
B zone V	1.80	1.24
C zone I	0.00	0.06, 0.53, 0.73
C zone II	1.00	1.07
C zone III	1.57	1.59
C zone IV	2.00	2.52
D zone I	0.00	0.00, 0.25
D zone II	1.00	1.00

*Relative to actinomycin D.

Ref:

L.C. Vining, F.J. Gregory and S.A. Waksman, Antibiotics and Chemotherapy, 5 (1955) 417–422.

9. **Paper**:

(Circular).

Solvent:

A. Isoamyl acetate:5% aq. sodium β-naphthalene sulfonate.

B. Dibutyl ether:1-butanol (5:1)/2% aq. sodium β-naphthalene sulfonate.

Detection:

Color.

R_f:

Photographs of circular chromatograms show comparisons and identity of actinomycin C, oncastatin C and actinomycin L.

Ref:

W. Woznicka, H. Niemczyk and A. Paszkiewicz, Medycyna Doswiadczalina i Mikrobiologia, 13 (1961) 47–52.

10. **Paper**:

(Circular) Toyo Roshi No. 50.

Solvent:

A. Isoamyl acetate:5% sodium naphthalene sulfonate (1:1).

B. As PC (4).

C. Ethyl acetate:2% β-naphthalene sulfonic acid:dibutyl ether (2:1:1).

Detection:

R_f:

R_D*

	Actinomycin		
Solvent	D	S_2	S_3
A	1.00 (std)	1.00	1.59
B	1.00 (std)	1.00	1.83
C	1.00 (std)	1.00	1.23

*Relative to actinomycin D.

Ref:

M. Furukama, A. Inoue and K. Asano, J. Antibiotics, 21 (1968) 568–570.

11. **Paper**:

(Circular).

Solvent:

As PC (2).

Detection:

As PC (2).

R_f:

Actinomycins S_1, S_2 and S_3 clearly separated.

Ref:

J. Kawamata and H. Fujita, J. Antibiotics, 13 (1960) 295–297.

12. **Paper**:

(Circular).

Solvent:

Amyl acetate:10% aq. sodium m-cresotinate (1:1).

Detection:

R_f:

Separation of actinomycin U complex.

Actinomycin	R_{C_2}*
U_1	0.32
U_2	0.45
U_3	0.73
U_4	1.18

*Relative to actinomycin C_2.

Ref:

G. Schmidt-Kastner, C. Hackman and J. Schmid, German Patent No. 1,126,563, March 29, 1962.

13. **Paper**:

(Circular) Whatman No. 3 mm. Useful for chromatography of tritiated actinomycin D.

Solvent:

As PC (7, no. 1).

Detection:

Radioautogram.

R_f:

Actinomycin-D-H[3] has an R_f of about 0.5

Ref:

Schwarz Bioresearcher 3 (1968) 1,3.

14. **Paper:**

(Circular).

Solvent:

n-Butyl acetate:di-n-butyl ether (3:1)/10% aq. sodium-m-cresotinate. Filter paper is dipped in the aq. layer, blotted and organic solvent phase used for development.

Detection:

Color.

R_f:

Actinomycin	R_{C_2}*
Z_0	0.35
Z_1	0.39
Z_2	0.78
Z_3	1.63
Z_4	2.36
Z_5	2.55
C_1	0.63
C_2	1.00
C_3	1.52
I_1	0.65
X_0	0.20
X_1	0.65
X_2	1.05

*Relative to C_2.

Ref:

R. Bossi, R. Hütter, W. Keller-Schierlein, L. Neipp and H. Zähner, Helv. Chim. Acta, 41 (1958) 1645–1652.

15. **Paper:**

(Circular).

Solvent:

A. Butanol:n-di-butyl ether (2:3)/10% aq. sodium-m-cresotinate.

B. As PC (14). Procedure for A and B same as PC (14).

Detection:

Color.

R_f:

Actinomycin	R_{C_2}*	
	Solvent 1	Solvent 2
C_0a	0.13	0.10
C_0	0.13	0.10
C_1	0.72	0.56
C_2	1.00	1.00
C_3	1.39	1.61
I_0a	–	0.12
I_0	0.49	0.27
I_1	0.74	0.63
I_2	1.00	0.97
I_3	–	1.34
X_0a	0.14	0.17
X_0	0.14	0.39
X_1	0.48	0.56
X_1a	–	0.71
X_2	0.72	0.98
X_3	0.93	1.49
X_4	1.11	1.90

*Relative to C_2.

Ref:

H. Brockmann and H. Gröne, Chem. Ber., 87 (1954) 1036–1051.

TLC.

1. **Medium:**

A. Alumina (Merck, G Grade).

B. Silica Gel (Merck G Grade).

Solvent:

A. Ethyl acetate:sym-tetrachloroethane: water (3:1:3, bottom layer).

B. Ethyl acetate:di-n-butyl ether:water (3:1:3, top layer).

C. Ethyl acetate:di-n-butyl ether:water (2:1:2, top layer).

D. Benzene:ethyl acetate:methanol (10:2.5:1).

E. Benzene:ethyl acetate:methanol (6:4:1).

F. Butan-1-ol:methanol:water (6:1:3).

G. Butan-1-ol:acetic acid:water (10:1:3).

H. Ethyl acetate:propan-2-ol:water (5:2:1).

Migration time ranged from 30 to 60 min.

Detection:

A. Bright orange color (E_{max} 440–450 nm).

B. UV light (E_{max} 240 nm).

R_f:

| | Solvent | R_f | | | | | | |
		C-group	C_1	C_2	C_3	F-group	F_1	F_2
Alumina	A	—	0.44	0.51	0.58	—	0.21	0.35
	B	—	0.40	0.46	0.53	—	0.23	0.29
	C	—	0.28	0.30	0.33	—	0.10	0.13
Silica gel	D	0.24	—	—	—	0.13	—	—
	E	0.43	—	—	—	0.33	—	—
	F	0.63	—	—	—	0.53	—	—
	G	0.70	—	—	—	0.50	—	—
	H	0.95	—	—	—	0.75	—	—

Ref:

G. Cassani, A. Albertini and O. Ciferri,
J. Chromatog. 13 (1964) 238–239.

ELPHO.

1. **Medium**:

Paper.

Buffer:

Pyridine:acetate, pH 6.5.

Detection:

Mobility:

Actinomycin, no movement; actinomycinic
acid, high mobility towards cathode;
actinomycin monolactone, one-half mobility
of the di-acid.

Ref:

As PC (5).

ACTINOSPECTACIN

PC.

1. **Paper**:

Eaton-Dikeman 613.

Solvent:

A. n-Butanol satd. with water.

B. n-Butanol with 2% (w/v) p-toluenesulfonic
acid.

C. n-Butanol with 2% (v/v) piperidine.

D. Methanol:water (4:1) with 1.5% (w/v)
sodium chloride vs. paper buffered with
1 M sodium sulfate-bisulfate, pH 2.0.

E. Ethanol:water (4:1) with 1.5% (w/v)
sodium chloride vs. paper buffered with
1 M sodium sulfate-bisulfate, pH 2.0.

F. Water (steaming).

G. Water, 5% ammonium chloride.

H. Water, 20% ammonium chloride.

All systems developed ascending at 28°C.

Detection:

Bioautography against *Bacillus subtilis*.

R_f:

Solvent	R_f
A	0.35
B	0.32
C	0.36
D	0.87
E	0.60
F	0.12
G	0.79
H	0.98

Ref:

A.C. Sinclair and A.F. Winfield, Antimicrobial Agents and Chemotherapy, 1961,
(1962) 503–506.

2. **Paper**:

Whatman No. 1.

Solvent:

A. n-Butanol:water (84:16, v/v).

B. n-Butanol:water plus 0.25% (w/v)
p-toluenesulfonic acid.

C. n-Butanol:acetic acid:water (2:1:1, v/v).

D. n-Butanol:water (84:16) with 2 ml
piperidine added to 98 ml of butanol:
water mixture.

E. n-Butanol:water (4:96, v/v).

F. n-Butanol:water (4:96) plus 0.25% (w/v)
p-toluenesulfonic acid.

Detection:

Bioautography against *Klebsiella pneumoniae*,
Bacillus subtilis and *Escherichia coli*.

R_f:

Solvent	R_f[*]
A	0.02
B	0.17
C	0.42
D	0.18
E	0.82
F	0.81

[*]Estimated from drawing.

Ref:

D.J. Mason, A. Dietz and R.M. Smith, Antibiot. and Chemotherapy, 11 (1961) 118–122.

ACTINOXANTHIN
ELPHO.
1. **Medium:**

Acrylamide gel (disc electrophoresis).
   Conditions:

Monomer concn. 15%; charge, 400 μg, current, 5 mA; time, 60 min; dye, nigrosin, 1.2 mg in 1000 ml of ethanol:acetic acid: water (5:1:4).
   Detection:

Bacillus subtilis; *Staphylococcus aureus* 209P.
   R_f:

Appears to move slightly toward anode.
   Ref:

A.S. Khoklov, B.Z. Cherches, P.D. Reshetov, G.M. Smirnova, I.B. Sorokina, T.A. Prokoptzeva, T.A. Koloditskoya and V.V. Smirnov, J. Antibiotics, 22 (1969) 541–544.

ADRIAMYCIN
PC.
1. **Paper:**

Whatman No. 1.
   Solvent:

A. n-Butanol satd. with pH 5.4 M/15 phosphate buffer.

B. Propanol:ethyl acetate:water (7:1:2 v/v).

C. Methylene chloride:methanol:water (100:20:2).
   Detection:
   R_f:

Solvent	R_f
A	0.10
B	0.25
C	0.17

Ref:

F. Arcamone, G. Cassinelli, G. Fantini, A. Grein, P. Orezzi, C. Pol and C. Spalla, Biotech. and Bioeng., 11 (1969) 1101–1110; F. Acramone, G. Cassinelli, A. diMarco and M. Gactani, U.S. Patent 3,590,028; June 29, 1971.

TLC.
1. **Medium:**

Kieselgel G layer buffered with 1% oxalic acid in water.
   Solvent:

A. n-Butanol:acetic acid:water (4:1:5).

B. Benzene:ethyl acetate:petroleum ether, b.p. 80–120°C (8:5:2).

C. Benzene:ethyl formate (1:2).
   Detection:
   R_f:

Solvent	R_f
A	0.33
B	0.0
C	0.0

Ref:

As PC (1).

ALBOCYCLINE
PC.
1. **Paper:**
   Solvent:

A. Wet butanol.

B. Aq. ammonium chloride 3%.

C. Aq. ammonium chloride 20%.

D. Aq. acetone.

E. Butanol:methanol:water (4:1:2).

F. Benzene:methanol (4:1).

G. Water.
   Detection:

Biological activity.
   R_f:

Solvent	R_f
A	1.00
B	0.52
C	0.35
D	1.00
E	1.00
F	1.00
G	0.67

Ref:

N. Bagahama, M. Suzuki, S. Awataguchi and T. Okuda, J. Antibiotics, 20 (1957) 261–266.

TLC.
1. **Medium:**

Silica Gel.
   Solvent:

A. Benzene.

B. n-Hexane:ethyl acetate (7:3).

C. Benzene:ethyl acetate (4:1).
D. Benzene:ethyl acetate (1:1).
E. Ether:isopropyl ether (1:1).
F. Isopropyl ether.
G. Chloroform.

Detection:
Biological activity.

R_f:

Solvent	R_f
A	0.90
B	0.28
C	0.28
D	0.63
E	0.57
F	0.33
G	0.04

Ref:
As PC (1).

ELPHO.
1. **Medium:**
Paper.
Conditions:
M/15 phosphate buffer, 10 v/cm, 2.5 h, pH 5.0 and 8.0.
Detection:
R_f:
At pH 5.0 or pH 8.0 albocycline did not move.
Ref:
As PC (1).

GLC.
1. **Apparatus:**
Column:
1.5 m packed with 5% SE-52.
Temperature:
180°C.
Carrier gas:
N_2, 90 ml/min.
Retention time:
6 min (est. from curve).
Ref:
As PC (1).

ALBOMYCIN
PC.
1. **Paper:**
Whatman No. 1 strips.
Solvent:

A. n-Butanol:water:acetic acid (4:2:1).
B. n-Butanol:water:acetic acid (1:2:1).
C. Methanol:0.1 N HCl (3:1).
D. n-Propanol:2.5% sodium chloride:acetic acid (10:8:1).
E. n-Butanol:ethanol:water:acetic acid (25:25:47:3).
F. Acetone:water:acetic acid (60:37:3).

Detection:
Bioautography against *Escherichia coli* W.

R_f:

Solvent	R_f
A	0.14, 0.33, 0.46
B	0.83
C	0.68
D	0.79
E	0.75, 0.92
F	0.71

Ref:
E.O. Stapley and R.E. Ormond, Science, 125 (1957) 587.

TLC.
1. **Medium:**
Solvent:

A. 1-Butanol:acetic acid:water (4:1:5), upper phase.
B. t-Butanol:0.004 N hydrochloric acid:satd. aq. sodium chloride soln. (2:1:1), upper phase; plate pre-treated with acetone:water:satd. aq. sodium chloride soln. (16:3:1).
C. Ethanol:water (2:1) containing 2% sodium chloride.
D. 1-Propanol:pyridine:water (15:1:10).
E. Pyridine:1-pentanol:water (7:7:6).
F. 2-Propanol:water (7:2); plate pre-treated with 0.2 M ammonium sulfate.

Detection:
Bioautography.

R_f:

Solvent	R_f	
	Albomycin δ_1	Albomycin δ_2
A	0.34	0.26
B	0.11	0.03
C	0.73	0.65
D	0.63	0.52
E	0.50	0.40
F	0.19	0.07

Ref:

H. Maehr and R.G. Pitcher, J. Antibiotics, 24 (1971) 830–834.

ALDGAMYCIN E
PC.
1. **Paper:**
   Solvent:
   A. n-Amyl acetate:dibutyl ether:acetic acid: water (20:6:1:10).
   B. Cyclohexane:secondary butanol:0.40% ammonium hydroxide (4:1:4).
   C. n-Heptane:tetrahydrofuran:n-amylacetate: 0.2 M aq. acetic acid (4:1:1:4).
   Detection:
   R_f:

Solvent	R_f
A	0.87
B	0.72
C	0.18

   Ref:

   M.P. Kunstmann, L.A. Mitscher and E.L. Patterson, Antimicrobial Agents and Chemotherapy, 1964 (1965) 87–90.

ALVEOMYCIN
PC.
1. **Paper:**
   Solvent:
   A. Phenol:butanol:water (5:4:9).
   B. Butanol:acetic acid:water (4:1:5).
   C. Butanol:aminopropanol:water (25:1:25).
   D. Butanol:phenol:water (3:3:4).
   Detection:

   R_f:

Solvent	R_f
A	0.50
B	0.13
C	0.50
D	0.85

   Ref:

   G. Schmidt-Kastner and J. Schmid, Chem. Abs. 60 (1964) 1542e. (Med. Chem. Abhandl. Med-Chem. Forschungsstraetten Farbenfabriken Bayer A.G., 7 (1963) 528–539).

AMAROMYCIN
PC.
1. **Paper:**

Solvent:
A. 3% aq. ammonium chloride.
B. Acetone.
C. Methanol.
D. Benzene.
E. Butyl acetate.
F. Butanol.
G. Petroleum ether.
Detection:
R_f:

Solvent	R_f
A	1.0
B	1.0
C	1.0
D	0.1
E	0.2
F	1.0
G	0.0

Ref:

T. Hata, Y. Sano, H. Tatsuta, R. Sugawara, A. Matsumae and K. Kanamori, J. Antibiotics, 8 (1955) 9–14.

AMBUTYROSINE
(chromatography of n-acetyl derivatives).
PC.
1. **Paper:**
   Solvent:
   1-Butanol:pyridine:5% boric acid (6:4:3).
   Detection:
   (Method of Pan and Dutcher). Spray paper with sodium hypochlorite (dil. 1 part 5.25% sodium hydrochlorite to 20 parts water). Dry. Spray with 95% ethanol. Dry. Spray with starch-iodide reagent (1% aq. soluble starch:1% aq. potassium iodide, 1:1). Acetylated spots show up as deep blue zones against a colorless background.
   R_f:
   Tetra-N-acetyl-ambutyrosine A   0.30–0.38
   Tetra-N-acetyl-ambutyrosine B   0.16–0.20
   Ref:

   Netherlands Patent No. 69,04408 (Sept. 29, 1969); S.C. Pan and J. Dutcher, Anal. Chem. 28 (1956) 836.

AMICETIN
PC.
1. **Paper:**

Solvent:
  A. 90% aq. 1-butanol.
  B. 1-Butanol satd. with water. Both solvents
     run descending.
Detection:
  Bioautography vs. *Mycobacterium avium*.
R_f:
Solvent	R_f
A	0.22
B	0.46
Ref:
  J.W. Hinman, E.L. Caron and C. DeBoer,
  J. Am. Chem. Soc. 75 (1953) 5864—5866.

2. **Paper:**
Solvent:
  1-Butanol satd. with 0.05 M pH 7.0
  phosphate buffer and paper strips impregnated
  with the buffer soln.
Detection:
  Bioautography vs. *E. coli* P-D 04863.
R_f:
  0.63
Ref:
  T.H. Haskell, A. Ryder, R.P. Forhardt,
  S.A. Fusari, Z.L. Jakubowski and Q.R. Baetz,
  J. Am. Chem. Soc. 80 (1958) 743—747.

AMIDINOMYCIN
PC.
1. **Paper:**
Solvent:
  Butanol:acetic acid:water (2:1:1).
Detection:
R_f:
  0.25—0.27.
Ref:
  S. Nakamura, H. Umezawa and N. Ishida,
  J. Antibiotics, 15 (1961) 163—164.

AMIDOMYCIN
PC.
1. **Paper:**
Solvent:
  A. Petroleum ether (b.p. 100—120°C) vs.
     paper impregnated with ethylene glycol.
  B. n-Amyl alcohol satd. with water.
  C. Ethanol:acetic acid:water (3:1:6).
  D. Ethanol:water (2:3).
Detection:
  Bioautography vs. *Candida albicans*.

R_f:
Solvent	R_f
A	0.86
B	0.90
C	0.36
D	0.89
Ref:
  W.A. Taber and L.C. Vining, Can. J.
  Microbiol., 3 (1957) 953—965.

3-AMINO-3-DEOXY-D-GLUCOSE
PC.
1. **Paper:**
Solvent:
  n-Butanol:pyridine:water:acetic acid
  (6:4:3:1).
Detection:
R_f:
Ref:
  S. Umezawa, K. Umino, S. Shibahara,
  M. Hamada and S. Omoto, J. Antibiotics,
  20 (1967) 355.

TLC.
1. **Medium:**
Solvent:
  A. Butanol:pyridine:water:acetic acid
     (6:4:3:1).
  B. 14% Aq. ammonia:methanol:chloroform
     (1:1:2), upper layer.
Detection:
  A. Ninhydrin.
  B. Bioautography vs. *Micrococcus pyogenes*
     var. *aureus* 209P.
R_f:
  One major and one minor zone result; major
  zone corresponds to 3-amino-3-deoxy-d-
  glucose. By ninhydrin method, major spot is
  brown and minor spot is purple.
Ref:
  S. Umezawa, U.S. Pat. 3,634,197; Jan. 11,
  1972.

AMPHOTERICINS
PC.
1. **Paper:**
  Whatman No. 1. Paper is soaked in 0.3 M
  potassium phosphate buffer, pH 3.0, and
  dried.
Solvent:
  80% Propanol. Antibiotics spotted (1 µg of

B, 30 μg of A) and papers equilibrated in tank with water vapor for 1 h, then developed 6—7 h. Longer periods of development resulted in destruction of antibiotics.

Detection:

Bioautography vs. *Candida albicans*.

R_f:

Amphotericin A 0.7

Amphotericin B 0.5

Ref:

W. Gold, H.A. Stout, J.F. Pagano and R. Donovick, Antibiotics Annual 1955—1956, 579—586.

2. **Paper:**

As chromin PC (1).

Solvent:

As chromin PC (1).

Detection:

As chromin PC (1).

R_f:

Amphotericin A 0.45.

Ref:

As chromin PC (1).

ANGOLAMYCIN

PC.

1. **Paper:**

Solvent:

A. 5% Aq. ammonium chloride.

B. Benzene:methanol (4:1).

C. pH 7.0 phosphate buffer, 1 M.

D. 0.05 N (0.175%) ammonia satd. with methyl iso-butyl ketone.

E. 1% Aq. ammonia.

F. 1% Ammonia satd. with methyl iso-butyl ketone.

All solvents developed ascending for 18—20 cm.

Detection:

R_f:

Solvent	R_f
A	0.75
B	0.88
C	0.26
D	0.48
E	0.49
F	0.71

Ref:

H. Koshiyama, M. Okanishi, T. Ohmori,

T. Miyaki, H. Tsukiura, M. Matsuzaki and H. Kawaguchi, J. Antibiotics, 16 (1963) 59—66.

TLC.

1. **Medium:**

Solvent:

A. Benzene:methanol (55:45).

B. Butanol:acetic acid:water (3:1:1).

Detection:

R_f:

Solvent	R_f
A	0.61
B	0.33

Ref:

N. Nishimura, K. Kumagai, N. Ishida, K. Saito, F. Kato and M. Azumi, J. Antibiotics, 18 (1965) 251—258.

ANTHELVENCINS

PC.

1. **Paper:**

Whatman No. 1.

Solvent:

Methanol:0.05 M sodium citrate buffer, pH 5.7 (7:3) vs. paper impregnated with same buffer.

Detection:

Bioautography vs. *Bacillus subtilis*.

R_f:

System useful for distinguishing anthelvencin from netropsin and distamycin A.

Ref:

G.W. Probst, M.M. Hoehn and B.L. Woods, Antimicrobial Agents and Chemotherapy, 1965 (1966) 789—795.

TLC.

1. **Medium:**

Cellulose.

Solvent:

n-Butanol:pyridine:acetic acid:water (15:10:1:12).

Detection:

A. Color: spray dried plates with 1% soln. of Ehrlich's reagent in acetone then heat 3—5 min at 90°C to develop a blue-violet color.

B. Bioautography vs. *Bacillus subtilis*.

R_f:

Ref:
As PC (1).

ANTHRAMYCIN
TLC.
1. **Medium:**
   Silica gel.
   Solvent:
   Ethyl acetate:methanol (4:1).
   Detection:
   R_f:
   0.50
   Ref:
   H. Aoki, N. Miyairi, M. Ajisaka and H. Sakai,
   J. Antibiotics 22 (1969) 201–206.

ANTICAPSIN
PC.
1. **Paper:**
   Solvent:
   A. n-Butanol satd. with water.
   B. n-Butanol satd. with water + 2% p-toluene-sulfonic acid.
   C. Methanol:0.1 N HCl (3:1).
   D. Propanol:pyridine:acetic acid:water (15:13:3:12).
   E. Methanol:0.05 M sodium citrate at pH 5.7 (70:30).
   Detection:
   Bioautography vs. *Streptococcus pyogenes* or *Salmonella gallinarum*.
   R_f:

Solvent	R_f
A	0.12
B	0.58
C	0.65
D	0.60
E	0.66

   Ref:
   R. Shah, N. Neuss, M. Gorman and
   L.D. Boeck, J. Antibiotics, 23 (1970)
   613–617.

ANTIMYCINS
PC.
1. **Paper:**
   Whatman No. 1.
   Solvent:
   Water:ethanol:acetone (7:2:1).

Detection:
Bioautography vs. *Saccharomyces cerevisiae* Y-30.
R_f:

Component	R_f
A_0	0.03
A_1	0.16
A_2	0.25
A_3	0.47
A_4	0.70
A_5	0.87
A_6	0.94

Ref:
D. Kluepfel, S.N. Sehgal and C. Vezina,
J. Antibiotics, 23 (1970) 75–80.

2. **Paper:**
   Eaton-Dikeman No. 613.
   Solvent:
   Water:ethanol:acetone (7:2:1). Develop ascending 21–24 h at 24–25°C.
   Detection:
   Bioautography.
   R_f:

Component	R_f
A_1	0.30
A_2	0.45
A_3	0.60
A_4	0.65

   Ref:
   W. Liu and K.M. Strong, J. Amer. Chem. Soc. 81 (1959) 4387–4390.

3. **Paper:**
   Eaton-Dikeman No. 613
   Solvent:
   Butanol:benzene (1:1).
   Detection:
   Bioautography vs. *Saccharomyces cerevisiae*.
   R_f:
   Antimycin B 0.05 (estimated from figure).
   Antimycin A 0.9 (estimated from figure).
   Ref:
   H.G. Schneider, G.M. Tener and F.M. Strong,
   Arch. Biochem. Biophys., 37 (1952) 147.

ANTIMYCOIN
PC.
1. **Paper:**
     As chromin, PC (1).
   Solvent:
     As chromin, PC (1).
   Detection:
     As chromin, PC (1).
   R_f:
     Antimycoin complex 0.45, 0.55.
     Antimycoin A, 0.55.
   Ref:
     As chromin, PC (1).

ANTIVIRAL substance from *Penicillium cyaneofulvum* Biourge.
ELPHO.
1. **Medium:**
     Paper.
   Buffer:
     Borate buffer, pH 8.6.
   Conditions:
     300 v, 6.8 mA, 2 h.
   Detection:
     Stain with mucicarmine (for acidic and
     neutral polysaccharides) or bromphenol blue
     (for S-H bonds).
   Mobility:
     Two bands appeared with each dye, one
     towards the anode, the other towards the
     cathode.
   Ref:
     P.M. Cooke and J.W. Stevenson, Can. J.
     Microbiol., 11 (1965) 913; D. Syeklocha,
     P.M. Cooke and J.W. Stevenson, *ibid*, 13
     (1967) 1481.

AQUAYAMYCIN
TLC.
1. **Medium:**
     Silica Gel G (E. Merck).
   Solvent:
     A. Water satd. butyl acetate.
     B. Ethyl acetate:chloroform (3:2).
     C. Chloroform:methanol (10:1).
     D. Benzene:methanol (10:1).
     E. Water.
   Detection:
   R_f:

Solvent	R_f
A	0.41
B	0.09
C	0.30
D	0.06
E	0.70

   Ref:
     M. Sezaki, T. Hara, S. Ayukama, T. Takeuchi,
     Y. Okami, M. Hamada, T. Nagatsu and
     H. Umezawa, J. Antibiotics, 21 (1968) 91.

2. **Medium:**
     MN-cellulose powder 300.
   Solvent:
     Water.
   Detection:
   R_f:
     0.66
   Ref:
     As TLC (1).

ELPHO.
1. **Medium:**
     Toyo filter paper No. 51.
   Buffer:
     Formic acid:acetic acid:water (25:75:900).
   Conditions:
     3300 V, 1.5 mA/cm, 15 min.
   Mobility:
   Ref:
     As TLC (1).

ARANOFLAVINS
TLC.
1. **Medium:**
     Silicic acid (Kieselgel G, Merck).
   Solvent:
     Ethyl acetate.
   Detection:
     Bioautography.
   R_f:
     Aranoflavin A 0.70.
     Aranoflavin B 0.45.
   Ref:
     K. Mizuno, T. Ando and J. Abe, J. Antibiotics, 23 (1970) 493–496.

ARISTEROMYCIN
PC.

1. **Paper:**
   Whatman No. 1.
   Solvent:
   A. n-Butanol satd. with water.
   B. Acetic acid:n-butanol:water (1:4:5).
   C. Pyridine:n-butanol:water (3:4:7).
   Detection:
   R_f:

Solvent	R_f
A	0.35
B	0.38
C	0.61

   Ref:
   T. Kusaka, H. Yamamoto, M. Shibata,
   M. Muroi, T. Kishi and K. Mizuno,
   J. Antibiotics, 21 (1968) 255.

TLC.
1. **Medium:**
   Silica Gel G, Merck.
   Solvent:
   Ethyl acetate:methanol (2:1).
   Detection:
   R_f:
   0.25.
   Ref:
   As PC (1).

ARMENTOMYCIN

PC.
1. **Paper:**
   Solvent:
   A. 1-Butanol:water (84:16); 16 h.
   B. 1-Butanol:water (84:16) + 0.25%
      p-toluene sulfonic acid; 16 h.
   C. 1-Butanol:acetic acid:water (2:1:1), 16 h.
   D. 2% Piperidine (v/v) in n-butanol:water
      (84:16); 16 h.
   E. 1-Butanol:water (4:96); 5 h.
   F. 1-Butanol:water (4:96) + 0.25%
      p-toluenesulfonic acid; 5 h.
   Detection:
   Bioautography vs. *Proteus mirabilis*.
   R_f:

Solvent	R_f[*]
A	0.25
B	0.42
C	0.65
D	0.42
E	0.85
F	0.80

   [*]Estimated from drawing.

Ref:
Netherlands Patent No. 66,04978;
Oct. 17, 1966.

ASCOCHOLIN α and β

TLC.
1. **Medium:**
   Silica Gel.
   Solvent:
   Benzene:methanol (4:1).
   Detection:
   Bioautography vs. *Candida albicans*.
   R_f:
   Ascocholin α 0.92
   Ascocholin β 0.67
   Ref:
   G. Tamura, S. Suzuki, A. Takatsuki, K. Ando
   and K. Arima, J. Antibiotics, 21 (1968) 539.

ASPERLIN

PC.
1. **Paper:**
   Solvent:
   A. 1-Butanol:water (84:16), 16 h.
   B. 1-Butanol:water (84:16) + 0.25%
      p-toluenesulfonic acid, 16 h.
   C. 1-Butanol:acetic acid:water (2:1:1), 16 h.
   D. 2% piperidine (v/v) in n-butanol:water
      (84:16), 16 h.
   E. 1-Butanol:water (4:96), 5 h.
   F. 1-Butanol:water (4:96) + 0.25%
      p-toluenesulfonic acid, 5 h.
   Detection:
   Bioautography vs. KB cells in agar. (KB cells
   are human epidermoid carcinoma cells.)
   R_f:

Solvent	R_f[*]
A	0.80
B	0.85
C	0.88
D	0.88
E	0.86
F	0.90

   [*]Estimated from drawing.

   Ref:
   A.D. Argoudelis and J.H. Coats, U.S. Patent
   No. 3,366,541, January 30, 1968.

ATROVENTIN

TLC.

1. **Medium:**
   Polyamide.
   Solvent:
   Acetone:acetic acid (5:1).
   Detection:
   Visible yellow color.
   R_f:

Compound	R_f
Atroventin	0.29
Atroventin monomethylether (deoxyherqueinone)	0.32

   Ref:
   As herqueinone TLC (1).

AUREOFUNGIN
PC.
1. **Paper:**
   Whatman No. 1.
   Solvent:
   A. Butanol:acetic acid:water (20:1:25).
   B. n-Propanol:water (4:1).
   C. Pyridine:ethyl acetate:water (2.5:6:7).
   D. Pyridine:ethyl acetate:acetic acid:water (5:5:1:3).
   E. Butanol:methanol:water (1:1:1.5).
   F. Butanol:methanol:water (4:1:2).
   Detection:
   R_f:

Solvent	R_f
A	0.64
B	0.57
C	0.19
D	0.78
E	0.94
F	0.46 (B minor), 0.65 (A major)

   Ref:
   G.R. Deshpande and N. Narasimhachari, Hindustan Antibiotic Bull., 9 (1966) 76–83.

AUREOTHRICIN
PC.
1. **Paper:**
   Whatman No. 1.
   Solvent:
   Carbon tetrachloride:acetic acid:water (8:3:2), organic phase, 4 h.
   Detection:
   Color; visible yellow spot.
   R_f:
   0.65

Ref:
J.H. Martin, W.C. Groth and W.K. Hausmann, Antimicrobial Agents and Chemotherapy, 1963 (1964) 130–133.

AVILAMYCIN
PC.
1. **Paper:**
   Solvent:
   Chloroform:benzene (7:3) vs. paper satd. with formamide as stationary phase.
   Detection:
   Bioautography vs. *Bacillus subtilis*.
   R_f:
   0.70
   Ref:
   F. Buzzetti, F. Eisenberg, H.N. Grant, W.K. Schierlein, W. Voser and H. Zahner, Experientia, 24 (1968) 320.

TLC.
1. **Medium:**
   Silica Gel G (Kieselgel G, Merck).
   Solvent:
   Chloroform:methanol (92:8).
   Detection:
   Concentrated sulfuric acid spray.
   R_f:
   0.62
   Ref:
   As PC (1).

AXENOMYCINS
TLC.
1. **Medium:**
   Silica Gel, buffered at pH 7.
   Solvent:
   n-Butanol:acetic acid:water (4:0.5:1).
   Detection:
   R_f:

Axenomycin A	0.49
Axenomycin B	0.61

   Ref:
   Netherlands patent no. 69,08269; published December 15, 1969.

AXENOMYCIN D
TLC.
1. **Medium:**
   Silica Gel.

Solvent:

Ethyl acetate:isopropanol:water (100:35:5).

Detection:

R_f:

0.35

Ref:

Belgian Patent 766,606; November 3, 1971.

AYAMYCINS

PC.

1. **Paper:**

Solvent:

n-Butyl ether:s-tetrachlorethane:10% aq.
sodium o-cresotinate (2:1:3).

Detection:

R_f:

Ayamycin	$R_f^\star$
A_1	0.05, 0.15
A_2	1.0
A_3	0.20, 0.80, 0.90

*Estimated from diagram.

Ref:

K. Sato, J. Antibiotics, 13 (1960) 321.

5-AZACYTIDINE

TLC.

1. **Medium:**

Silica Gel HF$_{254}$.

Solvent:

A. Methyl ethyl ketone:acetone:water
(15:5:2).

B. Chloroform:methanol (1:1).

C. Methanol.

Detection:

UV (254 nm); anisaldehyde spray; potassium
permanganate-sodium metaperiodate spray.

R_f:

Solvent	R_f
A	0.4
B	0.2
C	0.55

Ref:

M.E. Bergy and R.R. Herr, Antimicrobial
Agents and Chemotherapy, 1966 (1967)
625–630.

AZALOMYCINS

PC.

1. **Paper:**

Solvent:

Butanol:benzene:5% ammonium chloride
(1:9:10).

Detection:

Bioautography vs. *Sarcina lutea* or
Mycobacterium phlei.

R_f:

Azalomycin B   0.38

Ref:

M. Arai, J. Antibiotics, 13 (1960) 51.

2. **Paper:**

Solvent:

A. Water satd. n-butanol.

B. 20% Ammonium chloride.

C. 75% Phenol.

D. 50% Acetone.

E. Butanol, 40 ml:methanol, 10 ml:water,
20 ml:methyl orange, 1.5 g.

F. Butanol:methanol:water (40:10:20).
20 ml.

G. 80% benzene.

H. Water.

Detection:

Bioautography vs. *Candida albicans*.

R_f:

Solvent	Azalomycin F $R_f^\star$
A	0.55
B	0.0
C	0.0–0.1
D	0.95
E	0.7
F	0.7
G	0.0–0.2
H	0.0

*Estimated from diagram.

Ref:

As PC (1).

TLC.

1. **Medium:**

Silica Gel G (E. Merck).

Solvent:

Upper phase of sec-butanol:0.1 M phosphate
buffer, pH 6.0 (2:1). Spot 2–5 μg, develop
for 3 h at 20°C.

Detection:

A. Bioautography vs. *Candida albicans*
YU 1200.

B. Spray with 6N sulfuric acid and heat at
   120°C. Quantitative determination
   performed by densitometric scan using
   slit 0.5 mm wide × 6 mm long.

R_f:

Separates azalomycins F, F_3, F_4 and F_5.

Ref:

M. Arai and K. Hamano, J. Antibiotics, 23
(1970) 107–112.

ELPHO.
1. **Medium**:
   Paper.
   Buffer:
   1/150 M acetate buffer, pH 4.1.
   Conditions:
   500 V/34 cm, 0.2 mA/cm, 10 h.
   Detection:
   Bioautography vs. *Candida albicans*.
   Mobility:
   Moves slightly toward anode.
   Ref:
   As PC (1).

AZIRINOMYCIN
TLC.
1. **Medium**:
   Avicel microcrystalline cellulose (Brinkman).
   Solvent:
   n-Butanol:acetic acid:water (3:1:1).
   Detection:
   Ninhydrin, brom-thymol blue, iodine vapor
   or bioautography.
   R_f:
   0.82
   Ref:
   T.W. Miller, E.W. Tristram and F.J. Wolf,
   J. Antibiotics, 24 (1971) 48–50.

ELPHO.
1. **Medium**:
   Schleicher and Schuell SS-598 paper, 52 cm
   long.
   Buffer:
   0.165 M phosphate at pH 7.0.
   Conditions:
   600 V, 2.5 h, refrigerated.
   Detection:
   Bioautography vs. *Proteus vulgaris*.

Mobility:
12 cm from origin.
Ref:
E.O. Stapley, D. Hendlin, M. Jackson and
A.K. Miller, J. Antibiotics, 24 (1971) 42–47.

AZOMULTIN
PC.
1. **Paper**:
   Solvent:
   A. Water satd. n-butanol.
   B. 20% aq. ammonium chloride.
   C. 75% aq. phenol.
   D. 50% aq. acetone.
   E. Butanol:methanol:water (4:1:2) + methyl
      orange.
   F. Butanol:methanol:water (4:1:2).
   G. Benzene:methanol (4:1).
   H. Water.
   I. n-Propanol:pyridine:acetic acid:water
      (15:10:3:12).
   R_f:

Solvent	R_f
A	0.10
B	0.25
C	0.85
D	0.28
E	0.58
F	0.40
G	0.00
H	0.10
I	0.60

   Ref:
   Japanese Patent 6073/70, Feb. 28, 1970.

AZOTOBACTER CHROOCOCCUM **ANTIBIOTIC**
PC.
1. **Paper**:
   Solvent:
   A. Chloroform satd. with water.
   B. n-Butanol satd. with water.
   C. n-Butanol satd. with water + 2% piperidine.
   D. n-Butanol:pyridine:water (10:6:10).
   E. n-Butanol:acetic acid:water (2:1:1).
   F. n-Butanol satd. with water + 2% p-toluene/
      sulfonic acid.
   Detection:
   Bioautography vs. *Candida albicans*.

R_f:

Solvent	R_f
A	0.54
B	0.80
C	0.86
D	0.86
E	0.88
F	0.84

Ref:

E.N. Mishustin, A.N. Narimova,
Y.M. Khoklilova, S.N. Ovshtoper and
F.A. Smirnova, Microbiologia, 38 (1969)
87–90.

AZOTOMYCIN
PC.
1. **Paper:**
   Whatman No. 1.
   Solvent:
   A. 95% Ethanol:1 M ammonium acetate,
      pH 7.5 (75:30).
   B. Ethanol:t-butanol:88% formic acid:water
      (60:20:5:15).
   C. 93.8% Aq. n-butanol:40% aq. propionic
      acid (1:1).
   Detection:
   Bioautography vs. *Escherichia coli*,
   ninhydrin, UV.
   R_f:
   Solvent A, 0.62 (estimated from diagram).
   Ref:
   R.W. Brockman, R.F. Pittillo, S. Shaddix
   and D.L. Hill, Antimicrobial Agents and
   Chemotherapy, 1969 (1970) 56–62.

BACIMETHRIN
PC.
1. **Paper:**
   Solvent:
   A. n-Butanol:acetic acid:water (2:1:1).
   B. Water satd. n-butanol.
   C. Water satd. ethyl acetate.
   Detection:
   Bioautography; fluorescein reaction.
   R_f:

Solvent	R_f
A	0.52
B	0.37
C	0.27

Ref:

F. Tanaka, N. Tanaka, H. Yonehara and
H. Umezawa, J. Antibiotics, 15 (1962)
191–196.

BACITRACIN
PC.
1. **Paper:**
   Whatman No. 4.
   Solvent:
   Acetic acid:n-butanol:water (1:4:5).
   Detection:
   After treatment with 0.1% ninhydrin in
   n-butanol the components were localized by
   examination in visible and UV light.
   R_f:
   ∼ 0.6
   Ref:
   J. Prath, Acta Chemica Scandinavica, 6
   (1952) 1237–1248.

TLC.
1. **Medium:**
   Silica Gel G.
   Solvent:
   n-Butanol:acetic acid:water (4:1:2).
   Detection:
   A. Heat TLC plate at 110°C, 1 h and
      observe under UV light.
   B. Ninhydrin (0.0359 g in 10 ml n-butanol +
      0.41 ml acetic acid).
   R_f:

Bacitracin A	0.35
Bacitracin B	0.22

Ref:

P.A. Nussbaumer, Pharm. Acta Helv.,
40 (1965) 210–218.

ELPHO.
1. **Medium:**
   Paper; Munktell No. 20.
   Buffer:
   A. Acetate, pH 4.8, 0.1 M.
   B. Veronal, pH 8.6, 0.1 M.
   Conditions:
   8 V/cm, 5 h.
   Detection:
   Ninhydrin, bioautography.

Mobility:

One spot detected with both buffers. With buffer A, bacitracin moves toward cathode.

Ref:

As PC (1).

BAMICETIN

PC.

1. **Paper:**

   Solvent:

   As amicetin, PC (2).

   Detection:

   As amicetin, PC (2).

   R_f:

   0.22

   Ref:

   As amicetin, PC (2).

BANDAMYCIN A

PC.

1. **Paper:**

   Solvent:

   A. Water satd. n-butanol.
   B. 3% Aq. ammonium chloride.
   C. Phenol:water (4:1).
   D. Acetone:water (1:1).
   E. n-Butanol:methanol:water (4:1:2).
   F. Benzene:methanol (4:1).
   G. n-Butanol:acetic acid:water (74:3:25).
   All solvents were run ascending.

   Detection:

   R_f:

Solvent	R_f
A	0.96
B	0.89
C	0.94
D	0.96
E	0.96
F	0.96
G	0.95

   Ref:

   S. Kondo, J. Marie, J. Sakamoto and H. Yumoto, J. Antibiotics, 14 (1961) 365–366.

BANDAMYCIN B

PC.

1. **Paper:**

   Solvent:

   A. Water satd. n-butanol.

B. 15% Aq. ammonium chloride.
C. Phenol:water (4:1).
D. Acetone:water (1:1).
E. n-Butanol:methanol:water (4:1:2).
F. Benzene:methanol (4:1).
G. tert.-Butanol:acetic acid:water (74:3:25).
H. Ethyl ether satd. water.
I. Water.
All solvents were run ascending.

Detection:

R_f:

Solvent	R_f
A	0.97
B	0.76
C	0.97
D	0.95
E	0.97
F	0.94
G	0.95
H	0.95
I	0.77

Ref:

S. Kondo, T. Miyakawa, H. Yumoto, M. Sezaki, M. Shimura, K. Sato and T. Hara, J. Antibiotics, 15 (1962) 157–159.

BLASTICIDIN

PC.

1. **Paper:**

   Toyo No. 131, 1 × 16 cm.

   Solvent:

   A. Water satd. butanol.
   B. 3% Aq. ammonium chloride.
   C. 80% Aq. phenol.
   D. 50% Aq. acetone.
   E. Butanol:methanol:water (40:10:20) + 1.5 g methyl orange.
   F. Butanol:methanol:water (4:1:2).
   G. Benzene:methanol (4:1).

   Detection:

   R_f:

Solvent	R_f
A	0.30
B	0.00
C	1.00
D	0.80
E	0.75
F	0.70
G	0.00, 0.35

Ref:

K. Fukunaga, T. Misato, I. Ishii and
M. Asakawa, Bull. Agric. Chem. Soc. Japan,
19 (1955) 181—188.

BLASTICIDIN S
PC.
1. **Paper:**

Toyo Roshi No. 51.

Solvent:

n-Butanol:acetic acid:water (2:1:1),
ascending.

Detection:

A. UV light at 253.7 nm.

B. Spray with alkaline ferricyanide-nitro-
prusside reagent; blasticidin S appears as
a reddish-brown spot.

C. Bioautography vs. *Bacillus cereus* or
Piricularia oryzae.

R_f:

0.40

Ref:

H. Yonehara and N. Otake, Antimicrobial
Agents and Chemotherapy, 1965 (1966)
855—857.

TLC.
1. **Medium:**

Silica Gel (Kieselgel G).

Solvent:

Chloroform:methanol:ammoniacal water
(2:1:1), upper phase.

Detection:

As PC (1) B.

R_f:

Ref:

As PC (1).

BLEOMYCINS
PC.
1. **Paper:**

Solvent:

10% aq. ammonium chloride.

Detection:

R_f:

Bleomycin-Copper Chelates	R_f
Cu-At 1	0.92
Cu-Bt 1	0.71
Cu-At 2	0.83
Cu-Bt 2	0.72
Cu-At 3	0.85
Cu-At 4	0.85
Cu-Bt 3	0.71
Cu-At 5	0.86
Cu-Bt 4	0.72
Cu-Bt 5	0.70
Cu-At 6	0.88

Ref:

H. Umezawa, Y. Suhara, T. Takita and
K. Maeda, J. Antibiotics, 19 (1966) 210—215.

2. **Paper:**

Solvent:

As PC (1).

Detection:

R_f:

Bleomycin A   0.88—0.94

Ref:

French Patent 3.978M; June 3, 1964.

3. **Paper:**

Toyo No. 51.

Solvent:

As PC (1); ascending.

Detection:

Bioautography vs. *Mycobacterium phlei.*

R_f:

Bleomycin A   0.88—0.99

Bleomycin B   0.66—0.70

Ref:

H. Umezawa, K. Maeda, T. Takeuchi and
Y. Okami, J. Antibiotics, 19 (1966)
200—209.

TLC.
1 **Medium:**

Silica Gel G (Merck).

Solvent:

10% ammonium acetate:methanol (1:1).

Detection:

R_f:

Bleomycin-Copper Chelates	R_f
Cu-At 1	0.74
Cu-Bt 1	0.75
Cu-At 2	0.40
Cu-Bt 2	0.68
Cu-At 3	0.13
Cu-At 4	0.49

Cu-Bt 3	0.68
Cu-At 5	0.51
Cu-Bt 4	0.60
Cu-Bt 5	0.52
Cu-At 6	0.30

Ref:
As PC (1).

ELPHO.
1. **Medium:**
   Buffer:
   Formic acid:acetic acid:water (25:75:900),
   pH 1.8.
   Conditions:
   2000 V at 25 mA.
   Detection:
   Mobility:

Bleomycin-Copper Chelates	Relative Mobility
Cu-At 1	0.66
Cu-Bt 1	0.58
Cu-At 2	0.79
Cu-Bt 2	0.74
Cu-At 3	0.91
Cu-At 4	0.92
Cu-Bt 3	0.80
Cu-At 5	0.84
Cu-Bt 4	0.78
Cu-Bt 5	0.86
Cu-At 6	0.84

   Ref:
   As PC (1).

BLUENSOMYCIN
CCD.
1. **Solvent:**
   1-Butanol:water.
   Distribution coefficient:
   0.38 (p-toluenesulfonate salt).
   Ref:
   M.E. Bergy, T.E. Eble, R.R. Herr, C.M. Large
   and B. Bannister, Antimicrobial Agents and
   Chemotherapy, 1962 (1963) 614.

BOSEIMYCIN
PC.
1. **Paper:**
   Solvent:
   A. n-Propanol:pyridine:acetic acid:water
   (15:10:3:12).

B. Pyridine:acetic acid:water (50:35:15).
C. n-Butanol satd. with water + 0.25%
   p-toluenesulfonic acid.
D. n-Butanol satd. with water + 2%
   p-toluenesulfonic acid.
E. n-Butanol:acetic acid:water (2:1:1).
Detection:
R_f:

Solvent	R_f
A	0.14
B	0.25
C	0.02
D	0.08
E	0.07

Ref:
R.K. Sinha, J. Antibiotics, 23 (1970)
360–364.

TLC.
1. **Medium:**
   Silica Gel G.
   Solvent:
   A. As PC (1) A.
   B. As PC (1) B.
   C. As PC (1) E.
   Detection:
   R_f:

Solvent	R_f
A	0.75
B	0.68
C	0.09

   Ref:
   As PC (1).

ELPHO.
1. **Medium:**
   Paper.
   Buffer:
   A. 0.1 M acetate, pH 3.9.
   B. 0.1 M phosphate, pH 7.2.
   Conditions:
   2 h.
   Mobility:
   (as boseimycin HCl).
   A. 2.4 cm towards cathode.
   B. 3.8 cm towards cathode.
   Ref:
   As PC (1).

BOTTROMYCINS

TLC.

1. **Medium:**

   Silica Gel G.

   Solvent:

   Butanol:acetic acid:water (100:12:100), upper phase.

   Detection:

   Spray with 0.1% bromophenol blue.

   R_f:

   Bottromycin A   0.69

   Bottromycin B   0.64

   Ref:

   S. Nakamura, T. Chikaike, K. Karasawa, N. Tanaka, H. Yonehara and H. Umezawa, J. Antibiotics, 18 (1965) 47–52.

BRAMYCIN

PC.

1. **Paper:**

   Solvent:

   A. 30% Acetone.

   B. n-Hexane:benzene:ethyl acetate (1:1:1).

   Detection:

   Bioautography vs. *Piricularia oryzae.*

   R_f:

Solvent	R_f
A	0.32
B	0.78

   Ref:

   Y. Sakagami, H. Sekine, S. Yamabayashi, Y. Kitaura and A. Ueda, J. Antibiotics, 19 (1966) 99–103.

TLC.

1. **Medium:**

   Silica Gel G.

   Solvent:

   A. Methanol:ethyl acetate (100:15).

   B. Ethanol:water (4:1).

   Detection:

   As PC (1).

   R_f:

Solvent	R_f
A	0.70
B	0.69

   Ref:

   As PC (1).

BRESEIN

PC.

1. **Paper:**

   Solvent:

   A. t-Butanol:acetic acid:water (74:3:25).

   B. Acetic acid:ethyl acetate:water (6:88:6).

   C. Methanol:acetic acid:water (25:3:72).

   D. Acetone:acetic acid:water (20:6:74).

   E. Acetone:water (70:30).

   F. n-Butanol:acetic acid:water (79:6:15).

   G. t-Butanol:water (80:20).

   H. As D, but (80:3:17).

   I. As A, but (65:3:32).

   J. n-Butanol:ethanol:acetic acid:water (25:25:3:47).

   K. As A, but (70:6:24).

   L. As F, but (4:1:5).

   M. As D, but (60:13:17).

   N. As F, but (4:1:1).

   O. Phenol:n-butanol (1:1).

   P. As O, but (1:2).

   Q. As O, but (1:3).

   R. As O, but (4:1).

   S. Phenol:ethyl ether (4:1).

   T. Phenol:methanol (4:1).

   Detection:

   R_f:

Solvent	R_f
A	0.85
B	0.90
C	0.68
D	0.81
E	0.95
F	0.90
G	0.83
H	0.19
I	0.95
J	0.95
K	0.94
L	0.95
M	0.95
N	0.91
O	0.88
P	0.86
Q	0.90
R	0.78
S	0.75
T	0.84

   Ref:

   R.A. Radzhapov, G.G. Zharikova,

A.B. Silaev, G.S. Katrukha. Vestn. Mosk. Univ., Biol., Pochvoved. 1968, 23 (4), 42–7; Chem.Abs. 69 (1968) 109767f.

BULGERIN

PC.

1. **Paper:**
   Toyo Roshi No. 51.
   Solvent:
   A. n-Butanol:acetic acid:water (4:1:2).
   B. n-Propanol:pyridine:acetic acid:water (15:10:3:12).
   Detection:
   R_f:

Solvent	R_f
A	0.20
B	0.60

   Ref:
   J. Shoji, R. Sakazaki, M. Mayama, Y. Kawamura and Y. Yasuda, J. Antibiotics, 23 (1970) 295–299.

TLC.

1. **Medium:**
   Silica Gel GF.
   Solvent:
   A. Chloroform:methanol:17% aq. ammonia (2:1:1), upper layer.
   B. n-Butanol:ethanol:0.1 N hydrochloric acid (1:1:1).
   Detection:
   R_f:

Solvent	R_f
A	0.80
B	0.50

   Ref:
   As PC (1).

CANDICIDIN

PC.

1. **Paper:**
   Whatman No. 1.
   Solvent:
   A. Ethyl acetate:pyridine:water (4:3:2).
   B. n-Butanol:pyridine:water (6:4:5).
   C. Methanol:25% ammonium hydroxide: water (20:1:4).
   Detection:
   Bioautography vs. *Candida albicans*.

R_f:

Solvent	R_f
A	0.66
B	0.71
C	0.55

Ref:
R. Bosshardt and H. Bickel, Experientia 24 (1968) 422–424.

CAPREOMYCIN

PC.

1. **Paper:**
   Whatman No. 1 buffered with 0.05 M citrate buffer, pH 6.0.
   Solvent:
   Methanol:0.05 M citrate buffer, pH 6.0 (7:3),
   Detection:
   Bioautography vs. *Bacillus subtilis* ATCC 6633 at pH 8.0.
   R_f:
   Capreomycin II moves more rapidly than I.
   Ref:
   W.M. Stark, C.E. Higgins, R.N. Wolfe, M.M. Hoehn and J.M. McGuire, Antimicrobial Agents and Chemotherapy, 1962 (1963) 596–606.

2. **Paper:**
   As PC (1).
   Solvent:
   As PC (1).
   Detection:
   Bioautography vs. *Mycobacterium butyricum* at pH 8.0.
   R_f:
   After 30 h, capreomycin II separates from I; after 10 additional h, capreomycin II separates further into 2 components, IIA and IIB; with continuous flow for 80 h, capreomycin I separates into 2 components, IA and IB. Relative R_f's are IIB > IIA > IB > IA.
   Ref:
   W.M. Stark and L.D. Boeck, Antimicrobial Agents and Chemotherapy, 1964 (1965) 157–164.

TLC.

1. **Medium:**
   Silica Gel G (Kieselgel-G, Merck).

Solvent:

10% Aq. ammonium acetate:acetone:10% ammonium hydroxide (9:10:0.5).

Detection:

R_f:

0.15

Ref:

A. Negata, T. Ando, R. Izumi, H. Sakakibara, T. Take, K. Hayano and J. Abe, J. Antibiotics, 21 (1968) 681–687.

O-CARBAMYL-d-SERINE
PC.

1. **Paper:**
Solvent:

n-Butanol:acetic acid:water (4:1:5).

Detection:

Ninhydrin or biuret.

R_f:

0.20

Ref:

Y. Okami, K. Maeda, H. Kondo, T. Tanaka and H. Umezawa, J. Antibiotics, 15 (1962) 147–151.

2. **Paper:**
Solvent:

A. n-Butanol satd. with water:acetic acid (3:1).

B. 80% Phenol.

C. 77% Ethanol.

Detection:

R_f:

Solvent	R_f
A	0.18
B	0.39
C	0.20

Ref:

N. Tanaka, K. Sashikata, T. Wada, S. Sugawara and H. Umezawa, J. Antibiotics, 16 (1963) 217–221.

3. **Paper:**
Whatman No. 1.

Solvent:

A. Phenol:borate buffer pH 9.3
B. Phenol:phosphate buffer pH 11.2.
C. Pyridine:iso-amyl alcohol:water (8:4:7).
D. Butanol:formic acid:water (75:15:10).

Detection:

Ninhydrin.

R_f:

Solvent	R_f
A	0.41
B	0.27
C	0.33
D	0.08

Ref:

G. Hagemann, L. Penasse and J. Teillon, Biochim. Biophys. Acta, 17 (1955) 240–243.

CARBOMYCIN; cf. magnamycin
PC.

1. **Paper:**
Solvent:

A. Benzene vs. citrate buffer pH 4.6.
B. Butyl acetate vs. citrate buffer pH 4.6.

Detection:

R_f:

Solvent	R_f
A	0.09
B	0.58

Ref:

T. Osato, K. Yagishita and H. Umezawa, J. Antibiotics, 8 (1955) 161–163.

2. **Paper:**
Solvent:

A. Benzene:cyclohexane (1:1) vs. paper treated with formamide.
B. Benzene vs. paper treated with formamide.
C. Benzene:chloroform (3:1) vs. paper treated with formamide.
D. Benzene:chloroform (1:1) vs. paper treated with formamide.

Detection:

R_f:

Solvent	R_f	
	Carbomycin	Carbomycin B
A	0.25	0.45
B	0.76	0.89
C	0.98	0.98
D	0.98	0.98

Ref:

K. Murai, B.A. Sobin, W.D. Celmer and F.W. Tanner, Antibiotics and Chemotherapy, 9 (1959) 485–490.

3. **Paper:**
   Solvent:
   As angolamycin, PC (1), solvents A through F.
   Detection:
   R_f:

Solvent	R_f
A	0.75
B	0.88
C	0.26
D	0.48
E	0.49
F	0.71

   Ref:
   As angolamycin PC (1).

4. **Paper:**
   Solvent:
   As celesticetin PC (2) G.
   Detection:
   As celesticetin PC (2).
   R_f:
   0–0.28 (estimated from diagram).
   Ref:
   As celesticetin PC (2).

CCD.
1. **Solvent:**
   Benzene:acetate buffer, pH 4.5.
   Plates:
   60.
   Distribution:
   Carbomycin, K = 7.
   Carbomycin B, K = 12.
   Ref:
   F.A. Hochstein and K. Murai, J. Amer. Chem. Soc., 76 (1954) 5080–5083.
2. **Solvent:**
   Benzene:cyclohexane:95% ethanol:water (5:5:8:2).
   Plates:
   Distribution:
   Distribution coefficient:
   Carbomycin,　　0.41
   Carbomycin B,　0.67
   Ref:
   As PC (2).

CEFAZOLIN
PC.
1. **Paper:**
   Toyo No. 51A.
   Solvent:
   n-Butanol:acetic acid:water (5:1:4), upper layer.
   Detection:
   Potassium permanganate.
   R_f:
   0.69–0.71
   Ref:
   K. Kariyone, H. Harada, M. Kurita and T. Takano, J. Antibiotics, 23 (1970) 131–136.

2. **Paper:**
   Toyo No. 51.
   Solvent:
   n-Butanol:acetic acid:water (4:1:2), ascending, 16 h at room temperature.
   Detection:
   A. For radioactive antibiotic, developed papers exposed to X-ray films for 7–14 days.
   B. Bioautography vs. *Bacillus subtilis* ATCC 6633.
   R_f:
   0.75 (estimated from photographs)
   Ref:
   J. Kozatani, M. Okui, T. Matsubara and M. Nishida, J. Antibiotics, 25 (1972) 86–93.

TLC.
1. **Medium:**
   Silica Gel.
   Solvent:
   n-Butanol:acetic acid:water (6:3:2).
   Detection:
   Potassium permanganate.
   R_f:
   0.53–0.60
   Ref:
   As PC (1).

2. **Medium:**
   Eastman Chromagram Sheet No. 6061.
   Solvent:
   A. n-Butanol:acetic acid:water (4:1:5), upper phase.

B. n-Butanol:ethanol:water (4:1:5).
C. Methanol:n-propanol:water (6:1:2).

Detection:

Bioautography vs. *Bacillus subtilis*
ATCC 6633.

R_f:

A. 0.35 (estimated from photograph)
B, C not given.

Ref:

M. Nishida, T. Matsubara, T. Murakawa,
Y. Mine, Y. Yokota, S. Kuwahara and
S. Goto, Antimicrobial Agents and
Chemotherapy, 1969 (1970) 236–243.

3. **Medium:**

Silica Gel F_{254}.

Solvent:

A. As PC (2).
B. Ethyl acetate:acetic acid:water (4:2:1).

Detection:

As PC (2).

R_f:

Useful for detection of urine and bile
metabolites.

Ref:

As PC (2).

CELESTICETIN

PC.

1. **Paper:**

Solvent:

A. n-Butanol:water (81:19).
B. n-Butanol:water:p-toluenesulfonic acid
(81:18.7:0.25).
C. n-Butanol:water:glacial acetic acid
(50:25:25).
D. n-Butanol:water:piperidine (80:18:2).
E. Water:n-butanol (96:4).
F. Water:n-butanol:p-toluenesulfonic acid
(94:4:2).

Detection:

R_f:

Solvent	R_f*
A	0.55–0.65
B	0.45–0.55
C	0.75
D	0.80
E	0.60
F	0.75

*Estimated from diagram.

Ref:

H. Hoeksma, G.F. Crum and W.H. DeVries,
Antibiotics Annual (1954–1955) 837–841.

2. **Paper:**

Solvent:

A. n-Butanol satd. with water.
B. n-Butanol satd. with water + 0.25%
p-toluenesulfonic acid.
C. As PC (1) C.
D. n-Butanol satd. with water + 2%
piperidine.
E. As PC (1) E.
F. Water:n-butanol:p-toluenesulfonic acid
(96:4:0.25).
G. 1 M phosphate buffer, pH 7.0.

Detection:

Bioautography vs. *Bacillus subtilis*.

R_f:

Solvent	R_f*
A	0.7 –0.87
B	0.53–0.78
C	0.60–0.80
D	0.85
E	0.38
F	0.42–0.66
G	0.25–0.42

*Estimated from diagrams.

Ref:

C. DeBoer, A. Dietz, J.R. Wilkins, C.N. Lewis
and G.M. Savage, Antibiotics Annual
(1954–1955) 831–836.

TLC.

1. **Medium:**

Silica Gel G.

Solvent:

A. Methyl ethyl ketone:acetone:water
(186:52:20).
B. 2-Pentanone:methyl ethyl ketone:
methanol:water (2:2:1:1).
C. Chloroform:methanol (6:1).

Detection:

Bioautography vs. *Sarcina lutea*.

R_f:

	R_f Solvent		
	A	B	C
Desalicetin	0.11	0.22	0.23
Celesticetin B	0.41	0.54	0.52
Celesticetin C	0.43	0.66	0.59
Celesticetin D	0.34	0.39	0.53

Ref:

A.D. Argoudelis and T.F. Brodasky,
J. Antibiotics, 25 (1972) 194–196.

CCD.

1. **Solvent:**

1-Butanol:water:glacial acetic acid (4:5:1).

Distribution coefficient:

0.70

Ref:

As PC (1).

CENOCOCCUM **ANTIBIOTIC**

PC.

1. **Paper:**

Solvent:

Two dimensional chromatography.
Direction 1, methanol:ammonium hydroxide:
water (3:3:1); develop 130 min, dry 24 h.
Direction 2, benzene satd. with 10% acetic
acid, dry 25 h.

Detection:

A. Blue-green fluorescence under short
wavelength UV light.

B. Bioautography vs. *Bacillus cereus*.

R_f:

Direction 1   0.69
Direction 2   0.00

Ref:

L.F. Grand and W.W. Ward, Forest Science,
15 (1969) 286–288.

CEPHALOGLYCIN

cephaloglycin metabolites

PC.

1. **Paper:**

Whatman No. 1.

Solvent:

n-Butanol:acetic acid:water (3:1:1),
descending, 12–16 h.

Detection:

Air-dry chromatogram, steam lightly to
remove acetic acid; bioautography vs.
Sarcina lutea PCI 1001 using agar at pH 6.5.

R_f:

Desactyl cephaloglycin > cephaloglycin.

Ref:

M.M. Hoehn and C.T. Pugh, Appl.
Microbiol., 16 (1968) 1132–1133.

TLC.

1. **Medium:**

Eastman No. 6064 cellulose sheet.

Solvent:

Acetonitrile:ethyl acetate:water (3:1:1),
1.5 h.

Detection:

Bioautography vs. *Sarcina lutea* at pH 6.5.

R_f:

Desacetyl cephaloglycin lactone > desacetyl
cephaloglycin > cephaloglycin.

Ref:

As PC (1).

CEPHALOSPORINS

There are numerous cephalosporins including
derivatives. Certain of these which may be of
particular significance are indexed individually.

PC.

1. **Paper:**

Whatman No. 1 treated with either 0.05 M
sodium citrate buffer, pH 5.5 or M sodium
phosphate buffer, pH 6. Paper is dried at
37°C before use. Spot approximately 100 μg.

Solvent:

Methanol, dried over calcium oxide and
distilled.

Detection:

R_f:

Cephalosporin C   0.34
Cephalosporin N   0.44

Ref:

G.G.F. Newton and E.P. Abraham, Biochem.,
62 (1956) 651–658.

2. **Paper:**

Whatman No. 1. Spot 50–200 μg.

Solvent:

A. 1-Butanol:acetic acid:water (4:1:4).

B. 1-Propanol:water (7:3).

Detection:

A. Bioautography vs. *Staphylococcus aureus*
(Oxford strain NCTC 6571) or *Salmonella
typhi* (strain "Mrs S"; Felix and Pitt
1935).

B. Ninhydrin.

C. UV absorption at 230–400 nm (Corning
filter No. 9863). Cephalosporin C
chromophore appears as dark, light-
absorbing spot.

R_f:

Compound	$R_{glycine}$	
	Solvent A	Solvent B
Deacetyl cephalosporin C	0.57	0.60
Cephalosporin C	0.78	0.77
Cephalosporin C_C	0.85	0.98

Ref:

J.D'A. Jeffrey, E.P. Abraham and G.G.F. Newton, Biochem. J., 81 (1961) 591–596.

3. **Paper:**

Whatman No. 1.

Solvent:

1-Butanol:acetic acid:water (4:1:4).

Detection:

A. Bioautography vs. *Salmonella typhi* or *Staphylococcus aureus*.

B. UV light at 230–400 nm. Cephalosporin C_A derivatives show up as dark spots.

C. Ninhydrin. Derivatives appear as purple spots.

D. Compounds formed from cephalosporin C and sulfapyridine or sulfathiazole can be detected by spraying the paper with 0.2% $NaNO_2$ in 0.1 N HCl, drying at 60°C and then spraying with 1% (w/v) α-naphthylamine in 75% (v/v) acetic acid.

E. The cephalosporin C-nicotinamide derivative can be detected by suspending the paper for 1 h in vapor of 2-butanone: aq. ammonia soln. (sp. gr. 0.88) (1:1). It appears as a blue-white fluorescent spot when the paper is viewed in UV light at 365 nm.

R_f:

Cephalosporin C_A derived from	$R_{ceph\ c}$[*]
Nicotine	0.16
2-Aminopyridine	0.29
2-Amino-6-methylpyridine	0.60
Pyridine	0.31
Nicotinamide	0.30
2:4:6-Trimethylpyridine	0.54
2-Hydroxymethylpyridine	0.36
Quinoline	0.58
Sulphapyridine	0.55
Sulphadiazine	0.62
Sulphathiazole	0.74

3-Hydroxypyridine	0.36
iso-Nicotinic acid	0.20
Nicotinic acid	0.23
Picolinic acid	0.36
Pyridine-2:3-dicarboxylic acid	0.33

[*]$R_{ceph\ c}$: R_f compared to cephalosporin C.

Ref:

C.W. Hale, G.G.F. Newton and E.P. Abraham, Biochem. J., 79 (1961) 403–408.

4. **Paper:**

Whatman No. 1.

Solvent:

A. 1-Butanol:ethanol:water (4:1:5).

B. Ethyl acetate satd. with aq. sodium acetate buffer (0.1 M to Na) pH 5.2 vs. paper pre-treated with the buffer. Paper is soaked in buffer, blotted, air dried and used immediately. Solvent reaches bottom of paper in 3 h, but develop 18 h.

Detection:

Cephalosporin C, 7-ACA and related compounds converted to N-phenylacetyl derivatives by spraying dried chromatogram with pyridine in 50% acetone (v/v) until barely damp. Then, lightly spray with 2% (w/v) phenylacetyl chloride in acetone, and again with the pyridine solution until a spot of bromocresol green placed on the paper immediately turns blue (pH 5.0). Dry in air 3–5 min and bioautograph vs. *Staphylococcus aureus* (Oxford strain N.C.T.C. 6571).

R_f:

(Solvent A) Compound	R_f
Cephalosporin C	0.04
N-phenylacetyl cephalosporin C	0.13
Cephalosporin C_C	0.09
N-phenylacetyl cephalosporin C_C	0.23
Cephalosporin C_A (pyridine)	0.00
Cephalosporin C_A (pyridine) nucleus	0.07
Cephalosporin C nucleus (7-ACA)	0.14
N-phenylacetyl derivative of 7-ACA	0.40

Ref:

B. Loder, G.G.F. Newton and E.P. Abraham, Biochem. J., 79 (1961) 408–416.

5. **Paper:**
  Whatman No. 1.
  Solvent:
  A. 70% n-Propanol, descending.
  B. Methanol:n-propanol:water (6:2:1),
  18—20 h.
  Detection:
  Bioautography vs. *Bacillus subtilis*.
  R_f:
  A. Cephalosporins C and N move as a single
  zone but are well separated from penicillins
  G or V and cephalosporin P type.
  B. Cephalosporin P type runs off end of
  paper; others well separated.
  Ref:
  J.L. Ott, C.W. Godzeski, D. Pavey,
  J.D. Farran and D.R. Horton, Appl.
  Microbiol., 10 (1962) 515—523.

6. **Paper:**
  Solvent:
  Methanol buffered at pH 5.5 with 0.013 M
  citrate.
  Detection:
  Bioautography vs. *Salmonella typhimurium*,
  Bacillus subtilis, *Proteus vulgaris*,
  Staphylococcus aureus or *Sarcina lutea*.
  R_f:
  Cephalosporin N (synnematin B) moves as
  an elongated spot.
  Ref:
  B.H. Olson, J.C. Jennings and A.J. Junek,
  Science, 117 (1953) 76—78.

7. **Paper:**
  Solvent:
  A. 0.02 N acetic acid in 25% (v/v) ethanol.
  B. Diisopropyl ether satd. with 0.1 M
  potassium phosphate, pH 7.0.
  C. Amyl acetate satd. with 0.1 M potassium
  phosphate, pH 7.0.
  With solvents B and C the paper is treated
  with M potassium phosphate, pH 7.0, and
  dried before use.
  Detection:
  Bioautography vs. *Staphylococcus aureus*.
  R_f:

Antibiotic	R_f Solvent		
	A	B	C
Cephalosporin P_1	0.45	0.50	1.0
Cephalosporin P_2	0.45	–	–
Cephalosporin P_3	0.00	0.00	<0.05
Cephalosporin P_4	0.40	0.50	1.00
Cephalosporin P_5	0.20	–	–

Ref:
H.S. Burton and E.P. Abraham, Biochem. J.,
50 (1951—1952) 168—174.

8. **Paper:**
  Whatman No. 1.
  Solvent:
  A. 2-Butanone satd. with water used when
  chromatography is followed by bio-
  autography.
  B. 1-Butanol satd. with 5 N ammonium
  hydroxide for separation of biologically
  inactive radioactive metabolites.
  Detection:
  A. Bioautography vs. *Bacillus subtilis*.
  B. Radioactive spots indicated by using a
  scanner.
  R_f:
  Cephalothin, related cephalosporins and
  their radioactive metabolites can be
  detected by this method.
  Ref:
  H.R. Sullivan and R.E. McMahon, Biochem.
  J., (1967) 976—982.

9. **Paper:**
  Whatman No. 4 impregnated with 0.1 M
  acetate buffer (pH 4.6) before use.
  Solvent:
  Methyl ethyl ketone:acetonitrile:water
  (MEK) (84:8:8). A mixture of MEK and
  water (3:2) is placed in bottom of chamber
  to provide a solvent satd. atmosphere.
  Detection:
  Bacillus subtilis ATCC 6633.
  R_f:
  Desacetyl cephalothin > cephalothin.
  Ref:
  M.M. Hoehn, H.W. Murphy, C.T. Pugh and
  N.E. Davis, Appl. Microbiol., 20 (1970)
  734—736.

10. Quantitative Procedure.

Paper:

Whatman No. 1. An 8 × 20 in. sheet is slotted to give 17, ¼ in. wide strips spaced 1/8 in. apart. A 3½ in. margin is left intact at each end of the sheet along with a ¾ in. strip on each side. Samples are applied 4¼ in. from one end not to exceed 0.04 mg/ml of parent antibiotics, using 5 µl spots. Multiple applications of 5 µl made for dilute samples.

Solvent:

Water satd. methyl ethyl ketone. Develop for 3 h without prior equilibration.

Detection.

Bioautography vs. *Bacillus subtilis* ATCC 6633. A 1% inoculum of a standard spore suspension used in Difco Penassay Base Agar adjusted to pH 6.5. Use 200 ml agar per plate measuring 8¾ in. × 17½ in. Incubate overnight at 37°C. Measure max. zone widths and compare against standards at 0.05, 0.10 and 0.20 mcg plotted against zone widths on semi-logarithmic paper.

R_f:

Cephalosporin derivatives and their desacetyls and lactones moved; however, cephalosporin C itself and its desacetyl and lactone derivatives failed to move in this system.

Ref:

R.P. Miller, Antibiotics and Chemotherapy, 1962 (1963) 689–693.

TLC.

1. **Medium:**

Silica Gel G.

Solvent:

A. n-Butanol:glacial acetic acid (10:1) satd. with water.

B. n-Butanol:pyridine:glacial acetic acid: water (38:24:8:30).

C. Benzene:acetone (4:1).

D. Benzene:acetone (3:2).

E. Toluene:acetone (3:2).

F. Toluene:acetone (4:1).

G. Toluene:acetone (7:3).

H. Toluene:ethyl acetate (1:1).

I. Toluene:acetone (9:1).

Detection:

Color reaction. Spray with a soln. of 1 g ninhydrin in a mixture of 700 ml alcohol + 28 ml 2,4,6-collidine + 210 ml glacial acetic acid and heat at 90°C for 5–10 min.

R_f:

	Solvent	R_f
N-phthalyl-cephalosporin C-dibenzhydrylester	C	0.48
N-phthalyl-cephalosporin C-9-benzhydrylester	A	0.72
	B	0.68
N-phthalyl-cephalosporin C-9-benzhydrylester-1′-methylester	E	0.59
N-t-butyloxycarbonyl-cephalosporin C-dibenzylester	A	0.82
	D	0.72
	F	0.35
Cephalosporin-C-dibenzhydrylester	A	0.65
	B	0.78
	G	0.12
Cephalosporin-C-dibenzylester	A	0.51
	D	0.18
Iso-7-aminocephalosporanic acid-benzylester	A	0.72
	D	0.53
Piperidine-(6)-carbonic acid-(2)-benzylester	A	0.65
	F	0.08
7-Aminocephalosporanic acid-benzhydrylester	H	0.31
Iso-7-aminocephalosporanic acid-benzhydrylester	H	0.23
7-Aminocephalosporanic acid	B	0.48
Piperidine-(6)-carbonic acid-(2)-benzhydrylester	A	0.72
7-Aminocephalosporanic acid	A	0.08
	B	0.40
7-Phenylacetamidocephalosporanic acid	A	0.42
	B	0.62
7-Aminocephalosporanic acid-benzhydrylester	A	0.65
	B	0.74
	G	0.39
	F	0.33

N-phthalyl-D-α-aminoadipic
  acid-benzhydrylester-e-
  methylester   I   0.47
N-phthalyl-DL-α-amino-
  adipic acid-dimethylester   A   0.72
N-phthalyl-D-α-aminoadipic
  acid-e-methylester   A   0.63
                                            B   0.60

Ref:

B. Fechtig, H. Peter, H. Bickel and
E. Vischer, Helv. Chim. Acta, 51 (1968)
1108–1119.

2. **Medium:**

Diethylamino-ethyl cellulose.

Solvent:

Sodium acetate buffer, 0.05 M, pH 5.2.

Detection:

Color. Spray with ninhydrin reagent (0.3 g
ninhydrin, 100 ml of 1-butanol and 3 ml of
acetic acid).

R_f:

Cephalosporin C   0.2

Ref:

C.H. Nash and F.M. Huber, Appl. Microbiol.,
22 (1971) 6–10.

3. **Medium:**

Silica Gel.

Solvent:

A. n-Butanol:pyridine:acetic acid:water
   (42:24:4:30).
B. Ethyl acetate:n-butanol:pyridine:acetic
   acid:water (42:21:21:6:10).
C. n-Butanol:pyridine:acetic acid:water
   (34:24:12:30).

Detection:

Iodine vapor.

R_f:

	Solvent		
	A	B	C
Sodium salt of ethoxy-carbonyl-acetamido-cephalosporanic acid	0.32	0.35	0.52
Methoxy carbonyl-acetylamino-cephalosporanic acid	0.24	0.42	0.46

Ref:

H. Bickel, R. Bosshardt, E. Menard,
J. Mueller and H. Peter, U.S. Patent
3,557,104. January 19, 1971.

ELPHO.

1. **Medium:**

Whatman No. 1 paper.

Buffer:

Aq. collidine:acetate soln. 0.05 M to acetate,
pH 7.0.

Conditions:

17 V/cm, 2.5–4 h.

Detection:

As PC (3).

Mobility:

Cephalosporin C_A derived from	Electrophoretic mobility[*]
Nicotine	−1.4
2-Aminopyridine	−0.6
2-Amino-6-methylpyridine	−0.64
Pyridine	−0.4
Nicotinamide	−0.4
2,4,6 Trimethylpyridine	−0.4
2-Hydroxymethylpyridine	−0.4
Quinoline	−0.4
Sulphapyridine	+0.25
Sulphadiazine	+0.25
Sulphathiazole	+0.25
3-Hydroxypyridine	+0.75
iso-Nicotinic acid	+0.55
Nicotinic acid	+1.0
Picolinic acid	+0.75
Pyridine-2,3-dicarboxylic acid	+3.2

[*](+), migration towards anode; (−), migration
toward cathode.

Ref:

As PC (3).

2. **Medium:**

Whatman No. 1 paper.

Buffer:

A. Collidine:acetate, 0.05 M to acetate,
   pH 7.0.
B. Pyridine:acetate, 0.05 M to acetate,
   pH 4.5.
C. Acetic acid 10% (v/v), pH 2.2

Conditions:

14 V/cm, 2–5 h.

Detection:

As PC (2).

Mobility:

	Migration (cm) with solvent		
	A	B	C
Deacetylcephalo-sporin C	+4.3	+7.2	− 1.2
Cephalosporin C	+4.2	+6.8	− 0.6
Cephalosporin C_C	− 1.0	− 1.7	− 4.4
Cephalosporin C_A (pyridine)	− 1.0	− 1.7	—

Ref:

As PC (2).

3. **Medium:**

As ELPHO (2).

Buffer:

A. As ELPHO (2) A.
B. As ELPHO (2) B.
C. As ELPHO (2) B, but pH 4.0.
D. Formic acid, 10% (v/v), pH 1.5.
E. Acetic acid, 10% (v/v), pH 2.2.

Detection:

Bioautography vs. *Salmonella typhi*.

Mobility:

4. **Medium:**

Whatman No. 1 paper.

Buffer:

0.1 M ammonium carbonate, pH 9.0.

Conditions:

45 V/cm.

Detection:

A. UV light.
B. Ninhydrin spray.
C. 10% Aq. silver nitrate.
D. Ammoniacal silver nitrate (10 ml aq. 10% silver nitrate + 10 ml ammonium hydroxide + 80 ml methanol).
E. Starch-iodine (10 ml of 10 mM iodine in 3 mM potassium iodide + 9 ml aq. 2% soluble starch + 1 ml M phosphate buffer, pH 7).
F. Platinichloride reagent [27 ml M potassium iodide + 5 ml of 5% potassium platinum chloride (K_2PtCl_6) + 100 ml water].

Mobility:

Cephalosporin C moved 6 cm towards anode.

	Migration (cm) in buffer				
	A	B	C	D	E
Cephalosporin C	+5.2	+ 7.5	+7.2	− 3.2	− 0.4
N-phenylacetyl-cephalosporin C	+8.2	+12.0	—	—	—
Cephalosporin C_C	− 1.5	− 2.0	—	− 4.0	− 5.0
N-phenylacetyl-cephalosporin C_C	+3.4	—	—	—	—
Cephalosporin C_A (pyridine)	− 1.5	—	− 2.9	—	− 4.7
Cephalosporin C_A (pyridine) nucleus	− 1.5	—	− 9.8	—	− 9.9
Cephalosporin C_C nucleus	− 1.5	− 4.5	—	—	− 13.1
Penicillin nucleus (6-APA)	+7.5	+ 2.1	0.0	− 6.5	− 10.0
Cephalosporin C nucleus (7-ACA)	+7.5	+ 3.4	+1.0	− 4.5	− 4.0
N-phenylacetyl derivative of 6-APA (benzyl-penicillin)	+5.2	+ 7.5	—	—	—
N-phenylacetyl derivative of 7-ACA	+5.1	+ 7.5	—	—	—

Ref:

As PC (4).

Ref:
J.M.T. Hamilton-Miller, G.G.F. Newton and
E.P. Abraham, Biochem. J., 116 (1970)
371–384.

CCD.
1. **Solvent:**
Hexane:diisopropyl ether:acetone:0.5 M
potassium phosphate, pH 6.0 (25:8:25:25);
lower phase mobile.
Distribution coefficient:
Using a 15 tube distribution, most activity
was present in the central fractions (peak
activity tube No. 8).
Ref:
As PC (4).

CEPHALOSPORUM GRAMINIUS **ANTIBIOTIC**
PC.
1. **Paper:**
Solvent:
Butanol:acetic acid:water (4:1:5).
Detection:
R_f:
0.85
Ref:
G.W. Bruehl, R.L. Millar and B. Crunfer,
Can. J. Plant Sci., 49 (1969) 235–246.

CHALCIDIN
PC.
1. **Paper:**
Solvent:
A. Benzene:hexane:acetone (20:5:6),
descending.
B. Benzene:hexane:acetone (20:5:3).
Detection:
R_f:
A. 7 biologically active spots.
B. 3 biologically active spots in fraction II
and 2 in fraction III.
Ref:
G.F. Gause, M.G. Brazhnikova, V.A. Shorin,
T.S. Maksimova, O.L. Olkhovatova,
M.K. Kidinova, I.A. Vishnyakova,
N.S. Pevzner and S.P. Shapovalova,
Antibiotiki, 15 (1970) 483–486.

TLC.
1. **Medium:**
Silicic acid.
Solvent:
Benzene:acetone (5:1).
Detection:
R_f:
7 biologically active spots.
Ref:
As PC (1).

CHAMPAMYCINS
PC.
1. **Paper:**
Solvent:
A. Benzene:acetic acid:water (2:2:1),
ascending.
B. Pyridine:ethyl acetate:water (2.5:6:7),
upper phase, descending.
C. Isobutanol:pyridine:water (6:4:3),
descending.
D. Isobutanol:glacial acetic acid:water
(20:1:25), descending.
E. Pentanol:methanol:water (1:1:1.5),
descending.
F. Methanol:water:ammonium hydroxide
(20:4:1), descending.
G. n-Butanol:acetic acid:water (20:1:25).
Detection:
R_f:

Solvent	R_f Champamycin A	Champamycin B
A	0.00	0.33
B		0.87
C		0.96
D		0.91
E		0.39
F		0.94
G		0.70

Ref:
U.K. Rao and P.L. Narasimha Rao, Ind. J.
Exp. Biol., 5 (1967) 39–43.

CHAMPAVITIN
PC.
1. **Paper:**
Solvent:
As champamycins PC (1) A.
Detection:

R_f:

0.95

Ref:

As champamycins PC (1).

CHELOCARDIN

PC.

1. **Paper:**

Eaton-Dikeman No. 613, 5/16 in. wide strips.

Solvent:

A. Water satd. n-butanol.

B. As (A) + 2% w/v p-toluenesulfonic acid.

C. As (A) + 2% piperidine, w/v.

D. 80% Aq. methanol + 1.5% sodium chloride (w/v) vs. paper buffered with 0.05 M sodium bisulfate + 0.95 M sodium sulfate.

E. As (D), replacing methanol with ethanol.

F. Acetic acid:water:n-propanol (1:12.5:12.5).

All of above equilibrated with solvent for 3 h, developed 16 h ascending.

G. Water satd. with methyl isobutyl ketone + 2% (w/v), p-toluenesulfonic acid.

H. Water satd. with methyl isobutyl ketone.

I. As (H) + 1% (w/v) p-toluenesulfonic acid.

J. As (H) + 1% (v/v) piperidine.

K. Water:methanol:acetone (12:3:1) adjusted to pH 10.5 with ammonium hydroxide then to pH 7.5 with 30% phosphoric acid.

Systems G-K developed 3 h without prior equilibration, ascending.

Detection:

Bioautography vs. *Sarcina lutea* ATCC 9341.

R_f:

Solvent	R_f
A	0.13
B	0.79
C	0.51
D	0.80
E	0.90
F	0.81
G	0.22
H	0.12
I	0.18
J	0.34
K	0.26

Ref:

T.J. Oliver, J.F. Prokop, R.R. Bower and R.H. Otto, Antimicrobial Agents and Chemotherapy, 1962 (1963) 583–591.

CHLORAMPHENICOL

Chloramphenicol Derivatives

Chloramphenicol can be identified after chromatography (1) by bioautography, (2) by observation of a dark zone using ultraviolet light or (3) by reducing the nitro group to an aryl amino group which can be detected as a yellow spot by procedures outlined below.

PC.

1. **Paper:**

Whatman No. 1.

Solvent:

Water satd. n-butanol containing 2.5% acetic acid.

Detection:

Spray first with solution composed of 3 ml of 15% stannous chloride, 15 ml conc. HCl and 180 ml water. (Prepare fresh before use.) Air dry; spray again with solution composed of 1 g p-dimethylamino-benzaldehyde dissolved in a mixture of 30 ml ethanol, 30 ml conc. HCl and 180 ml n-butanol. Upon drying yellow zones appear.

R_f:

0.89

Ref:

A.J. Glazko, W.A. Dill and M.C. Rebstock, J. Biol. Chem., 183 (1950) 679.

2. **Paper:**

Whatman No. 1.

Solvent:

n-Butanol:water:acetic acid (4:5:1).

Detection:

As in 1.

R_f:

0.92

Ref:

V.H. Reber and E. Lichtenberg. Helv. Medica Acta, 20 (1953) 396.

3. **Paper:**

Whatman No. 1.

Solvent:

Stationary phase; sec. octyl alcohol. Mobile phase, McIlvaines buffer pH 6. Development time about 1 h.

Detection:

Dark zones are observed under UV. Quantitative estimation done by eluting with methanol and direct reading of UV absorption at 278 nm.

R_f:

Chloramphenicol, 0.30; -palimitate, 0.0; -stearate, 0.0; -succinate, 0.75.

Ref:

G. Sferruzza and R. Rangone, Il Farmaco, 18 (1943) 322.

4. **Paper:**

Arches 302 or Whatman No. 1.

Solvent:

A. Same as PC (2). Spot 5—20 ml containing 5—20 μg, ascending about 16 h at 20°C ± 1°C.

B. n-Butanol:pyridine:water (2:1:2), 8—10 h.

C. n-Butanol satd. with water on paper impregnated with M/5 monopotassium phosphate.

Detection:

Similar to PC (1) but second spray consists of p-dimethylaminobenzaldehyde, 1 g; conc. HCl, 20 ml; and 95% ethanol, Q.S. for 100 ml.

R_f:

A. 0.96   B. 0.96   C. 0.97

Ref:

M.R. Rousselet and R. Paris, Annales Pharm. Franc., 22 (1964) 249.

TLC.

1. **Medium:**

Silica Gel G.

Solvent:

A. Ethyl acetate satd. with water. Develop about 1 h.

B. n-Butanol saturated with water + 2.5% acetic acid. Develop about 4—5 h.

Detection:

As in PC (1). Heat plate in an oven at 100°C for 5 min after spraying on solution (1), then spray with (2). Sensitivity is 0.2 μg chloramphenicol.

R_f:

A. 0.90   B. 0.72

Ref:

M.M.J. Lachorine and G. Netien, Société de Pharmacie de Lyon, 9 (1963) 120.

2. **Medium:**

A. Silica Gel G; 1. Activated, 2. not activated.

B. Silica Gel G impregnated with pH 6

phosphate buffer; 1. activated, 2. not activated.

Solvent:

Chloroform:methanol. a. (90:10), b. (85:15), c. (80:20).

Detection:

A. Iodine vapor. Stand plate in a chamber with iodine for a few minutes; gives dark brown spots.

B. Spray plate with a 1% alcoholic solution of Rhodamine B.

C. UV lamp (254 nm) shows zones as dark spots.

R_f:

Solvent	Medium			
	A.1	A.2	B.1	B.2
a.	0.47	0.54	0.53	0.42
b.	0.65	0.65	0.66	0.64
c.	0.82	0.82	0.80	0.86

Ref:

M.A. Kassem, A.A. Kassem and A.E.M. El-Nimr, Pharm. Zeitung, 111 (1966) 1792.

3. **Medium:**

Silica Gel G. Mix 30 g Silica Gel G (Merck) with 60 ml water vigorously for 1 min and spread a 275 μ layer on a 20 × 20 cm glass plate. Air dry for 15 min at RT then for 30 min at 110°C in a drying oven and store in a desiccator over "Blaugel" (a drying agent).

Solvent:

Butanol:acetic acid:water (4:1:1).

Detection:

As PC (4). Useful for separation of chloramphenicol or its phthalate or succinate derivatives and their decomposition products.

R_f:

No numerical data presented.

Ref:

V.M. Sahll, H. Ziegler and M. Desch, Pharm. Zeitung, 44 (1965) 1542.

4. **Medium:**

Polyamide, according to Wang. E-poly-caprolactam powder (6 g) dissolved in 30 ml 80% formic acid and spread on a 18 × 25 cm glass plate. Dry overnight, heat at 100°C for 20 min. Layer = 55 mm thick.

Solvent:
    A. n-Butanol:chloroform:acetic acid
       (10:90:0.5).
    B. n-Butanol:water:acetic acid (82:18:0.5).

Detection:
    0.25% $SnCl_2$ in 1 N HCl; dry; follow with
    2% p-dimethylaminobenzaldehyde in 1.2 N
    HCl. Compounds appear as bright yellow
    spots after a few hours. Sensitivity:
    chloramphenicol 10 μg; palmitate, 40 μg;
    succinate, 30 μg.

R_f:

	System	
	A	B
chloramphenicol	0.35	0.80
chloramphenicol		
palmitate	0.95	0.90
chloramphenicol		
succinate	0.25	0.72

Ref:
    Y. Linn, K. Wang, T. Yang, J. Chromatogr.,
    21 (1966) 158; K. Wang, J. Chinese Chem.
    Soc., 8 (1961) 241.

GLC. (Quantitative)
1. **Apparatus:**
    Barber-Colman Model 5000 with FID, 5 mV
    recorder with 1/3 in./min chart speed.

Column:
    Glass, U-shaped, 6 ft × 3 mm ID packed
    with 5% SE-30 on Gas-Chrom. Q (80–100
    mesh).

Temperatures:
    Column, 240°C; detector, 250°C; injector,
    250°C.

Carrier gas:
    N_2 at 20 p.s.i. (50 ml/min) H_2 at 32 p.s.i.
    and air at 40 p.s.i.

Current:
    5×10^{-8} A f.s.d. (sens. 100, atten. 5).

Reagent solvent:
    200 mg m-phenylene dibenzoate dissolved in
    6 ml acetonitrile. 1 ml of N, O-bis (trimethyl-
    silyl) acetamide (BSA) is added and volume
    made up to 10 ml with acetonitrile; shake
    until uniform.

Derivative:
    Add 0.5 ml of reagent and stir vigorously.

Chromatography and calculations:
    One ml of each derivatized solution (= to

approx. 20 μg chloramphenicol) is injected
and peaks measured. Chloramphenicol
content is determined by direct comparison
of peak areas (chloramphenicol/internal
stand.) with chloramphenicol stand. treated
in an identical manner.

Ref:
    M. Margosis, J. Chromatogr., 47 (1970) 341.

CHLORTETRACYCLINE
See tetracyclines.

CHROMIN
PC.
1. **Paper:**
    Whatman No. 2.

Solvent:
    Ethanol:n-butanol:water (1:5:5), ascending
    18–24 h.

Detection:
    Bioautography vs. *Saccharomyces cerevisiae*.

R_f:
    0.55

Ref:
    C.P. Schaffner, I.D. Steinman, R.S. Safferman
    and H. Lechevalier, Antibiotics Annual,
    1957–1958, 869–873.

CHROMOMYCINS
PC.
1. **Paper:**
    Toyo No. 7. Immerse in glycerol:methanol
    (1:4), dry, briefly insert in excess of methanol,
    remove and dry in hot air current.

Solvent:
    A. Benzene:ethyl acetate (4:1 to 2:1).
    B. Diethyl ether:ethyl acetate (190:10 to
       170:30).
    C. Isopentyl acetate:n-butanol (9:1).
    D. Isopentyl acetate:acetone (19:1 to 14:1).

Detection:
    A. Bioautography vs. *Staphylococcus aureus*
       or *Bacillus subtilis*.
    B. Freshly prepared soln. of ferric chloride
       and potassium ferricyanide. Chromomycin
       A, BO_1, BO_2, B_p appear as bluish green
       spots against a yellow background.
       Remove excess reagent under tap water
       to fix blue spots.
    C. Spray with ethanol:2N alkali (1:1), dry

Solvent	Ratio	A Group					B Group				C Group
		A₁	A₂	A₃	A₄	A₅	O₁	O₂	P	F	
A	4:1			0.33 ± 0.05				0.00		0.00 ~ 0.02	0.00
	3:1			0.50 ± 0.05				0.00		0.00 ~ 0.02	0.00
	2:1			0.70 ± 0.05				0.00		0.00 ~ 0.02	0.00
B	185:15	0.60	0.50	0.35 ± 0.04	0.25	0.10		0.00		0.00	0.00
	170:30	0.70	0.60	0.50 ± 0.04	0.30	0.15		0.00		0.00	0.00
C	9:1			0.95 ± 1.00				0.75 ± 0.07		0.25 ± 0.04	0.00
D	19:1			0.90 ± 0.05			0.80	0.70	0.55	0.23 ± 0.04	0.00
	14:1			0.95 ± 0.05			0.87	0.78	0.65	0.30 ± 0.04	0.00

in air at room temperature and spray with 3% hydrogen peroxide. A_2, A_3, A_4 and A_5 appear as red spots, persisting for a few minutes.

D. UV light (wide range).

R_f:

See Table.

Ref:

K. Mizuno, J. Antibiotics, Ser. B, 13 (1960) 329–331.

2. **Paper**:

A. Acetylated Toyo No. 7.

B. Acetylated Whatman No. 1.

Solvent:

Butyl acetate:pyridine:water (1:5:10).

Detection:

UV light.

R_f:

Chromomycin A₃ derivative	R_f Toyo No. 7	What. No. 1	Fluorescence under UV light
A_3	0.53	0.57	orange
A_3-Formate	0.65	0.67	orange
A_3-Me	0.56	0.59	emerald green
A_3-Me-Ac	0.22	0.19	emerald green
A_3-Ac	0.32	0.26	emerald green

Ref:

K. Mizuno, J. Antibiotics, 16 (1963) 22–39.

TLC.

1. **Medium**:

Mix 30 g. Silica gel G (Merck, U.S.A.) and 60 ml Theorell's buffer soln. (pH 2.3, 0.07 M). Spread on a glass plate to form a 0.2 mm layer; dry at 100°C for 1 h.

Solvent:

Benzene:chloroform:methanol (1:2:1).

Detection:

R_f:

Chromomycin A_3 0.67 ± 0.1

Chromomycin A_3 hemisuccinate   0.40 ± 0.1

Ref:

K. Mizuno, N. Sugita, M. Asai and A. Miyaki, U.S. Patent 3,501,570; March 17, 1970.

CHROTHIOMYCIN
TLC.
1. **Medium:**
   Silica Gel.
   Solvent:
   A. Water satd. ethyl ether.
   B. Water satd. butanol.
   C. Ethyl acetate.
   D. Butyl acetate.
   E. Methanol.
   F. Butanol.
   G. Water.
   H. Benzene.
   I. Chloroform.
   Detection:
   Color. Gives purple spot.
   R_f:

Solvent	R_f
A	0.22
B	0.77
C	0.09
D	0.03
E	0.50
F	0.45
G	0.72
H	0.00
I	0.00

   Ref:
   S. Ayukawa, M. Hamada, K. Kojiri,
   T. Takeuchi, T. Hara, T. Nagatsu and
   H. Umezawa, J. Antibiotics, 22 (1969)
   303–308.

CINEROMYCIN B
GLC.
1. **Conditions:**
   Same as for albocycline GLC (1).
   Retention time:
   9 min (est. from curve).
   Ref:
   As albocycline PC (1).

CIRRAMYCINS
PC.
1. **Paper:**
   Solvent:
   A. Wet n-butanol.
   B. 3% Aq. ammonium chloride.
   C. 75% Phenol.
   D. 50% Acetone.
   E. Butanol:methanol:water:methyl orange
      (40 ml:10 ml:20 ml:1.5 g).
   F. Butanol:methanol:water (4:1:2).
   G. Benzene:methanol (4:1).
   H. Water.
   Detection:
   Bioautography vs. *Bacillus subtilis*.
   R_f:

Solvent	$R_f^\star$
A	0.9
B	0.75
C	0.95
D	0.95
E	0.95
F	0.95
G	0.4, 0.9 (trace)
H	0.1

   $\star$Estimated from drawing.

   Ref:
   H. Koshiyama, M. Okanishi, T. Ohmori,
   T. Miyaki, H. Tsukiura, M. Matsuzaki and
   H. Kawaguchi. J. Antibiotics, 16 (1963)
   59–66.

2. **Paper:**
   Solvent:
   Sorensen's buffer, pH 7.0.
   Detection:
   R_f:
   Cirramycin A   0.48
   Cirramycin B   0.15
   Ref:
   As PC (1).

3. **Paper:**
   Solvent:
   Solvents A-F same as for angolamycin
   PC (1).
   Detection:
   R_f:

Solvent	R_f Cirramycin A	Cirramycin B
A	0.73	0.70
B	0.66	0.94
C	0.48	0.15
D	0.86	0.60
E	0.74	0.78
F	0.84	0.85

   Ref:
   As PC (1).

4. Separation of components of cirramycin A.
   Paper:
   Solvent:
      0.05 N ammonium hydroxide satd. with
      methyl isobutyl ketone
   Detection:
      Bioautography vs. *Bacillus subtilis.*
   R_f:

Cirramycin A_1	0.84 (major zone)
Cirramycin A_2	0.89
Cirramycin A_3	0.75
Cirramycin A_4	0.67
Cirramycin A_5	0.86

   Ref:
      H. Koshiyama, H. Tsukiura, K. Fujisawa,
   M. Konishi, M. Hatori, K. Tomita and
   H. Kawaguchi, J. Antibiotics, 22 (1969)
   61–64.

5. **Paper:**
   Solvent:
      A. Stationary phase; formamide:methanol
      (1:1). Mobile phase, benzene:cyclohexane
      (1:1) satd. with formamide.
      B. Paper treated with 2% liquid paraffin.
      Stationary phase, butyl acetate. Mobile
      phase, M/15 Sorensen's buffer (pH 8)
      satd. with butyl acetate.
      C. Methyl isobutyl ketone:methyl ethyl
      ketone (4:1), ascending.
      D. Methyl isobutyl ketone, descending.
   Detection:

R_f:

Type of derivative	Derivative of cirramycin A_1	A	B	C	D
Esters of monobasic acids	Acetyl	0.45	–	–	0.87
	Triacetyl	0.93	–	0.98	–
	Propionyl	–	0.15	–	0.93
	Phenylacetyl	0.88	–	0.96	–
	Phenoxyacetyl	0.68	–	0.98	–
	Benzoyl	0.88	–	–	0.92
Esters of dibasic acids	Malcoyl	0	0.49	0.33	0.64
	Disuccinyl (III)	0	0.57	0.80	0.80
	Glutaryl	0	0.47	0.82	0.64
	Phthaloyl	0	0.48	0.33	0.68
Esters of amino acids	Leucyl	0	0.46	–	–
	Phenylglycyl	0	0.45	–	0.02
Esters of other acids	Methylsuccinyl (IV)	0.18	0.50	–	0.88
	β-sulfopropionyl	0	0.46	–	0.
	Methylsulfonyl	0.80	–	–	0.89
	Methylcarbamoyl	0	0.35	–	0.80
	Ethoxycarbonyl	0.61	0.30	–	0.89
Des-epoxy (II)	Depoxy (II)	–	0.35	–	0.78
	Depoxypropionyl	–	–	–	0.95
	Tetrahydro	–	0.88	–	0.90
N-Oxide	N-Oxide	0	0.78	0.76	–
	Succinyl N-oxide	0	0.78	–	0.31
Aldehyde modification	Aldoxime	–	0.64	–	–
	Hydantolnylimino	–	–	–	–
	Cirramycin A_1 (I)	0	0.51	0.28	0.73

Ref:

H. Tsukiura, M. Konishi, M. Saka,
K. Fujisawa, T. Ohmori, T. Hoshiya and
H. Kawaguchi, J. Antibiotics, 22 (1969)
100–105.

TLC.
1. **Medium:**
   Solvent:
   As angolamycin TLC (1).
   Detection:
   R_f:

Solvent	R_f Cirramycin A	Cirramycin B
A	0.23	0.58
B	0.40	0.47

   Ref:
   As angolamycin TLC (1).

CCD.
1. **Solvent:**
   A. Benzene:M/15 Sorensen's buffer (pH 5.8), 50 transfers.
   B. Benzene:M/15 Sorensen's buffer (pH 7.0), 50 transfers (used for repeated distribution of A component).
   C. Benzene:M/15 Sorensen's buffer (pH 4.5), 50 transfers (used for repeated distribution of B component).

   Distribution:

Solvent	Component	Peak Tube No.
A	Cirramycin A	5
	Cirramycin B	42
B	Cirramycin A	25
C	Cirramycin B	20

   Ref:
   As PC (1).

2. **Solvent:**
   Benzene:M/10 Sorensen's buffer (pH 7.0), 100 transfers.
   Distribution:
   Cirramycin A_1 found at tube No. 45. Cirramycin A_2 was distributed before A_1 peak. Cirramycin A_3, A_4 and A_5 appeared after the A_1 component.
   Ref:
   As PC (4).

CITROMYCIN
PC.
1. **Paper:**
   Solvent:
   A. Wet butanol.
   B. 20% Ammonium chloride.
   C. 75% Phenol.
   D. 50% Acetone.
   E. Butanol:methanol:water (4:1:2) + 1.5% methyl orange.
   F. Butanol:methanol:water (4:1:2).
   G. Benzene:methanol (4:1).
   H. Water.
   Detection:
   Bioautography vs. *Bacillus subtilis*.
   R_f:

Solvent	R_f
A	0.0
B	1.0
C	0.65
D	0–0.17
E	0.37–0.46
F	0–0.1
G	0.0
H	0–0.1

   Ref:
   Y. Kusakabe, Y. Yamauchi, C. Nagatsu,
   H. Abe, K. Akasaki and S. Shirato,
   J. Antibiotics, 22 (1969) 112–118.

TLC.
1. **Medium:**
   Alumina.
   Solvent:
   Ethanol:water (4:6).
   Detection:
   Bioautography vs. *Bacillus subtilis* PCI-219.
   R_f:
   0.5 (estimated from drawing)
   Ref:
   Y. Kono, S. Makino, S. Takeuchi and
   H. Yonehara, J. Antibiotics, 22 (1969)
   583–589.

COFORMYCIN
ELPHO.
1. **Medium:**
   Paper.
   Buffer:
   A. pH 5.0.
   B. pH 8.0.

Conditions:
400 V, 2.5 h.

Detection:

Mobility:
A. Moved toward cathode.
B. No movement.

Ref:
Japanese Patent No. 12278/70, published
May 4, 1970.

COLISAN

PC.

1. **Paper:**
Whatman No. 1.

Solvent:
n-Butanol:acetic acid:water (4:1:5),
descending, 24 h.

Detection:
Paper dipped into a satd. soln. of iodine in
petroleum ether (60–80°C).

R_f:
Elongated spot, 0.4–0.8.

Ref:
S.A. Leon and F. Bergmann, Biotech. and
Bioeng., 10 (1968) 429–444.

TLC.

1. **Medium:**
Silica Gel G.

Solvent:
A. n-Butanol:acetic acid:water (4:1:5).
B. Chloroform:methanol:water (65:36:8).
C. Benzene:chloroform:methanol:acetic
acid:water (15:15:23:7:7).

Detection:
A. Ninhydrin.
B. As PC (1).

R_f:

	Solvent	R_f
Colisan	A	0.38
Colisan	B	0.27
Colisan	C	0.75
Deaminated colisan	A	0.38
		(nin-
		hydrin–,
		iodine+)
Acetylated colisan		0.10
		(nin-
		hydrin–,
		iodine+)

Ref:
As PC (1).

ELPHO.

1. **Medium:**
Whatman No. 1 paper.

Buffer:
1 N acetic acid.

Conditions:
A. 1000 V, 1 hr. (Running tap water as
coolant.)
B. 3000 V, 1 hr.

Detection:
0.3% ninhydrin in acetone. Heat for 5 min
at 80°C.

Mobility:
A. 10 cm towards cathode.
B. 19 cm towards cathode.

Ref:
As PC (1).

COLISTIN

cf: Polymyxin E.

COMIRIN

PC.

1. **Paper:**

Solvent:
A. Water satd. amyl alcohol.
B. Water satd. n-butanol.
C. n-Butanol:pyridine:water (2:1:4).
D. Aq. ammonia (sp. gr. 0.88).
E. Water satd. phenol.
F. 60% Aq. dioxane (v/v).
G. 25% Aq. monoethyl amine (v/v).
H. 60% Pyridine-water (v/v).
I. Water.

Detection:
Bioautography vs. *Aspergillus flavus*.

R_f:

Solvent	R_f
A	0.05
B	0.16
C	0.42
D	0.75
E	0.81
F	0.88
G	0.92
H	0.96
I	0.00

61 COUMERMYCINS

Ref:

W.G.C. Forsythe, Biochem. J., 59 (1955) 500–506.

CCD.

1. **Solvent:**

n-Butanol:water containing 10% pyridine (1:5); ten-tube diagonal distribution.

Distribution:

Comirin was recovered from tubes 8–10.

Ref:

As PC (1).

COPIAMYCIN

PC.

1. **Paper:**

Solvent:

A. n-Butanol:methanol:water (4:1:2).
B. Pyridine:n-butanol:water (4:3:7).
C. 50% Acetone.
D. Benzene:methanol (4:1).
E. 75% Phenol.
F. 3% Ammonium chloride.
G. Water satd. with n-butanol.
H. n-Butanol:satd. with water.
I. Ethyl acetate:n-butanol (1:1).
J. t-Butanol:water (4:1).

Detection:

Bioautography vs. *Candida albicans*.

R_f:

Solvent	R_f*
A	0.75
B	0.95
C	0.7–0.9
D	0.2–0.4
E	0.95
F	0.05
G	0.02
H	0.4–0.6
I	0.2
J	0.65

*Estimated from drawing.

Ref:

T. Arai, S. Kuroda, H. Ohara, Y. Katoh and H. Kaji, J. Antibiotics, 18 (1965) 63–67.

TLC.

1. **Medium:**

Silica Gel G.

Solvent:

A. Acetic acid:n-butanol:water (6:25:25).
B. n-Butanol:methanol:water (4:1:2).

Detection:

R_f:

Solvent	R_f
A	0.4
B	0.5

Ref:

As PC (1).

2. **Medium:**

Aluminum oxide.

Solvent:

A. Pyridine:n-butanol:water (4:6:3).
B. Benzene:methanol (4:1).

Detection:

R_f:

Solvent	R_f
A	0.7
B	0.3

Ref:

As PC (1).

COUMERMYCIN

PC.

1. **Paper:**

Whatman No. 1. Equilibrate 1–2 h before development.

Solvent:

A. Paper dipped in capryl alcohol:methanol (1:5) blotted; developed with 0.1 M phosphate buffer, descending, 6.5 h.
B. As A, but developed 20–25 h.

Detection:

Bioautography vs. *Staphylococcus aureus*.

R_f:

	Solvent	R_f*
Coumermycin complex	A	0–0.1
Coumermycin D-1	B	0.1–0.3
Coumermycin D-2	B	0.4–0.6
Coumermycin D-3	B	0.7–0.9

*Estimated from drawing.

Ref:

J. Berger, A.J. Schocher, A.D. Batcho, B. Pecherer, O. Keller, J. Maricq, A.E. Karr, B.P. Vaterlaus, A. Furlenmeier and H. Speigelberg, Antimicrobial Agents and Chemotherapy, 1965 (1966) 778–785.

2. **Paper:**

S and S 589 Blue Ribbon; 1.3 cm wide strips.

Solvent:

0.1 M triethanolamine adjusted to pH 7.0
with glacial acetic acid (2:3).

Detection:

Bioautography vs. *Staphylococcus aureus*
ATCC 6538P.

R_f:

Coumermycin A_1 0.3—0.4

Ref:

J.G. Keil, I.R. Hooper, M.J. Cron,
H. Schmitz, D.E. Nettleton and J.C. Godfrey,
Antimicrobial Agents and Chemotherapy,
1968 (1969) 120—127.

TLC.

1. **Medium:**

Silica Gel G.

Solvent:

Glacial acetic acid:methanol:carbon tetrachloride (6:6:90), ascending, 15 cm.

Detection:

R_f:

Coumermycin D-1a	0.60
Coumermycin D-1b (c)	0.50
Coumermycin D-1d	0.40
Coumermycin D-2	0.35
Coumermycin D-3	0.30
Coumermycin D-4	0.25

Ref:

As PC (1).

CRANOMYCIN

PC.

1. **Paper:**

Toyo No. 50.

Solvent:

A. Water satd. n-butanol.
B. 1.5% Aq. ammonium chloride.
C. 75% Aq. phenol.
D. Acetone:water (1:1).
E. n-Butanol:methanol:water (4:1:2).
F. t-Butanol:acetic acid:water (74:3:25).
G. n-Butanol:acetic acid:water (4:1:1).
All of above developed ascending.

Detection:

Bioautography vs. *Sarcina lutea*.

R_f:

Solvent	R_f
A	0.97
B	0.76
C	0.98
D	0.96
E	1.0
F	0.97
G	0.08—0.11

Ref:

S.-I. Kondo, M.Shimura, M. Sezaki, K. Sato
and T. Hara, J. Antibiotics, 17 (1964)
230—233.

TLC.

1. **Medium:**

Silica Gel G.

Solvent:

A. Water satd. ethyl acetate.
B. Benzene:methanol (4:1).
C. Benzene:methanol:28% ammonium
hydroxide (80:20:1).
D. Benzene:methanol:acetic acid (80:20:1).
E. Water.
F. Water:28% ammonium hydroxide (100:1).
G. Water:acetic acid (100:1).

Detection:

Color: potassium permanganate solution.

R_f:

Solvent	R_f
A	0.06
B	0.17
C	0.49
D	0.08
E	0.18
F	0.58
G	0.23

Ref:

As PC (1).

CREMEOMYCIN

PC.

1. **Paper:**

Solvent:

A. 1-Butanol:water (84:16), 16 h.
B. 1-Butanol:water (84:16) + 0.25%
p-toluenesulfonic acid, 16 h.
C. 1-Butanol:acetic acid:water (2:1:1), 16 h.
D. 2% piperidine (v/v) in 1-butanol:water
(84:16), 16 h.
E. 1-Butanol:water (4:96), 5 h.

F. 1-Butanol:water (4:96) + 0.25% p-toluenesulfonic acid, 5 h.

Detection:

Bioautography vs. *Proteus vulgaris*.

R_f:

Solvent	R_f*
A	0.1—0.5
B	0.5
C	0.8
D	0.35—0.6
E	0.9
F	0.7—0.9

*Estimated from drawing.

Ref:

M.E. Bergy and T.R. Pyke, U.S. Patent
3,350,269, October 31, 1967.

CURAMYCIN

PC.

1. **Paper:**

    Solvent:

    As avilamycin, PC (1).

    Detection:

    As avilamycin, PC (1).

    R_f:

    0.60

    Ref:

    As avilamycin, PC (1).

2. **Paper:**

    As everninomicin PC (1).

    Solvent:

    As everninomicin PC (1).

    Detection:

    As everninomicin PC (1).

    R_f:

    0.42

    Ref:

    As everninomicin PC (1).

TLC.

1. **Medium:**

    As avilamycin, TLC (1).

    Solvent:

    As avilamycin, TLC (1).

    Detection:

    As avilamycin, TLC (1).

    R_f:

    0.43

    Ref:

    As avilamycin, PC (1).

CYANEIN

PC.

1. **Paper:**

    Solvent:

    A. Water.

    B. n-Butanol satd. with water.

    C. Ethyl acetate satd. with water.

    D. Benzene satd. with water.

    E. Iso-amyl acetate:methanol:formic acid:
    water (4:2:1:3), bottom layer.

    F. n-Butanol:methanol:water (4:1:5),
    bottom layer.

    G. Methanol:hexane (6:4), bottom layer.

    H. Benzene:cyclohexane:phosphate buffer
    of pH 7.4 (5:35:60), bottom layer.

    Detection:

    Bioautography vs. *Candida pseudotropicalis*.

    R_f:

Solvent	R_f
A	0.00
B	0.93
C	0.97
D	0.00
E	0.88
F	0.65
G	0.87
H	0.00

    Ref:

    V. Betina, P. Nemec, J. Dobias and Z. Barath,
    Folia Microbiol., 8 (1962) 353—357.

CYATHINS

TLC.

1. **Medium:**

    Silica Gel G, 0.5 mm thickness. Plates heated
    at 100°C for 30 min before use.

    Solvent:

    Benzene:acetone:acetic acid (75:25:1).

    Detection:

    Spray with 30% sulfuric acid.

    R_f:

Cyathin No. 1	0.67
Cyathin B	0.51
Cyathin B_3	0.56
Cyathin C_5	0.54
Cyathin A_3	0.27
Cyathin A_4	0.06

    Ref:

    B.N. Johri, J. Chromatog., 56 (1971)
    324—329.

CYCLAMIDOMYCIN
ELPHO.
1. **Medium**:
    Paper.
   Buffer:
    Formic acid:acetic acid:water (25:75:900).
   Conditions:
    3,300 V, 20 min.
   Detection:
    Bioautography vs. *Klebsiella pneumoniae*.
   Mobility:
    Cyclamidomycin moved 12.9 cm to cathode
    with R_m (L-alanine=1.0) of 1.29; two
    minor components at R_m 0.5, 1.90.
   Ref:
    S. Takahashi, M. Nakajima, Y. Ikeda,
    S. Kondo, M. Hamada, K. Maeda and
    H. Umezawa, J. Antibiotics, 24 (1971)
    902–903.

CYCLOSERINE
PC.
1. **Paper**:
   Solvent:
    Ethanol:water (4:1).
   Detection:
    Ninhydrin. Produces a brownish-yellow
    color.
   R_f:
    0.4
   Ref:
    D.A. Harris, M. Ruger, M.A. Reagon,
    F.J. Wolf, R.L. Peck, H. Wallick and
    H.B. Woodruff, Antibiotics and Chemo-
    therapy, 5 (1955) 183–190.

2. **Paper**:
   Solvent:
    A. Buffered phenol (pH 12).
    B. t-Butanol:acetic acid:water.
   Detection:
    A. Ninhydrin.
    B. Ferric chloride. Deep red color produced.
   R_f:

Solvent	R_f
A	0.60–0.65
B	0.60–0.65

   Ref:
    G.M. Shull and J.L. Sardinas, Antibiotics
    and Chemotherapy, 5 (1955) 398–399.

3. **Paper**:
    Whatman No. 3 MM.
   Solvent:
    A. n-Butanol:acetic acid:water (4:1:5).
    B. 77% Ethanol.
    C. Methyl ethyl ketone:pyridine:water
     (20:5:8).
    D. Isopropanol:ammonia:water (80:2:18).
   Detection:
   R_f:

Solvent	R_f
A	0.31
B	0.43
C	0.37 (streaking)
D	0.17

   Ref:
    F.C. Neuhaus and J.L. Lynch, Biochem., 3
    (1964) 472.

4. **Paper**:
    Whatman No. 1.
   Solvent:
    A. 80% ethanol.
    B. n-Butanol:water:acetic acid (3:1:1).
    C. 0.01 M phosphate buffer, pH 6.0:
     isopropanol (3:7).
    D. 75% Aq. methanol containing 2% sodium
     chloride.
    E. n-Propanol:2 N ammonium hydroxide
     (7:3).
    F. n-Butanol:acetic acid:water (8:2:5).
   Detection:
    A. Ninhydrin.
    B. Bioautography.
   R_f:

Solvent	R_f
A	0.36–0.42
B	0.32–0.36
C	0.41
D	0.66
E	0.22
F	0.22

   Ref:
    E.O. Stapley, T.W. Miller and M. Jackson,
    Antimicrobial Agents and Chemotherapy,
    1968 (1969) 268–273.

DANUBOMYCIN
PC.
1. **Paper**:

Solvent:

    A. n-Butanol satd. with water.

    B. n-Butanol satd. with water + 2% p-toluene-sulfonic acid + 2% piperidine.

    C. Methyl isobutyl ketone satd. with water.

    D. 80% Ethanol with 1.5% sodium chloride. Paper impregnated with 0.95 M sodium sulfate soln. and 0.05 M sodium bisulfate soln.

    E. Butanol:methanol:water (4:1:2).

    F. Water satd. with methyl isobutyl ketone.

    G. Water satd. with methyl isobutyl ketone + 1% p-toluenesulfonic acid.

    H. 75% Water + 25% of a mixture of methanol:acetone (3:1) adjusted to pH 10.5 with ammonia and neutralized with phosphoric acid to pH 7.5.

Detection:

    Bioautography vs. *Bacterium megatherium* or *Micrococcus pyogenes* var. *aureus*.

R_f:

Solvent	R_f
A	0.65
B	0.90
C	0.00
D	0.5
E	0.67
F	0.05, 0.70
G	0.80
H	0.05, 0.70

Ref:

    E. Gaumann and W. Voser, U.S. Patent No. 3,092,550. June 4, 1963.

CCD.

1. **Solvent:**

    A. Stage 1; petroleum ether, B.P. 40–70°C; benzene:methanol:water (5:5:8:2), 10 transfers.

    B. Stage 2; petroleum ether:benzene:absolute ethanol:water (7.5:2.5:7.5:2.5), 375 transfers.

Distribution:

    A. Danubamycin is found in tubes 4–10 and transferred to stage B.

    B. Danubamycin resolved into 4 components identified as B1, B2, B3, B4; maxima are in tubes 40, 64, 124 and 164, respectively.

Ref:

    As PC (1).

DAUNOMYCIN

PC.

1. **Paper:**

    As adriamycin, PC (1).

Solvent:

    As adriamycin, PC (1).

Detection:

R_f:

Solvent	R_f
A	0.20
	0.50
C	0.35

Ref:

    As adriamycin PC (1).

TLC.

1. **Medium:**

    As adriamycin TLC (1).

Solvent:

    As adriamycin TLC (1).

Detection:

R_f:

Solvent	R_f
A	0.4
B	0.0
C	0.0

Ref:

    As adriamycin PC (1).

DEOXYHERQUEINONE

See atroventin.

DESERTOMYCIN

PC.

1. **Paper:**

    Whatman No. 1 impregnated with MacIlvaines phosphate buffer at pH 2.2, 3, 4, 5, 6, 7, 8, 9 and 10. 10 µg antibiotic spotted.

Solvent:

    Distilled water.

Detection:

    A. Bioautography vs. *Bacillus subtilis* ATCC 6633.

    B. Alkaline potassium permanganate soln.

    C. Iodine vapor.

R_f:

    Varies according to pH. Most rapid movement at pH 2.2 decreasing to slightly off origin at pH 6 or 7, and increasing slightly to pH 10.

Ref:

    F. Sztariczkai and J. Uri, Microchim. Acta. (1963) 431–441.

DESMYCOSIN
PC.
1. **Paper:**
   Solvent:
   A. Methyl ethyl ketone vs. pH 4 buffered paper.
   B. Methyl ethyl ketone.
   C. n-Butanol satd. with water vs. pH 4 buffered paper.
   D. n-Butanol satd. with water.
   E. Water with 7% sodium chloride + 2.5% methyl ethyl ketone.
   F. Ethyl acetate satd. with water vs. pH 4 buffered paper.
   Detection:
   R_f:

Solvent	R_f
A	0.40
B	0.63
C	0.90
D	0.74
E	0.76
F	0.11

   Ref:
   R.L. Hamill and W.M. Stark, J. Antibiotics, 17 (1964) 133–139.

DETOXIN
PC.
1. **Paper:**
   Toyo-Roshi No. 51.
   Solvent:
   A. Water satd. n-butanol.
   B. Butanol:acetic acid:water (4:1:2).
   C. As B but (2:1:1).
   D. As B but (4:1:1).
   E. As B but (3:3:1).
   F. Butanol:formic acid:water (8:3:2).
   G. Butanol:ethanol:water (5:2:3).
   H. Butanol:methanol:water (4:1:2).
   I. Ethanol:acetic acid:water (33:5:62).
   J. Butanol:water:conc. HCl (5:1:1).
   K. Ethanol:ammonium hydroxide:water (80:4:16).
   L. Propanol:pyridine:acetic acid:water (15:10:3:12).
   Detection:
   R_f:

Solvent	R_f
A	0.43
B	0.86
C	0.89
D	0.81
E	0.91
F	0.55
G	0.77
H	0.53
I	0.84
J	1.00
K	0.80
L	0.93

Ref:
H. Yonehara, S. Aizawa, T. Hidaka, H. Sedo and N. Odake. 17th meeting, Japan Antibiotics Research Assn, March 24, 1967.

TLC.
1. **Medium:**
   Silica Gel G.
   Solvent:
   A. Ethanol:ammonium hydroxide:water (33:5:62).
   B. Butanol:methanol:water (2:1:1).
   C. Water satd. butanol.
   D. Acetone.
   Detection:
   R_f:

Solvent	R_f
A	0.67
B	0.60
C	0.085
D	0.00

   Ref:
   As PC (1).

ELPHO.
1. **Medium:**
   Buffer:
   A. Potassium chloride:HCl, pH 1.7.
   B. Potassium dihydrogen phosphate: disodium phosphate, pH 6.1.
   C. As B, but pH 7.5.
   D. As B, but pH 7.9.
   E. Sodium carbonate:sodium bicarbonate, pH 8.5.
   F. As E, but pH 9.0.
   Condition:
   10 mA/6 cm.

Detection:
Mobility:
Estimated relative mobility toward cathode or anode:

Buffer	Mobility
A	– 2.0
B	– 1.5
C	– 0.5
D	0.0
E	+ 0.5
F	+ 1.0

Ref:
As PC (1).

DEXTOCHRYSIN
TLC.
1. **Medium:**
   Silica Gel.
   Solvent:
   Ethyl acetate:methanol (4:1).
   Detection:
   R_f:
   0.46
   Ref:
   H. Aoki, N. Miyairi, M. Ajisaka and H. Sakai, J. Antibiotics, 22 (1969) 201–206.

DIANEMYCIN
PC.
1. **Paper:**
   Solvent:
   A. Water:ethanol:acetic acid (70:24:6).
   B. 10% Aq. propanol.
   Detection:
   Bioautography vs. *Bacillus subtilis*.
   R_f:

Solvent	R_f
A	0.28
B	0.77

   Ref:
   R.L. Hamill, M.M. Hoehn, G.E. Pittenger, J. Chamberlain and M. Gorman, J. Antibiotics, 22 (1969) 161–164.

TLC.
1. **Medium:**
   Silica Gel.
   Solvent:
   Ethyl acetate.
   Detection:
   Vanillin:sulfuric acid spray.

R_f:
0.25
Ref:
As PC (1).

DIAZOMYCINS
PC.
1. **Paper:**
   Solvent:
   80% Aq. isopropanol.
   Detection:
   R_f:

Diazomycin A	0.6
Diazomycin B	0.2
Diazomycin C	0.9

   (Estimated from drawing)
   Ref:
   K.V. Rao, S.C. Brooks, Jr., M. Kugelman and A.A. Romano, Antibiotics Annual (1959–1960) 943–949.

DIENOMYCIN
TLC.
1. **Medium:**
   Silica Gel.
   Solvent:
   Ethyl acetate:methanol (5:1).
   Detection:
   A. Color (Wood reagent). Plate heated to 100°C; sprayed while hot with a 1:1 mixture of 0.4% bromphenol blue in acetone and 2% silver nitrate soln. and allowed to cool. The blue-colored plate is immersed carefully into water without disturbing the surface. Water is changed, if necessary, until clearly stained blue spots appear on a light background.
   B. Ehrlich's reagent.
   C. Sulfuric acid.
   R_f:

Detection method	R_f				
A		0.27	0.40	0.48	
B		0.27	0.40	0.48	0.87
C	0.10	0.26	0.40	0.48	0.87

Ref:
S. Umezawa, T. Tsuchiya, K. Tatsuta, Y. Horiuchi and T. Usui, J. Antibiotics, 23 (1970) 20–27.

DIHYDROSTREPTOMYCIN
See streptomycin.

DISTAMYCIN A
PC.
1. **Paper:**
   Solvent:
   Butanol:acetic acid:water (2:1:1).
   Detection:
   R_f:
   0.52
   Ref:
   As kikumycin PC (1).

DIUMYCINS
PC.
1. **Paper:**
   Solvent:
   n-Propanol:n-butanol:0.5 N ammonium
   hydroxide (2:3:4).
   Detection:
   Bioautography.
   R_f:

   Diumycin A   0.32
   Diumycin B   0.45
   Ref:
   E. Meyers, D.S. Slusarchyk, J.L. Bouchard
   and F.L. Weisenborn, J. Antibiotics, 22
   (1969) 490—493.

CCD.
1. **Solvent:**
   As PC (1); 500 transfers.
   Distribution:
   Diumycin A was found in tubes 65—90;
   diumycin B, in tubes 130—160.
   Ref:
   As PC (1).

DORICIN
TLC.
1. **Medium:**
   Silica Gel.
   Solvent:
   Chloroform:methanol (100:15).
   Detection:
   R_f:
   0.1
   Ref:
   M. Bodanszky and J.T. Sheehan, Anti-

microbial Agents and Chemotherapy, 1963
(1964) 38—40.

CCD.
1. **Solvent:**
   Toluene:chloroform:methanol:water
   (5:5:8:2); 1500 transfers.
   Distribution:
   Distribution coefficient = 0.4.
   Ref:
   As PC (1).

ECHANOMYCIN
CCD.
1. **Solvent:**
   Carbon tetrachloride:chloroform:methanol:
   water (2.63:0.37:2.4:0.6); 82 transfers.
   Distribution:
   Echanomycin found in tube 35.
   Ref:
   E. Gaumann, V. Prelog and A. Wettstein,
   Swiss Patent 346,651. July 15, 1960.

ECHINOMYCIN
PC.
1. **Paper:**
   Solvent:
   di-n-Butyl ether:s-tetrachloroethane:10% aq.
   sodium o-cresotinate (2:1:3).
   Detection:
   R_f:
   0.13
   Ref:
   K. Katagiri, J. Shoii, T. Yoshida, J. Antibiotics, 15 (1962) 273.

2. **Paper:**
   Solvent:
   A. Petroleum ether:benzene:methanol:water
      (66.7:33.3:80:20).
   B. 25% Ethanol.
   C. Amyl acetate satd. with water.
   Detection:
   R_f:

	R_f
A	0.26
B	0.54
C	0.61

   Ref:
   T.S. Maksimova, I.N. Kovsharova,
   V.V. Proshlyakova, Antibiotiki, 10 (1965)
   298—304.

EDEINE

PC.

1. **Paper:**

    Whatman No. 3MM.

    Solvent:

    A. 1-Butanol:acetic acid:pyridine:water (6:3:2:3).

    B. Isopropanol:conc. ammonia:water (4:1:1).

    Detection:

    R_f:

	R_f	
Solvent	Edeine A	Edeine B
A	0.08	0.11
B	0.19	0.11

   Ref:

   T.P. Hettinger, Z.K. Borowski and L.C. Craig, Biochem., 7 (1968) 4153–4160.

ELPHO.

1. **Medium:**

    Paper.

    Buffer:

    pH 6.4.

    Conditions:

    Detection:

    Mobility:

    Cathodic mobility nearly equal to that of α, β-diamino propionic acid. Edeines A and B not resolved from each other.

    Ref:

    As PC (1).

2. For Resolution of edeine A.

    Medium:

    Cellulose acetate strips.

    Buffer:

    pH 6.4.

    Conditions:

    40 V/cm, 65 min, 0°C, 25 μg of edeine A/cm.

    Detection:

    Ninhydrin.

    Mobility:

    Edeine A resolved into 2 cationic compounds with the following mobility:

    Edeine A_1 23.2–24 cm

    Edeine A_2 22.0–23.0 cm

    Ref:

    T.P. Hettinger and L.C. Craig, Biochem., 9 (1970) 1224–1232.

CCD.

1. **Solvent:**

    88% Phenol:0.15 M ammonium acetate + 0.30 M acetic (1:1). Edeine distributed over first 30 tubes of a 500 tube CCD machine; distribution carried to 600 transfers.

    Distribution:

    Edeine A, tubes 240–290.

    Edeine B, tubes 120–170.

    Ref:

    As PC (1).

ENDOMYCINS

PC.

1. **Paper:**

    Whatman No. 1.

    Solvent:

    A. Water satd. n-butanol.

    B. As A vs. paper buffered with 0.1 N sodium carbonate.

    C. As A vs. paper buffered with 0.1 N sodium phosphate, pH 12.0.

    D. t-Butanol:water (4:1).

    E. n-Butanol:ethyl acetate (1:1) satd. with water.

    Detection:

    Bioautography vs. *Candida albicans*.

    R_f:

	R_f	
Solvent	Endomycin A	Endomycin B
A	0.04	0.37
B	0.03	0.25
C	0.10	0.38
D	0.30	0.70
E	0.03	0.29

   Ref:

   L.C. Vining and W.A. Taber, Can. J. Chem., 35 (1957) 1461–1466.

ENDURACIDIN

PC.

1. **Paper:**

    Whatman No. 1.

    Solvent:

    A. n-Butanol:acetic acid:water (4:1:5).

    B. n-Butanol:pyridine:water (4:3:7).

    Detection:

    R_f:

Solvent	R_f
A	0.45 ± 0.1
B	0.80 ± 0.1

Ref:
   M. Asai, M. Muroi, N. Sugita, H. Kawashima,
   K. Mizuno and M. Miyake, J. Antibiotics, 21
   (1968) 138–146.

CCD.
1. Solvent:
   As PC (1) A, 150 transfers.
   Distribution:
   Analyzed by determinations of biological
   activity against *Sarcina lutea* and UV
   absorption at 268 nm. K = 0.59.
   Ref:
   As PC (1).

ENHYGROFUNGIN
PC.
1. Paper:
   Solvent:
   A. 1-Butanol:water (84:16); 16 h.
   B. As A + 0.25% p-toluenesulfonic acid;
      16 h.
   C. 1-Butanol:acetic acid:water (2:1:1); 16 h.
   D. As A + 2% piperidine; 16 h.
   E. 1-Butanol:water (4:96); 5 h.
   F. As E + 25% p-toluenesulfonic acid; 64 h.
   Detection:
   Bioautography vs. *Saccharomyces cerevisiae*.
   R_f:

Solvent	R_f*
A	0.18–0.50
B	0.65
C	0.90
D	0.18–0.50
E	0.10–0.35
F	0.10–0.35

   *Estimated from drawing.
   Ref:
   Netherlands Patent 7008652. December 15,
   1970.

ENOMYCIN
ELPHO.
1. Medium:
   Paper.
   Buffer:
   Acetic acid:pyridine:water (8:40:952),
   pH 6.4.
   Conditions:
   Detection:

Mobility:
   Moved toward cathode as a single entity.
   Ref:
   Y. Suhara, M. Ishizuka, H. Naganawa,
   M. Hori, M. Suzuki, Y. Okami, T. Takeuchi
   and H. Umezawa, J. Antibiotics, 16 (1963)
   107–108.

ERICAMYCIN
TLC.
1. Medium:
   Silica Gel.
   Solvent:
   A. Ethyl acetate.
   B. Methanol:benzene (1:5).
   Detection:
   R_f:

Solvent	R_f
A	0.2–0.3
B	0.5–0.6

   Ref:
   Japanese Patent 30970/69. Published March
   18, 1969.

ERIZOMYCIN
PC.
1. Paper:
   Solvent:
   A. 1-Butanol:water (84:16); 16 h.
   B. As A + 0.25% p-toluenesulfonic acid;
      16 h.
   C. 1-Butanol:acetic acid:water (2:1:1); 16 h.
   D. As A + 2% piperidine; 16 h.
   E. 1-Butanol:water (4:96); 5 h.
   F. As E + 0.25% p-toluenesulfonic acid; 5 h.
   Detection:
   Bioautography vs. *Mycobacterium avium*.
   R_f:

Solvent	R_f*
A	0.7 –0.9
B	0.65–0.9
C	0.85
D	0.6 –0.83
E	0.05, streak to 0.8, 0.83
F	0.45–0.8

   *Estimated from drawing.
   Ref:
   R.R. Herr and F. Reusser, U.S. Patent No.
   3,367,833. February 6, 1968.

ERYTHROMYCIN
PC.
1. **Paper:**
   Solvent:
   Methanol:acetone:water (19:6:75).
   Detection:
   Bioautography vs. *Micrococcus pyogenes* var. *aureus* or *Bacillus subtilis*.
   R_f:
   Erythromycin   0.7
   Erythromycin B   0.6
   Ref:
   C.W. Pettinga, W.M. Starke and F.R. Van Abeele, J. Am. Chem. Soc., 76 (1954) 569–571.

2. **Paper:**
   Solvent:
   As celesticetin, PC (2), G.
   Detection:
   As celesticetin, PC (2).
   R_f:
   0.3–0.42 (estimated from drawing)
   Ref:
   As celesticetin, PC (2).

3. **Paper:**
   Solvent:
   As PC (1).
   Detection:
   R_f:
   Erythromycin C > erythromycin > erythromycin B.
   Ref:
   P.F. Wiley, R. Gale, C.W. Pettinga and K. Gerzon, J. Am. Chem. Soc., 79 (1957) 6074.

4. **Paper:**
   Solvent:
   A, B, C, D as carbomycin, PC (2), A, B, C, D.
   Detection:
   As carbomycin PC (2).
   R_f:

Solvent	R_f
A	0.00
B	0.02
C	0.24
D	0.50

   Ref:
   As carbomycin, PC (2).

5. Useful for chromatography of whole blood, serum, plasma, urine or saliva.
   Paper:
   Whatman No. 1.
   Solvent:
   Develop descending using absolute methanol for 1 h. Cut off upper portion of chromatogram 5 cm below point of application and develop descending, with the following solvent mixture. Dissolve 12.5 g of ammonium chloride and 100 g sodium chloride in 100 ml distilled water. Add 25 ml dioxane and 12.5 ml methyl ethyl ketone, dilute to 1 liter with distilled water and adjust to pH 5.7 with 1 N ammonium hydroxide.
   Detection:
   Bioautography vs. *Sarcina lutea* ATCC 9341.
   R_f:
   Erythromycin > propionyl erythromycin.
   Ref:
   V.C. Stephens, C.T. Pugh, N.E. Davis, M.M. Hoehn, S. Ralston, M.C. Sparks and L. Thompkins, J. Antibiotics, 22 (1969) 551–557.

TLC.
1. **Medium:**
   Silica Gel.
   Solvent:
   Methylene chloride:methanol:benzene: formamide (80:20:20:2.5). Quantity of formamide is varied according to laboratory humidity conditions. At a relative humidity of 20%, 5 vols. of formamide gives clear separation; higher humidity (30–40%) requires 3 or 2 vols. Development time is 30–40 min and is complete when solvent front is 10 cm from origin.
   Detection:
   A. Spray plate with 10% phosphomolybdic acid in ethanol; heat on a hot plate. Blue spots appear on a yellow background.
   B. Spray with 50% aq. sulfuric acid; heat on a hot plate. Charred zones result.
   R_f:
   Erythromycins A, B, A "Hemiketal", anhydroerythromycin and several erythromycin acetates can be separated.
   Ref:
   T.J. Anderson, J. Chromatog., 14 (1964) 127–129.

2. **Medium:**
   Talc.
   Solvent:
   Water:ethanol:ethyl acetate:acetic acid:25%
   ammonia (10:9:1:0.2:1).
   Detection:
   R_f:
   Erythromycin C > B; anhydroerythromycin
   same R_f as C.
   Ref:
   Z. Kotula and A. Kaminska, Med. Dosw.
   Microbiol., 19 (1967) 381–387; Chem. Abs.,
   68 (1968) 72292y.

3. **Medium:**
   Kieselgel G; Kieselguhr G (1:1, w/w). Dry
   at 110°C for 1 h and immerse for depth of
   1 cm in 15% formamide in acetone. Dry for
   several mins at room temperature and use
   directly.
   Solvent:
   A. Methylene chloride:n-hexane:ethanol
   (60:35:5).
   B. Methylene chloride:ethyl acetate:
   n-hexane:ethanol (40:40:15:5).
   Detection:
   A. Spray with 50% sulfuric acid.
   B. Spray with 1% cerium sulfate and 2.5%
   molybdic acid in 10% sulfuric acid and
   heat at 110°C for several mins. Spots are
   blue against a white background.
   R_f:

Solvent	R_f
A.	Erythrolosamine > erythromycin B = anhydroerythromycin A > erythromycin A = anhydro-erythromycin C > erythromycin C.
B.	Erythrolosamine > anhydro-erythromycin A > erythromycin B > anhydroerythromycin C > erythromycin A > erythromycin C.

   Ref:
   A. Banaszek, K. Krowicki and A. Zamojski,
   J. Chromatog., 32 (1968) 581–583.

4. **Medium:**
   Silica Gel G (Merck), 50 g in 100 ml of
   0.02 N aq. sodium acetate, 0.25 mm thick.
   Air-dry overnight.

Solvent:
Methanol:0.02 N aq. sodium acetate
(120:30).
Detection:
Spray with a soln. of glucose:85% phosphoric
acid:water:ethanol:n-butanol (2 g:10 ml:
40 ml:30 ml:30 ml). Heat 5 min at 150°C.
Prepare reagent fresh daily.
R_f:

	R_f	Color
Anhydroerythronolide	0.82	Red
Erythromycin estolate	0.65	Blue-gray
Erythromycin ethyl succinate	0.67	Blue-gray
Erythromycin ethyl carbonate	0.67	Blue-gray
Erythromycin	0.28	Blue-gray
Erythromycin stearate	0.28	Blue-gray
Erythromycin lactobionate	0.28	Blue-gray
Erythromycin gluceptate	0.28	Blue-gray
Anhydroerythromycin A	0.33	Blue-gray

Ref:
G. Richard, C. Radecka, D.W. Hughes and
W.L. Wilson, J. Chromatog., 67 (1972)
69–73.

ELPHO.
1. **Medium:**
   Whatman No. 1 paper.
   Buffer:
   Borate, pH > 8.
   Conditions:
   400 V, 4–6 h.
   Detection:
   Mobility:
   Erythromycin B > A > C.
   Ref:
   As TLC (2).

CCD.
1. **Solvent:**
   0.1 M phosphate buffer (pH 6.5):methyl
   isobutyl ketone:acetone (10:10:0.5);
   100 transfers.
   Distribution:

Erythromycin,	tubes 30–50
Erythromycin B,	tubes 60–80.

   Ref:
   As PC (1).

ESEIN
PC.
1. **Paper:**

Solvent:
- A. n-Butanol:acetic acid:water (2:1:1).
- B. As bresein, PC (1) N.
- C. Phenol satd. with 0.3% ammonium hydroxide.
- D. As bresein, PC (1) O.
- E. As bresein, PC (1) P.
- F. As bresein, PC (1) Q.
- G. As bresein, PC (1) R.
- H. As bresein, PC (1) S.
- I. As bresein, PC (1) T.

Detection:

R_f:

Solvent	R_f
A	0.92
B	0.88
C	0.70
D	0.60
E	0.64
F	0.67
G	0.60
H	0.62
I	0.66

Ref:

As bresein, PC (1).

EUROCIDIN

PC.

1. **Paper:**

Solvent:

n-Butanol:methanol:water (4:1:2).

Detection:

R_f:

0.64

Ref:

D. Brown, Naturwiss., 47 (1960) 474.

EVERNINOMICINS

PC.

1. **Paper:**

Whatman No. 1.

Solvent:

Benzene:petroleum ether (30–60°C): acetone (20:5:10); descending, 2 h.

Detection:

Bioautography vs. *Staphylococcus aureus* ATCC 6538P.

R_f:

Everninomicin A	0.0
Everninomicin B	0.17
Everninomicin C	0.28
Everninomicin D	0.62

Ref:

M.J. Weinstein, G.M. Luedemann, E.M. Oden and G.H. Wagman, Antimicrobial Agents and Chemotherapy, 1964 (1965) 24–32.

2. **Paper:**

Whatman No. 1.

Solvent:

- A. As PC (1); descending, 1.5 h.
- B. Toluene:n-butanol:water:petroleum ether, 30–60°C (20:1.5:7:1.5); descending, 4.5 h.
- C. Petroleum ether, 60–90°C:methanol: ethyl acetate:water (5:8:5:2), 2 h.
- D. Ligroin, 90–120°C:butyl acetate (3:7) satd. with 15% aq. 4-chloro-2-methyl phenoxyacetic acid sodium salt.

Detection:

Bioautography vs. *Staphylococcus aureus*.

Ref:

G.M. Luedemann and M.J. Weinstein, U.S. Patent 3,499,078. March 3, 1970.

R_f:

Solvent	R_f Component					
	A	B	C	D	E	F
A	0.00	0.14	0.28	0.64	0.74	0.74
B	0.00	0.19	0.42	0.61	0.71	0.71
C	0.00	0.08	0.26	0.60	0.82	0.82
D	—	0.11*	—	0.36*	0.16*	0.77*

*Front allowed to run off paper. Calculated as distance of zone from origin divided by distance from origin to end of paper.

TLC.

1. **Medium:**
   Silica Gel.
   Solvent:
   Benzene:acetone (60:40).
   Detection:
   A. Spray with sulfuric acid:methanol (1:1),
      heat at 105°C. Dark zones on white
      background.
   B. Dip plate in satd. soln. of iodine in
      petroleum ether, place in air stream to
      remove excess iodine. Brown zones
      appear.
   D. Bioautography vs. *Staphylococcus aureus*.
   R_f:
   Everninomicin D,   0.5 (estimated from
   photograph).
   Ref:
   As PC (1).

2. **Medium:**
   Silica Gel.
   Solvent:
   As TLC (1).
   Detection:
   As TLC (1), A, C.
   R_f:
   Not given. Method used to determine purity
   of everninomicin B column fractions.
   Ref:
   M.J. Weinstein, G.H. Wagman, E.M. Oden,
   G.M. Luedemann, P. Sloane, A. Murawski
   and J.A. Marquez, Antimicrobial Agents and
   Chemotherapy, 1965 (1966) 821–827.

3. **Medium:**
   Silica Gel G (E. Merck).
   Solvent:
   As TLC (1).
   Detection:
   Spray with sulfuric acid:methanol (85:15);
   heat to develop color.
   R_f:
   Everninomicin B   0.25
   Everninomicin D   0.45
   Ref:
   H.L. Herzog, E. Meseck, S. deLorenzo,
   A. Murawski, W. Charney and J.P. Rosselet,
   Appl. Microbiol., 13 (1965) 515–520.

4. **Medium:**
   Silica Gel fluorescent layer (Mallinckrodt
   Silicar TLC 7GF), 0.5 mm thick.
   Solvent:
   As TLC (1).
   Detection:
   UV light.
   R_f:
   Everninomicin E4*   0.18
   Everninomicin E3   0.25
   Everninomicin E2   0.32
   Everninomicin E1   0.40
   *Identical with everninomicin A–D.
   Ref:
   A. Sattler and C.P. Schaffner, J. Antibiotics,
   23 (1970) 210–215.

EXFOLIATIN

PC.

1. **Paper:**
   Solvent:
   As avilamycin, PC (1).
   Detection:
   As avilamycin, PC (1).
   R_f:
   0.58
   Ref:
   As avilamycin, PC (1).

TLC.

1. **Medium:**
   As avilamycin, TLC (1).
   Solvent:
   As avilamycin, TLC (1).
   Detection:
   As avilamycin, TLC (1).
   R_f:
   0.40
   Ref:
   As avilamycin, PC (1).

FERRAMIDO CHLOROMYCIN (FACM)

PC.

1. **Paper:**
   Solvent:
   A. Distilled water.
   B. 3% Ammonium chloride soln.
   C. Chloroform.
   D. Ethyl acetate:water (1:1).
   E. Acetone.

F. Methanol.

G. Ethanol:2% sodium chloride (3:1).

H. n-Butanol:water (1:1).

I. n-Butanol:acetic acid:water (4:1:5).

J. n-Butanol:acetic acid:water (2:1:1).

All solvents developed descending.

Detection:

R_f:

Solvent	R_f
A	0.05
B	0.00
C	0.00
D	0.00
E	0.76
F	0.89
G	0.48
H	0.85
I	0.23
J	0.45

Ref:

I.R. Shimi and S. Shoukry, J. Antibiotics, 19 (1966) 110–114.

FERRIMYCINS

PC.

1. **Paper:**

Whatman No. 1 paper impregnated with acetone:water:satd. aq. sodium chloride (6:3:1).

Solvent:

tert.-Butanol:0.004 N hydrochloric acid:satd. aq. sodium chloride (2:1:1).

Detection:

R_f:

Component	R_f
Ferrimycin A_1	0.59
Ferrimycin A_2	0.47

Ref:

E. Gaeumann, E. Vischer and H. Bickel, U.S. Patent 3,093,550. June 11, 1963.

2. **Paper:**

Solvent:

A. Butanol:glacial acetic acid:water (4:1:5), 10 h.

B. Butanol:butyl acetate:glacial acetic acid: water (100:30:13:143), 24 h.

C. As B but 60 h.

Detection:

Bioautography vs. *Staphylococcus aureus*.

R_f:

Solvent	R_f*			
	Component			
	A	A_1	A_2	B
A	0.4	0.4	0.4	0.6
B	0.1	0.1	0.1	0.5
C	0.4; 0.5	0.5	0.4	–

*Estimated from drawing.

Ref:

As PC (1).

ELPHO.

1. **Medium:**

Paper.

Buffer:

0.1M acetate buffer, pH 4.6.

Conditions:

500–4000 V.

Detection:

Mobility:

Ferrimycins A and B migrate towards cathode.

Ref:

As PC (1).

FERVENULIN

PC.

1. **Paper:**

Solvent:

A. 1-Butanol:water (84:16) + 0.25% p-toluenesulfonic acid.

B. 1-Butanol:acetic acid:water (2:1:1).

C. 1-Butanol:water (4:96).

Detection:

Bioautography vs. *Klebsiella pneumoniae*.

R_f:

Solvent	R_f*
A	0.50
B	0.75
C	0.75

*Estimated from drawing.

Ref:

C. DeBoer, A. Dietz, J.S. Evans and R.M. Michaels, Antibiotics Annual, 1959–1960, 220–226.

FILIPIN COMPLEX

TLC.

1. **Medium:**

Silica Gel HF_{254} (E. Merck). Prepare 60 g of silica gel HF_{254} suspended in 60 ml of 0.2 M

monopotassium phosphate and 60 ml of
0.2 M disodium phosphate. Air dry and
activate at 130°C for 2 h.

Solvent:

Methylene chloride:methanol (85:15).

Detection:

Fluorescence under 366 nm light. For
quantitation use densitometric measurement.

R_f:

Component	R_f
Filipin I	0.8
Filipin II	0.7
Filipin III	0.6
Filipin IV	0.5

Ref:

M.E. Bergy and T.E. Eble, Biochem., 7
(1968) 653—659.

FLAVOFUNGIN
PC.

1. **Paper:**

Solvent:

As flavomycoin, PC (1), A—K.

Detection:

R_f:

Solvent	R_f
A	0.79
B	0.85
C	0.95
D	0.72
E	0.89
F	0.81
G	0.12
H	0.01
I	0.02
J	0.45
K	0.07

Ref:

As flavomycoin, PC (1).

FLAVOMYCOIN
PC.

1. **Paper:**

Solvent:

A. Methanol:water:ammonia (80:16:4).
B. n-Butanol:methanol:water (4:1:2).
C. n-Propanol:acetic acid:water (60:4:4).
D. Dimethyl formamide:water (50:50).
E. Pyridine:butanol:water (4:6:5).
F. Dimethyl formamide:water:glacial acetic
acid (50:45:5).

G. Chloroform:tetrahydrofuran:formamide
(50:50:5).
H. Chloroform:methyl ethyl ketone:tetra-
hydrofuran:formamide (60:20:20:4).
I. Chloroform:methyl ethyl ketone:
formamide (66:33:4).
J. Benzene:methyl ethyl ketone (50:50,
formamide satd.).
K. Benzene:dioxane (50:50, formamide
satd.).

Detection:

R_f:

Solvent	R_f
A	0.90
B	0.88
C	0.94
D	0.77
E	0.86
F	0.84
G	0.55
H	0.42
I	0.33
J	0.69
K	0.21

Ref:

R. Schlegel and H. Thrum, J. Antibiotics, 24
(1971) 360—367.

2. **Paper:**

Schleicher and Schull 2043b.

Solvent:

Chloroform:tetrahydrofuran:formamide
(50:50:5), ascending 2.5 h, 7°C.

Detection:

Bioautography vs. *Penicillium notatum* P 36.

R_f:

0.5

Ref:

As PC (1).

FOLIMYCIN
PC.

1. **Paper:**

Solvent:

A. 40% Methanol in water.
B. 55% Methanol in water.
C. 20% n-Propanol in water.

Detection:

R_f:

Solvent	R_f
A	0.32
B	1.0
C	0.35

Ref:

As Ikutamycin, PC (1).

FORMYCINS

ELPHO.

1. **Medium:**

Toyo Roshi No. 51 paper.

Buffer:

A. Formic acid:acetic acid:water (5:75:900).

B. Phosphoric acid:monopotassium phosphate (pH 2.45, μ 0.06).

Conditions:

Solvent A: 3000 V/40 cm for 15 min.

Solvent B: 500 V/30 cm for 2 h.

Detection:

Mobility:

	Solvent
Formycin A Moves to anode 5.8 cm	A
Formycin A Moves to anode 7.5 cm	B
Formycin B Moves to anode 1.6 cm	A
Formycin B Moves to anode 0.3 cm	B

Ref:

Derwent Farmdoc No. 30580, Japanese Patent JA.759/68. January 11, 1968.

FOROMACIDINS

PC.

1. **Paper:**

Whatman No. 1 treated with a 2% aq. soln. of sodium m-cresotinate, blotted and used wet.

Solvent:

Dibutyl ether:butyl acetate (1:3) satd. with sodium m-cresotinate soln., 2–3 h.

Detection:

Dry at 100°C for 2–3 min: spray with 15% phosphoric acid, heat at 100°C. Blue-green colors result.

R_f:

Separates foromacidins A, B, and C.

Ref:

R. Corbaz, L. Ettlinger, E. Gaümann, W. Keller-Schierlein, F. Kradolfer, E. Kyburz, L. Neipp, V. Prelog, A. Wettstein and H. Zähner, Helv. Chim. Acta, 39 (1956) 304–317.

CCD.

1. **Solvent:**

Chloroform:0.2 M citrate buffer, pH 4.9 (1:1), 145 transfers.

Distribution:

Foromacidin A	Tubes 71–115
Foromacidin B	Tubes 39–70
Foromacidin C and D	Tubes 16–38

Ref:

As PC (1).

FUMIGACHLORIN

TLC.

1. **Medium:**

Kieselgel G (Merck).

Solvent:

A. Chloroform:ethyl acetate (3:1).

B. Carbon tetrachloride:ethyl acetate:acetic acid (100:30:1).

Detection:

R_f:

Solvent	R_f
A	0.65
B	0.42

Ref:

K. Atsumi, M. Takada, K. Mizuno and T. Ando, J. Antibiotics, 23 (1970) 223–224.

FUNGICHROMIN

PC.

1. **Paper:**

Whatman No. 1.

Solvent:

A. Methyl isobutyl ketone:1-butanol:water (50:15:3).

B. Methyl isopropyl ketone:water (satd. ca. 1.6%).

C. Methyl isopropyl ketone:1-butanol:water (50:10:3.5).

D. Methyl isopropyl ketone:methanol:water (50:1:0.4).

Detection:

The spots were detected by their intense greenish fluorescence in UV light.

R_f:

Solvent	R_f
A	0.73
B	0.35
C	0.76
D	0.47

Ref:
A.C. Cope, R.K. Bly, E.P. Burrows,
O.J. Ceder, E. Ciganek, B.T. Gillis,
R.F. Porter and H.E. Johnson, J. Amer.
Chem. Soc., 84 (1962) 2170–2178.

FURANOMYCIN
PC.
1. **Paper:**
Toyo Roshi No. 50.
Solvent:
A. n-Butanol:acetic acid:water (4:1:6, upper
phase).
B. n-Butanol satd. with 2 N ammonium
hydroxide.
C. Pyridine:acetic acid:water (10:7:3).
Detection:
Color spot.
R_f:

Solvent	R_f
A	0.35
B	0.12
C	0.69

Ref:
K. Katagiri, K. Tori, Y. Kimura,
T. Yoshida, T. Nagasaki and H. Minato,
J. Med. Chem., 10 (1967) 1149–1154.

TLC.
1. **Medium:**
Silica Gel G (Merck).
Solvent:
A. n-Propanol:water (7:3).
B. n-Butanol:acetic acid:water (3:1:1).
C. Chloroform:methanol:17% ammonia
(2:2:1, upper phase).
Detection:
R_f:

Solvent	R_f
A	0.41
B	0.41
C	0.64

Ref:
As PC (1).

FUSARIUM ANTIBIOTIC
TLC.
1. **Medium:**
Silica Gel F_{254}.

Solvent:
10% Ethyl acetate in benzene.
Detection:
UV absorption.
R_f:
0.45
Ref:
R.H. Evans, Jr., M.P. Kunstmann,
C.E. Holmlund and G.A. Ellestad, U.S.
Patent 3,546,074. December 8, 1970.

GATAVALIN
PC.
1. **Paper:**
Solvent:
n-Butanol:acetic acid:water (3:1:1).
Detection:
Bioautography vs. *Staphylococcus aureus*
FDA 209P.
R_f:
0.9
Ref:
N. Nakajima, S. Chihara and Y. Koyama,
J. Antibiotics, 25 (1972) 243–247.

GELBECIDIN
PC.
1. **Paper:**
Whatman No. 1.
Solvent:
A. Butanol:acetic acid:water (4:1:5).
B. Methanol:benzene (4:6).
Detection:
A. UV and visible light.
B. Bioautography.
R_f:

Solvent	R_f
A	0.94
B	0.80

Ref:
A. Aszalos, R.S. Robison, F.E. Pansy and
B. Berk, U.S. Patent 3,551,561. December
29, 1970.

TLC.
1. **Medium:**
Eastman Chromagram Sheets.
Solvent:
A. Methanol.
B. Methanol:chloroform (1:9).

Detection:
A. As PC (1), A.
B. As PC (1), B.

R_f:

Solvent	R_f
A	0.60
B	0.45

Ref:

As PC (1). German Patent No. 1942694; March 5, 1970.

GELDANAMYCIN

PC.

1. **Paper:**

Whatman No. 1.

Solvent:

A. 1-Butanol:water (84:16) + 2% p-toluene-sulfonic acid, 64 h.
B. 0.075 N ammonium hydroxide satd. with methyl isobutyl ketone, 5 h.
C. Benzene:methanol:water (1:1:2), upper phase, 5 h.
All systems developed descending.

Detection:

Bioautography vs. *Tetrahymena pyriformis.*

R_f:

Solvent	R_f
A	0.05; 0.4
B	0.05; 0.78
C	0.05; 0.6–0.7

Ref:

C. DeBoer, P.A. Meulman, R.J. Wnuk and D.H. Peterson, J. Antibiotics, 23 (1970) 442–447.

TLC.

1. **Medium:**

Silica Gel H (E. Merck).

Solvent:

Chloroform:methanol (9.5:0.5).

Detection:

A. Yellow color.
B. UV light.

R_f:

0.56

Ref:

As PC (1).

GENIMYCIN

CCD.

1. **Solvent:**

A. Butanol:methanol:hexane:borate buffer pH 7.5, 0.1 M (1:1:1:3).
B. Chloroform:methanol:borate buffer pH 5.6.

Distribution:

Solvent	
A	K = 1.22
B	K = 1.38

Ref:

Y.L. Severinets, V.M. Efimova, L.O. Bol'shakova, A.I. Karnaushkina, S.N. Solov'en and A.N. Egorenkova, Antibiotiki, 15 (1970) 5–9.

GENTAMICINS

PC.

1. **Paper:**

Whatman No. 1.

Solvent:

A. Methanol:water (4:1) + 3% sodium chloride vs. paper buffered with 0.95 M sodium sulfate + 0.05 M sodium bisulfate.
B. Propanol:pyridine:acetic acid:water (15:10:3:12).
C. Propanol:water:acetic acid (50:40:5).
D. Aq. phenol, 80%.

Detection:

Bioautography vs. *Staphylococcus aureus* ATCC 6538P.

R_f:

Solvent	R_f
A	0.59
B	0.26
C	0.10
D	0.30

Ref:

M.J. Weinstein, G.M. Luedemann, E.M. Oden and G.H. Wagman, Antimicrobial Agents and Chemotherapy, 1963 (1964) 1–7.

2. **Paper:**

Whatman No. 1.

Solvent:

Lower phase of chloroform:methanol:17% ammonium hydroxide (2:1:1). Upper phase placed in bottom of chamber several hours prior to use. Papers developed descending, ca. 5 h, 25°C. Solvent allowed to drip off end of paper.

Detection:

A. As PC (1).

B. Spray with 0.25% ninhydrin in pyridine: acetone (1:1). Heat at 105°C several min. Purple to blue spots result.

R_f:

Gentamicin $C_1 > C_2 > C_1a$.

Ref:

G.H. Wagman, J.A. Marquez and M.J. Weinstein, J. Chromatog., 34 (1968) 210–215.

3. **Paper:** (Quantitative)

Whatman No. 1 strips 1/4 in. wide ± 1/64 in.

Solvent:

As PC (2).

Detection:

As PC (1). Zone diameters are measured and compared to zone diameters of series of standards. Standard curves are constructed and conc. of each component determined from appropriate curve. Percentage of each component can be calculated for unknown samples.

R_f:

As PC (2).

Ref:

G.H. Wagman, E.M. Oden and M.J. Weinstein, Appl. Microbiol., 16 (1968) 624–627.

4. **Paper:** (Quantitative)

Whatman No. 4. Two replicate spots per sheet.

Solvent:

As PC (2) but used mixed phases to equilibrate chamber for 24 h prior to use.

Detection:

Modified Barrollier reagent. To 1 g ninhydrin add 0.1 g cadmium acetate, 3 ml water and 1.5 ml of glacial acetic acid and shake. Add to 100 ml n-propanol and shake until soln. is complete. Store in a brown bottle under refrigeration.

R_f:

As PC (2). Quantitative procedure: cut each paper in half lengthwise; spray one half with ninhydrin reagent and dry at 100°C for 1 min. Using this as a guide, cut other half of

paper in segments representing 3 gentamicin components. Cut each segment into small strips and put into separate 125 ml flasks, add 50 ml of 0.1 M potassium phosphate buffer, pH 8.0, and shake 30 min. Decant, allow paper to settle, pipet 4 ml of clear soln. in a 25 ml volumetric flask and bring to volume with same buffer. Assay each soln. by microbiological plate assay vs. *Staphylococcus* epidermidis. The percentage of each fraction is calculated as follows:

$$\% \, C_1 \;=\; \frac{A_1}{504} \times \frac{100}{B}$$

$$\% \, C_1a \;=\; \frac{A_1a}{626} \times \frac{100}{B}$$

$$\% \, C_2 \;=\; \frac{A_2}{656} \times \frac{100}{B}$$

where:

A_1 = concentration of the assayed C_1 soln. in mcg/ml.

A_1a = concentration of the assayed C_1a soln. in mcg/ml.

A_2 = concentration of the assayed C_2 soln. in mcg/ml.

$$B = \frac{A_1}{504} + \frac{A_1a}{626} + \frac{A_2}{56}$$

504, 626 and 656 are the activities of C_1 sulfate, C_1a sulfate, and C_2 sulfate, respectively, compared to the gentamicin sulfate standard.

Ref:

N. Kantor and G. Selzer, J. Pharm. Sci., 57 (1968) 2170–2171.

5. **Paper:** (Quantitative)

Schleicher and Schuell No. 589 blue ribbon chromatographic paper cut to size 20 × 58 cm (along grain).

Solvent:

As PC (1).

Detection:

After development, strips containing the antibiotic are treated with ninhydrin reagent, developed, and color intensities read on an integrating scanner from which component proportions can be determined. Results are in excellent agreement with the microbiological method. (Integrating scanner-instrument used for the determina-

Comparison of intensity of ninhydrin reactions on chromatograms
for individual components of the gentamicin complex

Derivative	Component	Relative intensity of ninhydrin spot	Factor, reciprocal of intensity
Base	C_1	0.518	1.93
	C_1a	1.000	1.00
	C_2	0.578	1.73
Sulfate	C_1	0.397	2.52
	C_1a	1.000	1.00
	C_2	0.485	2.06

tions to be described was the model RB
Analytrol, manufactured by Beckman
Instruments, Inc., Fullerton, California.)
Comparison of ninhydrin reactivity for each
of the gentamicin base component standards
showed that the intensity of color varied
with $C_1a > C_2 > C_1$. This was true also for
the sulfates, but the ratios were somewhat
different. For the free bases, if C_1a is
assigned a ninhydrin peak value of 1.00,
then an equal quantity of C_2 results in a less
intense color reaction and a value of 0.58
(58% of the intensity of color for an equal
weight of C_2 compared to C_1a). For the C_1
component the value is 0.52.

R_f:

$C_1 > C_2 > C_1a$.

Ref:

G.H. Wagman, J.V. Bailey and M.M. Miller,
J. Pharm. Sci., 57 (1968) 1319–1322.

6. **Paper:**

Whatman No. 1.

Solvent:

A. Chloroform:methanol:17% ammonium
hydroxide (2:1:1), lower phase,
descending, 16 h, 25°C. Solvent allowed
to drip off paper.

B. 2-Butanone:tert.-butanol:methanol:conc.
ammonium hydroxide (16:3:1:6),
descending, 16 h.

Detection:

Bioautography vs. *Staphylococcus aureus*
ATCC 6538P.

R_f:

	A*	B** (R_fB_1)
Gentamicin A_1	0.0	0.36
Gentamicin A	0.0	0.41
Gentamicin B	9.0	0.52
Gentamicin X	13.5	0.55
Gentamicin B_1	27.0	1.00

* mm from origin.

$$**R_fB_1 = \frac{\text{distance component from origin}}{\text{distance } B_1 \text{ from origin}}$$

Ref:

G.H. Wagman, J.A. Marquez, J.V. Bailey,
D. Cooper, J. Weinstein, R. Tkach and
P. Daniels, J. Chromatog., 70 (1972)
171–173.

TLC.

1. **Medium:**

MN Cellulose 300. Mix 1 part cellulose
powder with 6 parts water and prepare plates
250 μ thick. Dry at 100°C, 20 min.

Solvent:

n-Propanol pyridine:acetic acid:water
(15:10:3:12).

Detection:

Ninhydrin.

R_f:

0.35, 0.28, 0.20

Ref:

Y. Ito, M. Namba, N. Nagahama,
T. Yamaguchi and T. Okuda, J. Antibiotics,
17 (1964) 218–219.

2. **Medium:**

Silica Gel.

Solvent:

Chloroform:methanol:conc. ammonium
hydroxide:water (1:4:2:1).

Detection:
  A. Ninhydrin spray. Developed plates dried at 100°C and sprayed with pyridine; reheat to aid removal of ammonia traces.
  B. Bioautography vs. *Staphylococcus aureus*. The pyridine and heat treatments of the plates are omitted.

R_f:

Component	R_f
Gentamicin A	0.60
Gentamicin C_1a (D)	0.69
Gentamicin C_1	0.71
Gentamicin C_2	0.76

Ref:
  H. Maehr and C.P. Schaffner, J. Chromatog., 30 (1967) 572–578.

3. **Medium:**
  Silica Gel G.
Solvent:
  Chloroform:methanol:17% ammonium hydroxide (2:1:1), lower phase.
Detection:
  A. 0.25% Ninhydrin in pyridine-acetone and consequent heating at 105°C for several min. The zones appear as purple or blue spots against a white background.
  B. Starch-potassium iodine reagent spray with which the zones show up as dark blue spots against a white background.
  C. Bioautography vs. *Staphylococcus aureus* ATCC 6538P.
R_f:
  $C_1 > C_2 > C_1a$
Ref:
  G.H. Wagman, J.A. Marquez and M.J. Weinstein, J. Chromatog., 34 (1968) 210–215.

4. **Medium:**
  DC-Alufolien strips (Merck).
Solvent:
  1-Butanol:methanol:glacial acetic acid:water (1:1:1:2).
Detection:
  A. Bioautography.
  B. Ninhydrin.

R_f:

Spot No.	R_f	Color	Antibacterial action
1	0.26	Gray-blue	+
2	0.38	Bluish-purple	+
3	0.51	Bluish-purple	–
4	0.55	Pale pink	–
5	0.62	(a) Reddish-blue	(+)
		(b) Bluish-purple	+
6	0.73	Bluish-purple	–
7	0.76	Bluish-purple	–

Ref:
  U. Ullmann, Arzneimittelforsch., 21 (1971) 263–267.

5. **Medium:**
  ChromAR Sheet 500.
Solvent:
  Lower phase of chloroform:methanol:conc. ammonium hydroxide (1:1:1), ascending, 50 min.
Detection:
  Bioautography vs. *Staphylococcus aureus* ATCC 6538P.
R_f:

	R_f
Gentamicin A_1	0.10
Gentamicin A	0.16
Gentamicin B	0.22
Gentamicin X	0.28
Gentamicin B_1	0.40

Ref:
  As PC (6).

GEOMYCIN
PC.
1. **Paper:** (Circular)
  Schleicher and Schuell 2043b.
Solvent:
  A. Butanol:formic acid:water (2:1:1), 4.75 h.
  B. As A, but (3:3:2), 5.75 h.
  C. Butanol:acetic acid:water (1:2:1), 7.3 h.
  D. Butanol:pyridine:acetic acid:water (15:10:3:12), 4.3 h.
Detection:
  Ninhydrin.
R_f:

Solvent	R_f
A	Single band
B	Single band
C	Single band
D	Two bands

Ref:
H. Brockmann and H. Musso, Chem. Ber., 87 (1954) 1779–1799.

GLEBOMYCIN
PC.
1. **Paper:**
   Solvent:
   A. 100 ml of 80% aq. methanol + 10.5 ml piperidine (adjusted to pH 9.09–9.5 with acetic acid), ascending.
   B. Methanol:water:glacial acetic acid (80:15:5), ascending.
   C. 50% Acetone, ascending.
   D. Wet n-butanol containing 2% p-toluene-sulfonic acid, descending.
   E. Wet n-butanol containing 2% p-toluene-sulfonic acid and 2% piperidine, descending.
   F. Wet n-butanol containing 2% p-toluene-sulfonic acid, 2% piperidine and 2% lauric acid, descending.
   Detection:
   R_f:

Solvent	R_f	cm from origin at 24 h
A	0.74	
B	0.66	
C	0.83	
D		3.0
E		2.6
F		5.6

Ref:
B.B. Clyman, C.W. Carlson and H.W. Taylor, Jr., U.S. Patent 3,142,671; July 28, 1964.

GLIOTOXIN
PC.
1. **Paper:**
   Solvent:
   Butanol:acetic acid:water (4:2:1), descending.
   Detection:
   R_f:
   0.75

Ref:
G. Nanda, A. Pal and P. Nandi, Curr. Sci., 38 (1969) 518–519.

GLUCONIMYCIN
PC.
1. **Paper:**
   Whatman No. 1.
   Solvent:
   A. Distilled water.
   B. Ethyl acetate.
   C. Ethyl acetate:ethanol:water (5:2.5:2.5).
   D. Chloroform.
   E. Chloroform:ethanol:water (5:2.5:2.5).
   F. Ethyl acetate:petroleum ether:water (5:2.5:2.5).
   G. Chloroform:petroleum ether:water (5:2.5:2.5).
   H. Petroleum ether:ethanol:water (5:2.5:2.5).
   I. Petroleum ether.
   J. n-Butanol:petroleum ether:water (5:2.5:2.5).
   K. n-Butanol:acetic acid:water (4:1:5).
   All solvents developed descending.
   Detection:
   R_f:

Solvent	R_f
A	0.75
B	0.95
C	0.48
D	0.91
E	0.89
F	0.89
G	0.89
H	0.96
I	0.00
J	0.94
K	0.95

Ref:
I.R. Shimi and A. Dewedar, Archiv für Mikrobiologie, 54 (1966) 246–252.

GOUGEROXYMYCIN
PC.
1. **Paper:**
   Toyo No. 51.
   Solvent:
   A. Methanol:water:2.5% acetic acid (3:1:0.5).

B. Water satd. n-butanol.

C. Methanol.

D. 50% Acetone.

E. Phosphate buffer pH 9.0 satd. with n-butanol.

F. Water.

G. Ethanol.

Detection:

R_f:

Solvent	R_f
A	0.72
B	0.54
C	0.49
D	0.76
E	0.73
F	0.00
G	Tailing spot

Ref:

E.L. Wang, N. Kanda and H. Umezawa, J. Antibiotics, 22 (1969) 211–214.

TLC.

1. **Medium:**

Silica Gel (Wakogel B-O).

Solvent:

A. Methanol:water:2.5% acetic acid (3:1:0.5).

B. Methanol:1 N ammonium hydroxide (2:1).

C. Water satd. n-butanol:methylcellosolve (1:1).

D. Methanol:dioxane (1:1).

E. Methanol:water:2.5% acetic acid (3:1:0.5).

F. Ethanol.

G. Chloroform.

Detection:

R_f:

Solvent	R_f
A	0.4
B	0.37
C	0.00
D	0.00
E	0.55
F	0.00
G	0.00

Ref:

As PC (1).

ELPHO.

1. **Medium:**

Paper.

Buffer:

Formic acid:acetic acid:water (25:75:900).

Conditions:

3,500 V/42 cm. 65 mA/20 cm, 15 min.

Detection:

Mobility:

Remains at origin.

Ref:

As PC (1).

GRAMICIDIN

TLC.

For gramicidin J.

1. **Medium:**

A. Silica Gel G (Merck 7731), 0.45–0.65 mm thick. Dry plates at 100–110°C before use.

B. Cellulose MN 300 (Machery, Nagel Co. D-516). Dry plates at room temperature for 12 h.

Solvent:

A. n-Butanol:acetic acid:water (3:1:6).

B. n-Butanol:acetic acid:water:2 N ammonia (30:10:60) and 1 ml ammonia added to upper layer.

C. As A, but (20:3:20).

D. As A, but (60:15:20).

E. n-Propanol:water:benzene:diethylene glycol:acetic acid (75:25:5:1.5:1, v/v).

F. n-Butanol satd. with water + 20% acetic acid and 10% pyridine.

G. Toluene:acetic acid:water (10:10:1).

H. n-Butanol:pyridine:water (15:15:10).

I. Isopropanol:1 N ammonia:water (20:10:10).

J. Isopropanol:formamide:2 N ammonia: water (20:10:2:10).

K. Acetone:water:acetic acid:2 N ammonia (15:5:1:2).

Detection:

Ninhydrin. Heat plates at 80–110°C and spray with 0.3–0.5% soln. of ninhydrin in water satd. n-butanol.

R_f:

Medium	Solvent	R_f Gramicidin J
A	A	0.39
	B	0.50
	C	0.46
	D	0.57
	E	0.76

	F	0.71
	G	0.32
	H	0.15
	I	0.84
	J	0.21
B	C	0.91
	K	0.95

Ref:

K. Obojska, Acta, Polon. Pharm., 27 (1970) 285—288.

ELPHO.
1. Medium:
Buffer:

Formic acid:acetic acid:water (4:15:180), pH 1.9.

Conditions:

15 cm × 40 cm, 600 V, 2 h.

Detection:

Ninhydrin.

Mobility:

(4-5-δ-Aminovaleric acid) gramicidin S moves to cathode 11.8 cm (slightly faster than gramicidin S).

Ref:

I. Muramatsu, S. Sofuku and A. Hagitani, J. Antibiotics, 25 (1972) 189—190.

CCD.
1. Solvent:

Water:methanol:chloroform:benzene (7:23:15:15), 100 transfers.

Distribution:

Peak in tubes 46 and 47.

Ref:

J.D. Gregory, L.C. Craig, J. Biol. Chem., 172 (1948) 839—840.

GRISEIN
PC.
1. Paper:

Whatman No. 1.

Solvent:

A. n-Butanol:water:acetic acid (4:2:1).
B. n-Butanol:water:acetic acid (1:2:1).
C. Methanol:0.1 N hydrochloric acid (3:1).
D. n-Propanol:2.5% sodium chloride:acetic acid (10:8:1).
E. n-Butanol:ethanol:water:acetic acid (25:25:47:3).
F. Acetone:water:acetic acid (60:37:3).

Detection:

Bioautography vs. *Escherichia coli W.*

R_f:

Solvent	R_f
A	0.14, 0.37, 0.46
B	0.83
C	0.68
D	0.78
E	0.97
F	0.75

Ref:

E.O. Stapley and R.E. Ormond, Science, 125 (1957) 587.

GRISEOFULVINS
PC.
1. Paper:
Solvent:

A. Water satd. butanol:ammonium hydroxide (20:1), vs. chloroform stationary phase.
B. Butanol satd. water, vs. ethyl acetate stationary phase.
C. Butanol:ethanol:water (5:1:4), vs. ethyl acetate stationary phase.
D. Butanol satd. water, vs. methyl ethyl ketone stationary phase.

Detection:

UV fluorescence.

R_f:

Solvent	R_f
A	0.40
B	0.22
C	0.37
D	0.24

Ref:

E.G. McNall, Arch. Dermatol., 81 (1960) 657—661.

2. Paper:
Solvent:

Benzene:cyclohexane:methanol:water (5:5:6:4), organic phase; add 0.5% acetic acid after separation.

Detection:

UV light gives blue fluorescent spots.

R_f:

	R_f
Griseofulvin	0.90
4-demethylgriseofulvin	0.70
Griseofulvin acid	0.20
6-demethylgriseofulvin	0.15

Ref:

B. Boothroyd, E.J. Napier and
G.A. Somerfield, Biochem. J., 80 (1961)
34–37.

3. **Paper:**

Whatman No. 1.

Solvent:

Benzene:cyclohexane:methanol:water
(5:5:6:4), organic phase; add 0.5% acetic
acid after separation.

Detection:

UV absorption.

R_f:

	R_f	
Griseofulvin	0.9	(bright fluorescence)
6-demethylgriseofulvin	0.15	(dark blue fluorescence)

Ref:

M.J. Barnes and B. Boothroyd, Biochem. J.,
78 (1961) 41–43.

TLC.

1. **Medium:**

Silica Gel HF$_{254}$ (Merck).

Solvent:

A. Butyl acetate:acetone (4:1).
B. Chloroform:methanol (98:2).

Detection:

5% potassium carbonate, 0.2% potassium
permanganate.

R_f:

	Solvent	R_f
(−) Dehydrogriseofulvin	A	0.47
(+) Griseofulvin		0.49
(−) Dehydrogriseofulvin	B	0.65
(+) Griseofulvin		0.68

Ref:

A. Segal and E.H. Taylor, J. Pharm. Sci., 57
(1968) 874–876.

2. **Medium:**

Silica Gel.

Solvent:

Chloroform:ether:acetone:acetic acid
(65:20:15:0.5).

Detection:

The standards are visible as dark spots on
the green background under 253 nm light.

R_f:

Ref:

P.A. Harris and S. Riegelman, J. Pharm. Sci.,
58 (1969) 93–96.

3. **Medium:**

Solvent:

Chloroform:acetic acid:water (4:1:1).

Detection:

As TLC (2).

R_f:

Ref:

W.L. Chiou and S. Riegelman, J. Pharm. Sci.,
58 (1969) 1505–1510.

4. **Medium:**

Cellulose Strips (Eastman MN-Polygram
300/UV).

Solvent:

Hexane:ethyl acetate:methanol:water
(70:30:15:6), lower phase.

Detection:

UV light.

R_f:

Component	R_f
Dehydro-1-thiogriseofulvin	0.78
(+)-1-thiogriseofulvin	0.92
(+)-5′-hydroxy-1-thiogriseofulvin	0.65

Ref:

H. Newman, P. Shu and W.W. Andres, U.S.
Patent 3,532,714; October 6, 1970; U.S.
Patent 3,616,237; October 26, 1971.

5. **Medium:**

Kieselgel G-HR.

Solvent:

Chloroform:acetone (93:7).

Detection:

First under long-wave UV light and then in
normal light after being sprayed with 50%
sulfuric acid and heat at 110°C for 30 min.

R_f:

Ref:

R.J. Cole, J.W. Kirksey and C.E. Holaday,
Appl. Microbiol., 19 (1970) 106–108.

GLC.

1. **Apparatus:**

Shimadzu Model GC-LB gas chromatograph
equipped with a differential hydrogen F.I.D.
system.

Column:

A 150 cm (75 cm × 2) × 4 mm I.D. U-shaped stainless steel column is packed in a vertical position by tapping and is preconditioned overnight at 260°C before use. Packings are 1.5% SE-30 (methyl silicone; General Electric Co.) on acid-washed and silanized Chromosorb W, 80 to 100 mesh (Johns-Manville Co.), and 1.5% QF-1 (fluorinated alkyl silicone; Dow Corning Corp.) on acid-washed and silanized Anakrom, 80 to 100 mesh (Analabs Inc), both prepared by the soln.-coating technique.

Temperature:

Operating conditions are as follows: column and injection port temperature, 230°C; detector temperature, 240°C.

Carrier gas:

Nitrogen as carrier gas at 17.5 ml/min (2 kg/sq. cm) at inlet.

Sample preparation:

A quantity of suspension or a finely pulverized sample equivalent to 3 to 15 mg of griseofulvin.

Calculations:

A series of synthetic mixtures is prepared for injection by accurately adding 1 to 8 mg of pure griseofulvin to 1 ml of a soln. containing 2 mg per ml diphenylphthalate (internal standard) in acetone. At the fixed sensitivity and range of the instrument, approximately 1 μl of each mixture is injected into the chromatograph. The peak areas are determined by planimeter and/or by triangulation. By plotting the weight ratios against the peak area ratios of griseofulvin to diphenylphthalate, a straight line passing through origin was obtained for the calibration curve. Approximately 1 to 2 μl of soln. is injected, the ratio of the peak areas again determined, and the amount of griseofulvin is calculated by comparison with the calibration curve.

Relative retention times

	1.5% Se-30	1.5% QF-1
Diphenylphthalate (internal standard)	1.00[*]	1.00[**]
Griseofulvin	1.84	3.25
Isogriseofulvin	2.40	5.15

[*] Retention time: 5.5 min.
[**] Retention time: 5.2 min.

Ref:

S. Iguchi, M. Yamamoto and T. Goromaru, J. Chromatog., 24 (1966) 182–185.

2. **Apparatus:**

Barber Coleman series 5000 gas chromatograph equipped with a hydrogen FID and disc integrator.

Column:

Glass column.

Supports:

The liquid phases used were 1% QF-1 and 1 to 2% SE-30 coated onto Anakrom ABS 80 mesh (Analab Corp., Hamden, Conn.).

Relative retention times[*]

	SE-30	QF-1
Griseofulvin	6.31	0.81

[*]Retention time relative to cholestone.

Ref:

As TLC (6).

GRISEOLUTEINS
PC.

1. **Paper:**

Toyo Roshi No. 51.

Solvent:

n-Butanol:acetic acid:water (4:1:1).

Detection:

A. Bioautography.
B. 15% Hydrochloric acid.
C. 10% Sodium hydroxide.

R$_f$:

Compound	R$_f$	Detection B	C
Griseolutein A	0.84–0.86	Orange	Orange Pink
Griseolutein B	0.89–0.94	Yellow	No color change

Ref:

K. Yagishita, J. Antibiotics, 13 (1960) 83—96.

2. **Paper:**

Whatman No. 1. Impregnate with aq. buffer (usually 0.25M, pH 6 phosphate) satd. with methyl isobutyl ketone.

Solvent:

Buffer satd. methyl isobutyl ketone, descending.

Detection:

Bioautography vs. *Bacillus subtilis*.

R_f:

Component	R_f
Griseolutein A	0.5—0.55
Griseolutein B	0.07—0.1

Ref:

F. Tausig, F.J. Wolf and A.K. Miller, Antimicrobial Agents and Chemotherapy, 1964 (1965) 59—64.

HALOMICIN
PC.

1. **Paper:**

Solvent:

A. Benzene:chloroform (93:7) satd. with formamide. Chromatographic paper, prior to use, is dipped in 25% methanolic formamide, blotted and air dried for 5 min to remove methanol, 2 h.

B. Benzene:methanol (9:1).

C. Methanol:water (80:20) containing 3% sodium chloride. The paper is buffered with a soln. of 0.95 M sodium sulfate + 0.05 M sodium bisulfate and dried prior to developing, 4—6 h.

D. Propanol:acetic acid:water (50:5:40), 18 h.

E. Butanol:acetic acid:water (4:1:5), 18 h.

F. Propanol:pyridine:acetic acid:water (15:10:3:12), 18 h.

G. Phenol:water (80 g:20 ml), 18 h.

System A developed descending, B—G, ascending.

Detection:

Bioautography vs. *Staphylococcus aureus* ATCC 6538P.

R_f:

Solvent	R_f
A	Halomicin A, 0.0, B, 0.35, C, 0.60, D, 0.75
B	1.0
C	0.78—1.0
D	0.95
E	1.0
F	1.0
G	1.0

Ref:

G.M. Luedemann and M.J. Weinstein, U.S. Patent 3,511,909; May 12, 1970.

M.J. Weinstein, G.M. Luedemann, E.M. Oden and G.H. Wagman, Antimicrobial Agents and Chemotherapy, 1967 (1968) 435—441.

HAMYCIN
PC.

1. **Paper:**

Whatman No. 1.

Solvent:

A. Water satd. n-butanol, descending, 16 h.

B. n-Butanol:pyridine:water (1:0.6:1), ascending, 16 h.

C. 50% Aq. acetone, ascending, 10 h.

D. Methanol:water:ammonium hydroxide (20:4:1), descending, 5.5 h.

E. 60% Aq. isopropanol, ascending, 16 h.

Detection:

Bioautography vs. *Saccharomyces cerevisiae*.

R_f:

Solvent	R_f
A	0.26
B	0.75
C	0.77
D	0.67; 0.44
E	0.99

Ref:

P.V. Divekar, V.C. Vora and A.W. Khan, J. Antibiotics, 19 (1966) 63—64.

2. **Paper:**

Solvent:

A. Butanol:acetic acid:water (20:1:25).

B. n-Propanol:water (80:20).

C. Pyridine:ethyl acetate:water (2.5:6:7).

D. Pyridine:ethyl acetate:acetic acid:water (5:5:1:3).

E. Butanol:methanol:water (1:1:1.5).

F. Butanol:methanol:water (4:1:2).

Detection:

R_f:

Solvent	R_f
A	0.59
B	0.56
C	0.17
D	0.69
E	0.95
F	0.31; 0.64

Ref:

G.R. Deshpande and N. Narasimhachari, Hindustan Antibiotic Bull., 9 (1966) 76–83.

HERQUEICHRYSIN

TLC.

1. **Medium:**

   Polyamide.

   Solvent:

   Acetone:acetic acid (5:1).

   Detection:

   A. Visible yellow color.

   B. Ethanolic ferric chloride (gives deep brown color with desmethyl herqueichrysin).

   R_f:

	R_f
Herqueichrysin	0.73
Desmethylherqueichrysin	0.67

   Ref:

   N. Narasimhachari and L.C. Vining, J. Antibiotics, 25 (1972) 155–162.

HIKIZIMYCIN

PC.

1. **Paper:**

   Toyo Roshi No. 51.

   Solvent:

   A. 3% Ammonium chloride.

   B. 50% Acetone.

   C. 80% Phenol.

   D. Wet butanol.

   E. Butanol:methanol:water (40:20:20) + 1.5 g methyl orange.

   F. Butanol:acetic acid:water (1:1:1).

   G. Propanol:pyridine:acetic acid:water (15:10:3:12).

   All systems developed ascending.

   Detection:

   Bioautography vs. *Pseudomonas fluorescens*.

R_f:

Solvent	R_f
A	1.0
B	0.10
C	0.08
D	0.00
E	0.25
F	0.40
G	0.35

Ref:

K. Uchida, T. Ichikawa, Y. Shimauchi, T. Ishikura and A. Ozaki, J. Antibiotics, 24 (1971) 259–262.

ELPHO.

1. **Medium:**

   Toyo Roshi No. 51.

   Buffer:

   M/30 Sorensen phosphate buffer, pH 5.0.

   Conditions:

   300 V/35 cm, 2.0–2.5 mA/5 cm, 1.5 h, 15°C.

   Detection:

   Mobility:

   4.1 cm to the cathode.

   Ref:

   As PC (1).

HISTIDOMYCIN

ELPHO.

1. **Medium:**

   Schleicher and Schuell No. 598 paper.

   Buffer:

   0.25 M sodium phosphate buffer, pH 7.

   Conditions:

   600 V for 6 h.

   Detection:

   Mobility:

   Histidomycin A migrates as anion, 7.5 cm. Histidomycin B does not migrate.

   Ref:

   E.A. Kaczka, T.W. Miller, F. Tausig and F.J. Wolf, Antimicrobial Agents and Chemotherapy, 1966 (1967) 603–605.

   T.C. Demny, U.S. Patent 3,657,418; April 18, 1972.

HODYDAMYCIN

PC.

1. **Paper:**

Solvent:
- A. Ethyl acetate.
- B. Ethyl acetate:water (1:1).
- C. Ethyl acetate:petroleum ether:water (5:2.5:5).
- D. Ethyl acetate:ammonia (1:1).
- E. Ethyl acetate:acetic acid (1:1).
- F. 3% Ammonium chloride.
- G. Distilled water.
- H. 0.5% Disodium phosphate.
- I. n-Butanol.
- J. n-Butanol:petroleum ether:water (5:2.5:5).
- K. n-Butanol:ethanol:water (5:2.5:5).
- L. n-Butanol:acetic acid:water (4:1:5).
- M. Chloroform.
- N. Chloroform:ethanol:water (5:2.5:5).
- O. Chloroform:petroleum ether:water (5:2.5:5).
- P. Chloroform:water (1:1).
- Q. Chloroform:ammonia (1:1).
- R. Chloroform:acetic acid (1:1).
- S. Petroleum ether.
- T. 0.5% Sodium carbonate.

Detection:

R_f:

Solvent	R_f
A	1.00
B	0.92
C	0.40
D	1.00
E	1.00
F	0.00
G	0.00
H	0.00
I	0.78
J	0.45
K	0.60
L	1.00
M	1.00
N	0.60
O	0.55
P	1.00
Q	1.00
R	1.00
S	0.00
T	0.00

Ref:

I.R. Shimi, A. Dewedar and S. Shoukry, J. Antibiotics, 23 (1970) 388–393.

HOLOMYCIN

PC.

1. **Paper:**

   Solvent:
   - A. Stationary phase: formamide; mobile phase: benzene.
   - B. Stationary phase: sodium meta-cresotinate; mobile phase: a 3:1 mixture of n-butyl acetate and di-n-butyl ether.

   Detection:

   R_f:

	R_{th}*	
	Solvent	
	A	B
Holomycin	0.10	0.78
Propionyl holothin	0.28	1.50
Butyryl holothin	0.52	1.87

   *R_{th} = distance relative to thiolutin (= 1.00).

   Ref:

   E. Gaeumann, V. Prelog and E. Vischer, U.S. Patent 3,014,922; December 26, 1961.

HON (δ-hydroxy-γ-oxo-L-norvaline)

PC.

1. **Paper:**

   Solvent:
   n-Butanol:acetic acid:water (4:2:1), ascending.

   Detection:
   Ninhydrin reagent.

   R_f:
   0.22

   Ref:
   S. Tatsuoka, A. Miyake, H. Hitomi, J. Ueyanagi, H. Iwasaki, T. Yamaguchi, K. Kanazawa, T. Ataki, K. Tsuchiya, F. Hiraiwa, K. Nakazawa and M. Shibata, J. Antibiotics, 14 (1961) 39–43.

HONDAMYCIN

PC.

1. **Paper:**

   Solvent:
   - A. Benzene:water:acetic acid (1:1:0.2).
   - B. Ethanol:n-hexane (1:2).
   - C. Water:acetone (75:25).
   - D. 16% Aq. soln. n-propanol.

   All systems developed ascending.

Detection:
R_f:

Solvent	R_f
A	0.62
B	0.65
C	0.41
D	0.19

Ref:
Y. Sakagami, A. Ueda, S. Yamabayashi,
Y. Tsurumaki and S. Kumon, J. Antibiotics,
22 (1969) 521–527.

TLC.
1. **Medium:**
   Silica Gel.
   Solvent:
   A. Ethanol:water (4:1).
   B. Ethyl acetate:methanol (100:15).
   C. Benzene:ethyl acetate (1:1).
   Detection:
   R_f:

Solvent	R_f
A	0.75
B	0.82
C	0.42

   Ref:
   As PC (1).

CCD.
1. **Solvent:**
   Methanol:water:chloroform:carbon tetra-
   chloride (3:1:1.5:4).
   Distribution:
   K = 0.35
   Ref:
   As PC (1).

HORDECIN
PC.
1. **Paper:**
   Whatman No. 3MM. Impregnate paper with
   20% formic acid for 24 h; evaporate formic
   acid and wash paper with doubly distilled
   water.
   Solvent:
   n-Butanol:acetone:water (5:1:2).
   Detection:
   UV light and yellow fluorescences.
   R_f:
   0.93

Ref:
I.S. Ezhov and N.V. Novotel'nov,
Prikladnaya Biokhimiya i Mikrobiologiya, 3
(1967) 178–183.

HORTADINES
TLC.
1. **Medium:**
   Microcrystalline cellulose.
   Solvent:
   n-Butanol:acetic acid:water (4:1:5), upper
   phase.
   Detection:
   A. Diazotized nitraniline.
   B. Bromocresol green.
   C. Sakaguchi reagent.
   R_f:
   Hordatine A   0.54
   Hordatine B   0.53
   Ref:
   A. Stoessl, U.S. Patent 3,475,459; October
   28, 1969.

HYDROXYMYCIN
PC.
1. **Paper:**
   Whatman No. 1.
   Solvent:
   A. n-Butanol:acetic acid:water (2:1:2).
   B. n-Butanol:water:p-toluenesulfonic acid
      (15:15:0.7).
   C. n-Butanol:piperidine:p-toluenesulfonic
      acid (98:2:2).
   D. Methanol:soln. of 2% sodium chloride
      (2:1), with paper buffered at pH 2.4 with
      sodium bisulfate.
   Detection:
   A. Ninhydrin.
   B. Bioautography vs. *Bacillus subtilis*.
   R_f:

Solvent	R_f
A	0.01
B	0.07
C	0.01
D	0.46

   Ref:
   G. Hagemann, G. Nominé and L. Pénasse,
   Ann. Pharm. Franc., 16 (1958) 585–596.

ELPHO.
1. **Medium:**
   Paper.
   Buffer:
   Phosphate buffer 0.1 M at pH 4.6.
   Conditions:
   240 V, 120 mA (11.4×10^{-5} cm/sec/V/cm).
   Detection:
   Bioautography vs. *Bacillus subtilis.*
   Mobility:
   Homogeneous zone.
   Ref:
   As PC (1).

CCD.
1. **Solvent:**
   Acetone:water:chloroform (3:1:1.8),
   25 transfers.
   Distribution:
   Peak is in tube 22.
   Ref:
   As PC (1).

HYDROXYSTREPTOMYCIN
(cf Streptomycin)
PC.
1. **Paper:**
   Whatman No. 4.
   Solvent:
   Wet butanol containing 2% p-toluenesulfonic acid and 2% piperidine.
   Detection:
   Bioautography vs. *Staphylococcus aureus.*
   R_f:
   Ref:
   F.H. Stodola, O.L. Shotwell, A.M. Borud, R.G. Benedict and A.C. Riley, Jr., J. Amer. Chem. Soc., 73 (1951) 2290.

HYGROMYCIN
CCD.
1. **Solvent:**
   A. Equilibrate n-butanol:water:glacial acetic acid (1:1:0.4).
   B. n-Amyl alcohol:water:glacial acetic acid (1:1:0.4).
   Distribution:

Solvent	K
A	1.0
B	0.3

Ref:
R.L. Mann, R.M. Gale and F.R. van Abeele, Antibiotics Annual, 1953–1954, 167–170.

HYGROSTATIN
PC.
1. **Paper:**
   Solvent:
   Water satd. butanol.
   Detection:
   Bioautography vs. *Candida albicans.*
   R_f:
   0.41
   Ref:
   M. Arai, J. Antibiotics, 13 (1960) 51.

ELPHO.
1. **Medium:**
   Buffer:
   pH 4.1 1/150 M acetate buffer.
   Conditions:
   500 V/34 cm. 0.2 mA/cm. 10 h.
   Detection:
   Mobility:
   Migrates toward cathode.
   Ref:
   As PC (1).

IKUTAMYCIN
PC.
1. **Paper:**
   Toyo No. 51.
   Solvent:
   A. 40% Aq. methanol.
   B. 40% Aq. ethanol.
   C. 20% Aq. n-propanol.
   D. Water satd. butanol.
   E. 3% Ammonium chloride.
   F. Butanol:methanol:water (4:1:2).
   G. 55% Aq. methanol.
   Detection:
   Bioautography vs. *Piricularia oryzae.*
   R_f:

Solvent	R_f
A	0.62
B	1.00
C	0.35
D	0.37
E	0.00
F	0.91
G	1.00

Ref:

Y. Sakagami, A. Ueda and S. Yamabayashi,
J. Antibiotics, 20 (1967) 299–307.

TLC.

1. **Medium:**

Silica Gel.

Solvent:

A. Ethyl acetate.

B. n-Hexane:ethyl acetate (1:1).

C. n-Hexane:ethyl acetate (3:7).

D. Chloroform:methanol (15:1).

E. Methanol:tetrahydrofuran (10:1).

F. Benzene:ethanol (1:1).

G. Benzene:acetone (1:1).

H. Benzene:methanol (1:1).

I. Acetone:ethanol (9:1).

Detection:

As PC (1).

R_f:

Solvent	R_f
A	0.31
B	0.00
C	0.13
D	0.00
E	0.77
F	0.53
G	0.30
H	0.79
I	0.79

Ref:

As PC (1).

ILICICOLINS

TLC.

1. **Medium:**

Silica Gel.

Solvent:

A. n-Hexane:acetone (3:1).

B. Benzene:ethyl acetate (7:1).

Detection:

R_f:

	R_f Solvent	
	A	B
Ilicicolin A	0.60	0.67
Ilicicolin B	0.44	0.50
Ilicicolin C	0.37	0.44
Ilicicolin D	0.31	0.43
Ilicicolin E	0.31	0.39
Ilicicolin F	0.23	0.27
Ilicicolin G	0.35	0.27
Ilicicolin H	0.09	0.055

Ref:

S. Hayakawa, H. Minato, K. Katagiri,
J. Antibiotics, 24 (1971) 653–654.

ITURINE

PC.

1. **Paper:**

Solvent:

A. Pyridine:butanol:water (2:3:1.5).

B. n-Butanol:acetic acid:water (4:5:1).

Detection:

R_f:

Useful for detection of fraction B and
impurities.

Ref:

L. Delcambe, Bull. Soc. Chim. Belges, 73
(1965) 315–328.

ELPHO.

1. **Medium:**

Paper.

Buffer:

A. Collidine 0.1 N:acetic acid 0.1 N (3:1.85),
pH 7.0.

B. Pyridine 0.1 N:acetic acid 0.1 N (1:1),
pH 5.2.

C. Acetic acid:water (1:10), pH 2.3.

Conditions:

500 V, 12 mA, 2.5 h.

Detection:

A. Pauly reagent.

B. Bioautography vs. *Penicillium notatum*.

Mobility:

Purified fraction B is immobile; impurities
move to positive pole.

Ref:

As PC (1).

JANIEMYCIN

PC.

1. **Paper:**

Whatman No. 1.

Solvent:

A. n-Butanol:acetic acid:water (4:3:7).

B. n-Butanol:pyridine:water (4:3:7).

Detection:

R_f:

Solvent	R_f
A	0.13
B	0.85

Ref:

E. Meyers, F.L. Weisenborn, F.E. Pansy, D.S. Slusarchyk, M.H. von Saltza, M.L. Rathnum and W.L. Parker, J. Antibiotics, 23 (1970) 502—507.

ELPHO.

1. Medium:
   Buffer:
   pH 3.3 in the presence of 40% formamide.
   Conditions:
   Detection:
   Saframin O, cathodic indicator; apalon, electroosmotic indicator.
   Mobilities:
   + 85 (major); + 44 (minor); + 12 (minor).
   Ref:
   As PC (1).

JOSAMYCIN

PC.

1. Paper:
   Toyo No. 50.
   Solvent:
   A. Benzene:chloroform (1:1).
   B. Benzene:ethyl acetate satd. with water (9:1).
   C. Benzene:acetone (95:5).
   D. Carbon tetrachloride:chloroform (1:1).
   Detection:
   R_f:

Solvent	R_f
A	0.49
B	0.68
C	0.65
D	0.76

Ref:

T. Osono, Y. Oka, S. Watanabe, Y. Numazaki, K. Moriyama, H. Ishida and K. Suzaki, J. Antibiotics, 20 (1967) 174—180.

2. Paper:
   Solvent:
   Benzene:chloroform (1:1).
   Detection:

R_f:
   0.49
   Ref:
   H. Umezawa and T. Osono, U.S. Patent 3,636,197; January 18, 1972.

TLC.

1. Medium:
   A. Alumina G (Merck).
   B. Silica Gel (Merck).
   Solvent:
   A. Ethyl acetate.
   B. n-Butanol:acetic acid:water (3:1:1).
   Detection:
   R_f:

Solvent	R_f
A	0.67
B	0.64

Ref:
   As PC (1).

2. Medium:
   Kieselguhr G 0.5 mm.
   Solvent:
   Benzene:acetone (2:1).
   Detection:
   Coloration: 20% sulfuric acid.
   R_f:
   0.69
   Ref:
   S. Omura, Y. Hironaka and T. Hata, J. Antibiotics, 23 (1970) 511—513.

3. Medium:
   A. Silica Gel.
   B. Alumina.
   Solvent:
   A. n-Butanol:acetic acid:water (3:1:1).
   B. Ethyl acetate.
   Detection:
   R_f:

Solvent	R_f
A	0.64
B	0.66

Ref:
   As PC (2).

JULYMYCINS

TLC.

1. Medium:

Silica Gel (Merck). Metal-free silica gel prepared as follows: the silica gel (Merck; less than 0.08 mm for chromatography) was washed with 6 N hydrochloric acid being warmed at 90–100°C to remove contaminating metal ions which interfere with the chromatography in forming metal chelate compounds with B-11. After usual water-washing to remove the absorbed hydrochloric acid, the gel was washed repeatedly with boiling water until the chlor ion test became negative. The washed gel was then dried at 110°C before use. Thin-layer plate: 10% of gypsum was mixed with the metal free silica gel and used to prepare plates by the usual method.

Solvent:
A. Chloroform:methanol (9:1).
B. Benzene:ethyl formate:formic acid (3:2:1).

Detection:

R_f:

	R_f Julymycin					
Solvent	B-0	B-I	B-II	S.V.	B-III	B-IV
A	0.85	0.65	0.45	0.35	0.25	0–0.1
B	–	0.50	0.40	0.40	0.45	–

Ref:
J. Shoji, Y. Kimura and K. Katagiri, J. Antibiotics, 17 (1964) 156–160.

JUVENIMICINS

PC.

1. **Paper:**
Toyo Roshi No. 51.

Solvent:
A. Aq. 0.05 N ammonium hydroxide satd. with methyl ethyl ketone.
B. Methyl isobutyl ketone:methyl ethyl ketone (4:1).
C. Methyl isobutyl ketone.
D. M/15 phosphate buffer, pH 8.0, satd. with n-butyl acetate. Paper impregnated with 2% liquid paraffin.
E. Benzene:cyclohexane (1:1) satd. with formamide. Paper impregnated with formamide:methanol (1:1).
F. Aq. 0.05 N ammonium hydroxide satd. with n-butyl ethyl ketone.

Detection:

R_f:

Solvent	R_f
A	0.74
B	0.68
C	0.57
D	0.60
E	0.02
F	0.70

Ref:
German Offenlegungsschrift No. 2,034,245; February 25, 1971.

TLC.

1. **Medium:**
A. Spotfilm F.
B. Silica Gel.

Solvent:
Chloroform:methanol:7% aq. ammonia (40:12:20).

Detection:

R_f:

	R_f Medium	
	A	B
Juvenimicin A group A_1	0.85	–
Juvenimicin A group A_2	0.80	–
Juvenimicin A group A_3	0.70	0.70
Juvenimicin A group A_4	0.65	
Juvenimicin B group B_1	0.50	–
Juvenimicin B group B_2	0.40	–
Juvenimicin B group B_3	0.33	–
Juvenimicin B group B_4	0.25	–

Ref:
As PC (1).

2. **Medium:**
Aluminum oxide.

Solvent:
Ether.

Detection:

R_f:

	R_f
Juvenimicin A_1	0.65
Juvenimicin A_2	0.80
Juvenimicin A_3	0.80
Juvenimicin A_4	0.29

Ref:
As PC (1).

KALAFUNGIN
PC.
1. **Paper:**
   Whatman No. 1.
   Solvent:
   A. 1-Butanol:water (84:16), 16 h.
   B. 1-Butanol:water (84:16) + 0.25%
      p-toluenesulfonic acid, 16 h.
   C. 1-Butanol:acetic acid:water (2:1:1), 16 h.
   D. 1-Butanol:water (84:16) + 2% piperidine,
      16 h.
   E. 1-Butanol:water (4:96), 5 h.
   F. 1-Butanol:water (4:96), + 0.25% p-toluene-
      sulfonic acid, 5 h.
   Detection:
   Bioautography vs. *Saccharomyces
   pastorianus* subsp. *arbignensis* ATCC 2366.
   R_f:

Solvent	R_f
A	0.80
B	0.80
C	0.85
D	0.70
E	0.60
F	0.60

   Ref:
   L.E. Johnson and A. Dietz, Appl. Microbiol.,
   16 (1968) 1815–1821.

TLC.
1. **Medium:**
   Silica Gel HF$_{254}$ (E. Merck), prepared by
   suspending 0.2 M disodium phosphate:0.2 M
   monopotassium phosphate (1:1), pH 6.7.
   The plates were activated at 120–130°C for
   2 h prior to use.
   Solvent:
   Ethyl acetate:cyclohexane (1:1).
   Detection:
   A. UV light (254 nm).
   B. Potassium permanganate-sodium
      metaperiodate spray.
   R_f:
   0.4
   Ref:
   M.E. Bergy, J. Antibiotics, 21 (1968)
   454–457.

KANAMYCINS
PC.
1. **Paper:**

Solvent:
   Water satd. n-butanol + 2% p-toluenesulfonic acid.
Detection:
   Bioautography vs. *Bacillus subtilis*.
R_f:
   0.1 –0.26 (major)
   0.21–0.37 (minor)
Ref:
   K. Maeda, M. Ueda, K. Yagishita, S. Kawaji,
   S. Kondo, M. Murase, T. Takeuchi, Y. Okami
   and H. Umezawa, J. Antibiotics, 10 (1957)
   228–230.

2. **Paper:**
   Solvent:
   2% p-Toluenesulfonic acid (monohydrate) in
   water satd. n-butanol.
   Detection:
   R_f:
   0.21–0.26 (major); 0.00, 0.37 (minor).
   Ref:
   H. Umezawa, M. Ueda, K. Maeda,
   K. Yagishita, K. Kondo, Y. Okami,
   R. Utahara, Y. Osato, K. Nitta and
   T. Takeuchi, J. Antibiotics, 10 (1957)
   181–188.

3. **Paper:**
   Whatman No. 1.
   Solvent:
   n-Butanol:water:2% p-toluenesulfonic acid.
   Detection:
   The dye used to locate the position of the
   kanamycins on paper chromatograms,
   commonly called "chromato red", is made
   by coupling diazotized para-rosaniline with
   1-naphthol-4-sulfonic acid. The developed
   strips are dried thoroughly at room or higher
   temperatures before being dipped into a
   0.1–0.5% aq. soln. of this dye. The stained
   strips are hung vertically, and the excess dye
   is removed by several washes alternately
   with warm water and methanol.
   R_f:

	R_f
Kanamycin A	0.13–0.18
Kanamycin B	0.26–0.28
Kanamycin C	0.20–0.24

   Ref:
   J.W. Rothrock, R.T. Goegelman and
   F.J. Wolf, Antibiotics Annual 1958–1959,
   796–803.

4. **Paper:**
   Whatman No. 1.
   Solvent:
   Water satd. butanol containing 2% p-toluene-sulfonic acid.
   Detection:
   As PC (3).
   R_f:

	R_f
Kanamycin A	0.15—0.22
Kanamycin B	0.25—0.40
Kanamycin C	0.20—0.30

   Ref:
   J.W. Rothrock and I. Putter, U.S. Patent 3,032,547; September 12, 1958.

5. **Paper:**
   Toyo Roshi No. 50.
   Solvent:
   0.4% Aq. ammonium chloride and 20% methanol:water.
   Detection:
   Bioautography vs. *Bacillus subtilis*.
   R_f:
   Kanamycin methanesulfonate, 1.0.
   Ref:
   H. Umezawa, M. Murase and S. Yamazaki, J. Antibiotics, 12 (1959) 341—342.

6. **Paper:**
   A. Schleicher and Schuell 589 Blue Ribbon.
   B. Toyo No. 50.
   Solvent:
   n-Butanol:water:2% p-toluenesulfonic acid.
   Detection:
   Ninhydrin reaction.
   R_f:

	R_f	
Kanamycin A	0.35	(Paper A)
Kanamycin B	0.60	(Paper A)
Kanamycin C	0.21—0.26	(Paper B)

   Ref:
   D.A. Johnson and G.H. Hardcastle, Jr., U.S. Patent 2,967,177; January 3, 1961.

7. **Paper:**
   Toyo Roshi No. 51.
   Solvent:
   A. Ethanol:conc. ammonium hydroxide: water (8:1:1).
   B. n-Butanol:conc. ammonium hydroxide: water (8:1:1).
   C. n-Butanol:acetic acid:water (4:1:4), upper layer.
   D. n-Butanol:pH 7.0, M/15 phosphate buffer (3:1), upper layer. Filter paper was treated with the buffer.
   E. n-Octanol:water:conc. ammonium hydroxide (5:4:1), upper layer.
   All solvents developed ascending.
   Detection:
   A. UV absorption.
   B. Bioautography vs. *Bacillus subtilis*

R_f:

	R_f Solvent				
	A	B	C	D	E
Tetra-N-benzylkanamycin	0.858	0.845	0.760	0.175	0.545
Tetra-N-phenylethylkanamycin	0.889	1.000	0.964	0.286	0.710
Tetra-N-phenylpropylkanamycin	0.910	1.000	0.974	0.252	0.761
Tetra-N-cinnamylkanamycin	0.889	1.000	0.976	0.218	0.671
Tetra-N-2-hydroxybenzylkanamycin Na$_2$	0.815	0.695	0.646	0.030	0.355
Tetra-N-3-hydroxybenzylkanamycin	0.737	0.423	0.544	0.038	0.020
Tetra-N-2-methoxybenzylkanamycin	0.868	0.859	0.704	0.107	0.360
Tetra-N-4-methoxybenzylkanamycin	0.843	0.648	0.687	0.068	0.139
Tetra-N-2,4-dimethoxybenzylkanamycin	0.868	0.916	0.832	0.077	0.296
Tetra-N-2-chlorobenzylkanamycin	0.864	1.000	0.769	0.727	0.707
Tetra-N-4-chlorobenzylkanamycin	0.884	1.000	0.966	0.489	0.688
Tetra-N-2,4-dichlorobenzylkanamycin	0.902	1.000	0.962	0.987	0.705
Tetra-N-4-methylbenzylkanamycin	0.900	0.920	0.954	0.316	0.725
Tetra-N-4-isopropylbenzylkanamycin	0.942	1.000	0.974	0.496	0.801
Tetra-N-3-nitrobenzylkanamycin	0.779	0.636	0.704	0.084	0.055
Tetra-N-2-hydroxy-3-methoxybenzyl-kanamycin-Na$_2$	0.674	0.316	0.588	0.084	0.105
Kanamycin A	0.079	0.000	0.000	0.000	0.000

Ref:
A. Fujii, K. Maeda and H. Umezawa,
J. Antibiotics, 21 (1968) 340–349.

TLC.
1. **Medium:**
Silica Gel G.
Solvent:
Methanol:water:conc. ammonium hydroxide
(20:4:1).
Detection:
10% Sulfuric acid spray and heat.
R_f:

	R_f
Tetra-N-benzylkanamycin	0.83
Tetra-N-phenylethylkanamycin	0.82
Tetra-N-phenylpropylkanamycin	0.81
Tetra-N-cinnamylkanamycin	0.80
Tetra-N-2-hydroxybenzylkanamycin Na$_2$	0.85
Tetra-N-3-hydroxybenzylkanamycin	0.85
Tetra-N-2-methoxybenzylkanamycin	0.84
Tetra-N-4-methoxybenzylkanamycin	0.78
Tetra-N-2,4-dimethoxybenzyl-kanamycin	0.77
Tetra-N-2-chlorobenzylkanamycin	0.86
Tetra-N-4-chlorobenzylkanamycin	0.82
Tetra-N-2,4-dichlorobenzyl-kanamycin	0.84
Tetra-N-4-methylbenzylkanamycin	0.85
Tetra-N-4-isopropylbenzylkanamycin	0.83
Tetra-N-3-nitrobenzylkanamycin	0.80
Tetra-N-2-hydroxy-3-methoxybenzyl-kanamycin Na$_2$	0.65
Kanamycin A	0.03

Ref:
As PC (7).

GLC.
1. **Apparatus:**
F and M Model 400 with F.I.D.
Column:
Glass column, 3 mm × 1830 mm (6 ft)
packed with 3% OV-1 on Gas Chrom Q,
100/120 mesh (Applied Science Laboratories,
Inc., State College, Pa.).
Gases:
Hydrogen 40 ml/min, air 600 ml/min, and
carrier gas (helium) 70 ml/min. Chart speed
0.25 in/min.

Temperatures:
Column, conditioned at 330°C for 1 h; oven
temperature, 300°C, flow at 200 and 250°C,
injection, 300°C.
Internal standard-silylation reagent:
For kanamycin a soln. containing 8 mg of
trilaurin and 25 μl of N-tri-methyl-silyl-
diethylamine/ml of Tri-Sil Z is prepared.
Reference standard:
A water soln. containing 10.0 mg of
kanamycin sulfate reference standard/ml.
Sample:
Samples are prepared in the same way as the
reference standard.
Silylation procedures:
One ml of the internal standard-silylation
reagent is added to the sample and the
reference standard vials using a tuberculin
syringe. Vials are heated in a 75°C oil bath
for 45 min, swirling occasionally.
Separation of kanamycins:
Order of elution is (1) aminoglucosyl deoxy-
streptamine (2) kanamycin B, (3) kanamycin
A.
Ref:
K. Tsuji and J.H. Robertson, Anal. Chem.,
42 (1970) 1661–1663.

KANCHANOMYCIN
TLC.
1. **Medium:**
Solvent:
A. Acetone:methanol:acetic acid (1:1:1).
B. 1-Butanol:methanol:10% citric acid
(4:2:2).
C. 1-Butanol:acetic acid:methanol (3:1:1).
D. Benzene:ethyl acetate:methanol
(10:2.5:1).
E. Water.
Detection:
R_f:

Solvent	R_f
A	0.73
B	0.65
C	0.46
D	0.10
E	0.00

Ref:
T.F. Kuimova, K. Fukushima, S. Kuroda and
T. Arai, J. Antibiotics, 24 (1971) 69–76.

KASUGAMYCIN

PC.

1. **Paper:**

   Toyo No. 51.

   Solvent:

   A. Butanol:acetic acid:water (2:1:1).

   B. Butanol:ethanol:water:ammonia
      (4:1:4.9:0.1).

   C. Butanol:acetic acid:water (6.3:1:2.7).

   D. Butanol:acetic acid:water (2:1:1).

   Detection:

   R_f:

Solvent	R_f
A	0.28
B	0.07
C	0.06
D	0.29

   Ref:

   H. Umezawa, Y. Okami, T. Hashimoto,
   Y. Suhara, M. Hamada and T. Takeuchi,
   J. Antibiotics, 18 (1965) 101–103.
   H. Umezawa, Y. Okami, T. Takeuchi,
   M. Hamada, U.S. Patent 3,358,001;
   December 12, 1967.

TLC.

1. **Medium:**

   Avicel.

   Solvent:

   A. n-Propanol:pyridine:water:acetic acid
      (15:10:12:3).

   B. Methyl acetate:2-propanol:ammonium
      hydroxide (45:105:60).

   Detection:

   Ninhydrin spray.

   R_f:

Solvent	R_f
A	0.35
B	0.20

   Ref:

   M.J. Cron, R.E. Smith, I.R. Hooper,
   J.G. Keil, E.A. Ragan, R.H. Schreiber,
   G. Schwab and J.C. Godfrey, Antimicrobial
   Agents and Chemotherapy, 1969 (1970)
   219–224.

ELPHO.

1. **Medium:**

   Buffer:

   Formic acid:acetic acid:water (25:75:900),
   pH 1.8.

Conditions:

3,000 V/40 cm at 10°C, 15 min.

Detection:

Mobility:

Moves to cathode 3.7 cm.

Ref:

H. Umezawa, Y. Okami, T. Hashimoto,
Y. Suhara, M. Hamada and T. Takeuchi,
J. Antibiotics, 18 (1965) 101–103.

KETOMYCIN

PC.

1. **Paper:**

   MN 212.

   Solvent:

   Methanol:water (90:10).

   Detection:

   R_f:

   Ref:

   W. Keller-Schierlein, K. Poralla and
   H. Zähner, Arch. Mikrobiol., 67 (1969)
   339–356.

TLC.

1. **Medium:**

   Kieselgel G.

   Solvent:

   A. Butanol:acetic acid:water (80:20:20).

   B. Ethyl acetate:water:formic acid
      (200:60:5), organic phase.

   Detection:

   R_f:

   Ref:

   As PC (1).

KIDAMYCIN

PC.

1. **Paper:**

   Toyo No. 50.

   Solvent:

   A. Acetonitrile.

   B. n-Butyl acetate:dibutyl ether (3:1).

   C. n-Butanol:methanol:water (4:1:2).

   All solvents developed ascending.

   Detection:

   R_f:

Solvent	R_f
A	0.14
B	0.71
C	0.68

Ref:
  N. Kanda, J. Antibiotics, 24 (1971)
  599—606.

TLC.
1. **Medium:**
     A. Silica Gel (Merck Kieselgel G).
     B. Schleicher and Schull No. 288 aluminum
        oxide paper.
   Solvent:
     A. Ethanol:14% ammonia water (4:1).
     B. Ethanol:pyridine (4:1).
     C. Water satd. ethyl acetate.
   Detection:
   R_f:

	R_f Medium	
Solvent	A	B
A	0.81	—
B	0.06	—
C	—	0.10

   Ref:
     As PC (1).

KIKUMYCIN
PC.
1. **Paper:**
   Solvent:
     Butanol:acetic acid:water (2:1:1).
   Detection:
   R_f:

Component	R_f
Kikumycin A	0.04
Kikumycin B	0.72

   Ref:
     M. Kikuchi, K. Kumagai, N. Ishida, Y. Ito,
     T. Yamaguchi, T. Furumai and T. Okuda,
     J. Antibiotics, 18 (1965) 243—250.

2. **Paper:**
   Solvent:
     A. Wet butanol.
     B. 3% Ammonium chloride.
     C. 80% Phenol.
     D. 50% Acetone.
     E. Butanol:methanol:water (4:1:2), 1.5%
        methyl orange.
     F. Butanol:methanol:water (4:1:2).
     G. Benzene:methanol (4:1).
     H. Water.

   I. Pyridine.
   J. Butanol satd. water:propanol:acetic acid:
      water (10:15:3:12).
Detection:
R_f:

	R_f Component	
Buffer	A	B
A	0.00	0.00
B	0.12	0.12
C	1.00	1.00
D	0.00	0.10
E	0.50	0.60
F	0.10	0.40
G	0.00	0.00
H	0.02	0.05
I	0.02	0.00
J	0.50	0.50

Ref:
  As PC (1).

ELPHO.
1. **Medium:**
     Paper.
   Buffer:
     A. pH 5.0.
     B. pH 8.0.
   Conditions:
     250 V/30 cm, 2.5 h.
   Detection:
   Mobility:
     A. Moves toward cathode.
     B. Moves toward cathode.
   Ref:
     As PC (1).

KINAMYCIN
TLC.
1. **Medium:**
     Kieselgel G (Merck).
   Solvent:
     Chloroform:ethyl acetate (3:2).
   Detection:
   R_f:

	R_f
Kinamycin A	0.89
Kinamycin B	0.82
Kinamycin C	0.47
Kinamycin D	0.39

Ref:

S. Ito, T. Matsuya, S. Omura, M. Otani, A. Nakagawa, H. Takeshima, Y. Iwai, M. Ohtani and T. Hata, J. Antibiotics, 23 (1970) 315–317.

2. Medium:

Kieselgel G (Merck) treated with 2% sulfuric acid.

Solvent:

A. Benzene:acetone (5:1).
B. Chloroform:ethyl acetate (3:2).

Detection:

A. UV lamp.
B. Visible color.

R_f:

Solvent	R_f Component			
	A	B	C	D
A	0.60	0.60	0.25	0.25
B	0.89	0.82	0.47	0.39

Ref:

T. Hata, S. Omura, Y. Iwai, A. Nakagawa, M. Otani, S. Ito and T. Matsuya, J. Antibiotics, 24 (1971) 353–359.

KIRROMYCIN

TLC.

1. Medium:

A. Kieselgel.
B. Aluminum oxide.

Solvent:

A. Benzyl alcohol.
B. Ethyl acetate:methanol (1:1).
C. Ethyl acetate:methanol:formic acid (17:2:1).
D. 1-Propanol:water:conc. ammonium hydroxide (7:2:1).

Detection:

R_f:

Medium	Solvent	R_f
A	A	0.57
	B	0.80
	C	0.63
	D	0.59
B	C	0.45
	D	0.33

Ref:

H. Wolf and H. Zähner, Arch. Mikrobiol., 83 (1972) 147–154.

KOBENOMYCIN

PC.

1. Paper:

Toyo No. 51.

Solvent:

A. t-Butanol:acetic acid:water (2:1:1).
B. n-Butanol:acetic acid:water (4:1:5), upper phase.
C. Acetone:water (1:1).

All systems developed ascending.

Detection:

R_f:

Solvent	R_f
A	0.60
B	0.15
C	0.83

Ref:

S. Okamoto, M. Mayama, Y. Tanaka, K. Tawara, N. Shimaoka, H. Kato, H. Nishimura, M. Ebata and H. Ohtsuka, J. Antibiotics, 21 (1968) 320–326.

TLC.

1. Medium:

Silica Gel G.

Solvent:

A. n-Butanol:acetic acid:water (4:1:2).
B. n-Butanol:ethanol:0.1 N hydrochloric acid (1:1).
C. n-Butanol:pyridine:acetic acid:water (15:10:3:10).
D. Chloroform:methanol:17% ammonium hydroxide (2:1:1), upper phase.
E. Ethanol:water (4:1).

Detection:

R_f:

Solvent	R_f
A	0.30
B	0.50
C	0.75
D	1.00
E	0.57

Ref:

As PC (1).

ELPHO.

1. Medium:

Toyo Paper No. 51.

Buffer:

pH 2.0, 5.0, 6.0, 7.0, 8.0 and 11.4 buffer solns.

Conditions:
   300 V for 3 h.
Detection:
Mobility:
   Moves slightly to anode at pH 11.4; moves slightly to cathode at other pH values.
Ref:
   As PC (1).

KOMAMYCINS
TLC.
1. **Medium:**
   Solvent:
      A. n-Butanol:acetic acid:water (3:1:1).
      B. Phenol:water (4:1).
      C. Methanol:water (17:3).
      D. n-Propanol:water (7:3).
   Detection:
   R_f:

	R_f Component	
Solvent	A	B
A	0.40	0.40
B	0.52	0.40
C	0.52	0.44
D	0.63	0.63

Ref:
   Japanese Patent No. 2338IR; March 27, 1970.

KUJIMYCIN
TLC.
1. **Medium:**
      A. Silica Gel.
      B. Alumina.
   Solvent:
      A. Benzene:acetone (1:1).
      B. Ethyl acetate.
   Detection:
      Bioautography vs. *Sarcina lutea*.
   R_f:

Component	Medium	Solvent	R_f
Kujimycin A	A	A	0.46
	B	A	0.12
		B	0.38
Kujimycin B	A	A	0.62
	B	A	0.55
		B	0.65

Ref:
   S. Omura, S. Namiki, M. Shibata, T. Muro, H. Nakayoshi and J. Sawada, J. Antibiotics, 22 (1969) 500–505.

KUNDRYMYCIN
TLC.
1. **Medium:**
      Silica Gel.
   Solvent:
      Methanol:toluene:formic acid (95:5:0.5).
   Detection:
      Bioautography vs. *Bacillus subtilis* ATCC 6633.
   R_f:
      0.78
   Ref:
      J.A. Bush, C.S. Cassidy, K.E. Crook, Jr., and L.B. German, J. Antibiotics, 24 (1971) 143–148.

LACTENOCIN
PC.
1. **Paper:**
   Solvent:
      A. Methyl ethyl ketone on pH 4 buffered paper.
      B. Methyl ethyl ketone.
      C. n-Butanol satd. with water on pH 4 buffered paper.
      D. n-Butanol satd. with water.
      E. Water with 7% sodium chloride and 2.5% methyl ethyl ketone.
      F. Ethyl acetate satd. with water on pH 4 buffered paper.
   Detection:
   R_f:

Solvent	R_f
A	0.20
B	0.38
C	0.75
D	0.60
E	0.86
F	0.05

Ref:
   R.L. Hamill and W.M. Stark, J. Antibiotics, 17 (1964) 133–139.

LAGOSIN
PC.
1. **Paper:**
      Whatman No. 1.
   Solvent:
      A. Methyl isobutyl ketone:1-butanol:water (50:15:3).

B. Methyl isopropyl ketone:water (satd. ca. 1.6%).

C. Methyl isopropyl ketone:1-butanol:water (50:10:3.5).

D. Methyl isopropyl ketone:methanol:water (50:1:0.4).

Detection:

UV light; greenish fluorescence.

R_f:

Solvent	R_f
A	0.72
B	0.35
C	0.76
D	0.47

Ref:

A.C. Cope, R.K. Bly, E.P. Burrows, O.J. Adar, E. Ciganek, B.T. Gillis, R.F. Porter and H.E. Johnson, J. Am. Chem. Soc., 84 (1962) 2170–2178.

LARGOMYCIN

TLC.

1. **Medium:**

A. Silica Gel.

B. Aluminum oxide.

System:

A. Ethanol:ammonium hydroxide:water (8:1:1).

B. n-Butanol:methanol:water (4:1:2).

Detection:

R_f:

	R_f Medium	
Solvent	A	B
A	0.95	—
B	—	0.74

Ref:

T. Yamaguchi, T. Kashida, K. Nawa, T. Yajma, T. Miyagishima, Y. Ito, T. Okuda, N. Ishida and K. Kumagai, J. Antibiotics, 23 (1970) 373–381.

LASPARTOMYCIN

PC.

1. **Paper:**

Solvent:

A. Benzene:methanol (4:1).

B. n-Butanol satd. with water.

C. n-Butanol:pyridine:water (2:1:1).

All systems developed ascending.

Detection:

R_f:

Solvent	R_f
A	0.70
B	0.45
C	0.41

Ref:

H. Naganawa, M. Hamada, K. Maeda, Y. Okami, T. Takeuchi and H. Umezawa, J. Antibiotics, 21 (1968) 55–62.

2. **Paper:**

Toyo No. 51.

Solvent:

A. 1-Butanol satd. with water.

B. 5% ammonium chloride.

C. 1-Butanol:acetic acid:water (4:1:2).

D. 1-Butanol:pyridine:water (2:1:1).

E. 1-Butanol:pyridine:acetic acid:water (20:5:5:10).

F. Benzene:methanol (4:1).

All solvents developed ascending.

Detection:

Bioautography.

R_f:

Solvent	R_f
A	0.45
B	0.23
C	0.91
D	0.41
E	0.80
F	0.70

Ref:

H. Umezawa, M. Hamada, H. Naganawa, T. Takeuchi, K. Maeda and Y. Okami, U.S. Patent 3,639,582; February 1, 1972.

TLC.

1. **Medium:**

Silica Gel.

Solvent:

A. 1-Butanol satd. with water.

B. Acetic acid:chloroform (2:1).

C. Sec.-butanol:formic acid:water (75:15:10).

D. n-Propanol:acetic acid:chloroform (1:4:2).

E. 1-Butanol:acetic acid:water (4:1:2).

F. 1-Butanol:pyridine:water (2:1:1).

Detection:
  Permanganate.
R_f:

Solvent	R_f
A	0.14
B	0.13
C	0.45
D	0.16
E	0.58
F	0.78

Ref:
  As PC (1).

2. **Medium:**
  Silica Gel.
Solvent:
  A. n-Butanol:satd. with water.
  B. Acetic acid:chloroform (2:1).
  C. n-Butanol:acetic acid:water (4:1:2).
  D. n-Butanol:pyridine:water (2:1:1).
Detection:
  A. Decolorization of permanganate.
  B. Bioautography.
R_f:

Solvent	R_f
A	0.14
B	0.13
C	0.58
D	0.76

Ref:
  As PC (1).

LATERIOMYCIN F
PC.
1. **Paper:**
  A. Whatman No.1.[*]
  B. Arches No. 302.[*]
  C. Toyo Roshi No. 51.[*]
  [*]Impregnate papers with McIlvaines buffer, pH 4.8.
Solvent:
  A. n-Butanol satd. with water.
  B. n-Butanol satd. with water, phosphate
    buffer pH 5.6.
  C. n-Butanol:acetic acid:water (4:1:5).
  D. Acetone:benzene:water (12:3:2).
Detection:
R_f:

Solvent	Paper	R_f
A	A	0.8–0.9
A	B	0.8–0.9
A	C	0.8–0.9
B	A	0.65–0.95
C	A	0.75–0.95
D	A	0.75–0.99

Ref:
  French Patent No. 1,523,522; March 31,
  1967. E. Higashide, T. Hasegawa, M. Shibata,
  T. Kishi, S. Harada and K. Mizuno, U.S.
  Patent 3,660,567; May 2, 1972.

TLC.
1. **Medium:**
  Silica Gel G (Merck).
Solvent:
  Ethyl acetate:methanol (10:1), ascending.
Detection:
R_f:
  0.2–0.45
Ref:
  As PC (1).

LEMACIDINE
PC.
1. **Paper:**
Solvent:
  Ethanol:water (3:1) + 2% sodium chloride.
Detection:
R_f:

	R_B[*]
Lemacidine B_1	0.34
Lemacidine B_2	0.61
Lemacidine B_3	1.00

$$^\star R_B = \frac{\text{distance zone moved}}{\text{distance } B_3 \text{ moved } (= 1.00)}$$

Ref:
  E. Gaeumann, F. Benz, U.S. Patent
  3,089,816; May 14, 1963.

LEMONOMYCIN
PC.
1. **Paper:**
  Whatman No. 1.
Solvent:
  Pyridine:chloroform:acetic acid:water
    (140:35:10:30), upper phase.
Detection:
  Bioautography vs. *Bacillus subtilis* on agar
  medium, pH 6.

R_f:

0.40

Ref:

H.A. Whaley, E.L. Patterson, M. Dann,
A.J. Shay and J.N. Porter, Antimicrobial
Agents and Chemotherapy, 1964 (1965)
83–86.

LEUCINAMYCIN

PC.

1. **Paper:**

Toyo No. 51A.

Solvent:

A. Wet n-butanol, ascending.

B. 1.5% Ammonium chloride, ascending.

C. 50% Aq. acetone, ascending.

D. n-Butanol:methanol:water (4:1:2),
ascending.

E. n-Butanol:acetic acid:water (4:1:5),
upper phase, descending.

Detection:

R_f:

Solvent	R_f
A	0.09
B	0.40
C	0.86
D	0.50
E	0.31

Ref:

K. Mizuno, Y. Ohkubo, S. Yokoyama,
M. Hamada, K. Maeda and H. Umezawa,
J. Antibiotics, 20 (1967) 194–199.

ELPHO.

1. **Medium:**

Toyo No. 51.

Buffer:

Formic acid:acetic acid:water (25:75:900),
pH 1.8.

Conditions:

3500 V/46 cm. 50 mA/20 cm, for 20 min.

Detection:

Mobility:

0.35 towards cathode.

Ref:

As PC (1).

LEUCOMYCIN

PC.

1. **Paper:**

Solvent:

A. Citrate buffer of pH 4.6 and benzene.

B. Citrate buffer of pH 4.0 and butyl acetate.

Detection:

Bioautography vs. *Bacillus subtilis*.

R_f:

Solvent	R_f
A	0.40
B	0.60

Ref:

T. Osato, K. Yagashita and H. Umezawa,
J. Antibiotics, 8 (1955) 161–163.

2. **Paper:**

Solvent:

A. Benzene.

B. n-Butanol.

C. Methanol.

D. Acetone.

E. Ethyl acetate.

F. Ether.

G. Petroleum ether.

H. Chloroform.

I. 3% Aq. ammonium chloride.

Detection:

Bioautography vs. *Bacillus subtilis* 219.

R_f:

Solvent	R_f
A	0.17
B	0.84
C	0.73
D	1.00
E	0.83
F	0.86
G	0.00
H	0.90
I	0.83

Ref:

Y. Sano, J. Antibiotics, 7 (1954) 93–97.

TLC.

1. **Medium:**

Kieselgel G 0.5 mm.

Solvent:

Benzene:acetone (2:1).

Detection:

Coloration:20% sulfuric acid.

R_f:

0.69

Ref:

S. Omura, Y. Hironaka and T. Hata,
J. Antibiotics, 23 (1970) 511–513.

CCD.
1. **Solvent:**
    A. Benzene:M/15 sodium phosphate buffer
       pH 6.5:methanol (5:2:5).
    B. Benzene:M/15 sodium citrate buffer
       pH 4.9:chloroform:methanol (10:9:8:20).
    C. Chloroform:M/15 sodium acetate buffer
       pH 4.5:acetone (1:2:2).
   Distribution:

	Coefficient Solvent		
	A	B	C
Leucomycin A_1	0.92	0.33	1.86
Leucomycin A_2	2.33	0.14	3.00

   Ref:

T. Watanabe, H. Nishida, J. Abe and
K. Satake, Bull. Chem. Soc. Japan, 33
(1960) 1104–1108.

LEUCOPEPTIN
PC.
1. **Paper:**
    Toyo No. 50.
   Solvent:
    A. Water satd. n-butanol.
    B. 1.5% Aq. ammonium chloride.
    C. 75% Aq. phenol.
    D. 50% Aq. acetone.
    E. n-Butanol:methanol:water (4:1:2).
    F. Water.
    G. t-Butanol:acetic acid:water (74:3:25).
    H. n-Butanol:acetic acid:water (4:1:2).
    All systems developed ascending.
   Detection:
    Bioautography vs. *Bacillus subtilis*.
   R_f:

Solvent	R_f
A	0.05
B	0.26
C	0.97
D	0.47
E	0.54
F	0.13
G	0.61
H	0.47

Ref:

S. Kondo, M. Sezaki, M. Shimura, K. Sato
and T. Hara, J. Antibiotics, 17 (1964)
262–263.

LEUCYLNEGAMYCIN
ELPHO.
1. **Medium:**
   Buffer:
    Formic acid:acetic acid:water (25:75:900).
   Conditions:
    3,500 V for 20 min.
   Detection:
    A. Ninhydrin.
    B. Red tetrazolium.
    C. Rydon-Smith reactions (starch-potassium
       iodide).
   Mobility:
    14.3 cm to cathode with Km (relative
    mobility against alanine) 1.24.
   Ref:
    S. Kondo, H. Yamamoto, K. Maeda and
    H. Umezawa, J. Antibiotics, 24 (1971)
    732–734.

LEUPEPTIN
TLC.
1. **Medium:**
    Silica Gel G.
   Solvent:
    Butanol:butyl acetate:acetic acid:water
    (4:2:1:1).
   Detection:
    A. Sakaguchi reagent.
    B. Starch-potassium iodide reagent.
   R_f:
   Ref:
    S. Kondo, K. Kawamura, I. Iwatsuki,
    J. Iwanaga, T. Aoyagi, M. Hamada, T. Hara,
    K. Maeda, T. Takeuchi and H. Umezawa,
    164th Antibiot. Res. Assn; May 26,
    1972.

LEVOMYCIN
PC.
1. **Paper:**
   Solvent:
    A. n-Butanol:water.
    B. n-Butanol:10% acetic acid.
    C. Methyl isopropyl ketone.

D. Methyl isopropyl ketone:2% toluene-
   sulfonic acid.
E. Methyl isopropyl ketone:2% piperidine.

Detection:

R_f:

Solvent	R_f
A	0.94
B	0.95
C	0.55
D	0.63
E	0.84

Ref:

H.E. Carter, C.P. Schaffner and D. Gottlieb,
Arch. Biochem. Biophys., 53 (1954) 282.

2. **Paper:**

Solvent:

Di-n-butyl ether:s-tetrachloroethane:10% aq.
sodium o-cresotinate (2:1:3).

Detection:

R_f:

0.13

Ref:

K. Katagiri, J. Shoii, T. Yoshida, J. Antibiotics, 15 (1962) 273.

3. **Paper:**

Solvent:

A. Petroleum ether:benzene:methanol:
   water (66.7:33.3:80:20).
B. 25% Ethanol.
C. Amyl acetate satd. with water.

Detection:

R_f:

Solvent	R_f
A	0.26
B	0.32
C	0.60

Ref:

T.S. Maksimova, I.N. Kovsharova,
V.V. Proshlyakova, Antibiotiki, 10 (1965)
298–304.

LEVORIN A

PC.

1. **Paper:**

Whatman No. 1.

Solvent:

A. Acetic acid:pyridine:water (4:3:2).
B. n-Butanol:pyridine:water (6:4:5).
C. Methanol:25% ammonia:water (20:1:4).

Detection:

Bioautography vs. *Candida albicans*.

R_f:

Solvent	R_f
A	0.66
B	0.71
C	0.55

Ref:

R. Bosshardt and H. Bickel, Experientia, 24
(1968) 422–424.

LICHENIFORMIN

PC.

1. **Paper:**

Whatman No. 4.

Solvent:

Collidine:lutidine:aq. 2N ammonia (1:1:2).

Detection:

A. Ninhydrin spray.
B. Bioautography vs. *Staphylococcus aureus*.
C. Bioautography vs. *Mycobacterium phlei*.

R_f:

Licheniformin C > B > A.

Ref:

R.K. Callow and T.S. Work, Biochem. J., 51
(1952) 558–567.

LINCOMYCIN

PC.

1. **Paper:**

Solvent:

A. 1-Butanol:water (84:16), 16 h.
B. 1-Butanol:water (84:16) + 0.25%
   p-toluenesulfonic acid, 16 h.
C. 1-Butanol:acetic acid:water (2:1:1), 16 h.
D. 1-Butanol:water (84:16) + 2% piperidine,
   16 h.
E. 1-Butanol:water (4:96), 5 h.
F. 1-Butanol:water (4:96) + 0.25%
   p-toluenesulfonic acid, 5 h.

Detection:

Bioautography vs. *Sarcina lutea*.

R_f:

Solvent	R_f*
A	0.40–0.50
B	0.40–0.45
C	0.70
D	0.60–0.81
E	0.81–0.95
F	0.90

*Estimated from drawing.

Ref:

D.J. Mason, A. Dietz and C. Deboer, Anti-microbial Agents and Chemotherapy, 1962 (1963) 554–559.

2. **Paper:**

Whatman No. 1.

Solvent:

n-Butanol:water:isoamyl alcohol:dichloro-acetic acid (100:75:50:1).

Detection:

R_f:

S-ethyl homolog of lincomycin   0.50

Ref:

E.L. Patterson, J.H. Hash, M. Lincks, P.A. Miller, N. Bohonos, Sci., 146 (1964) 1691–1692.

3. **Paper:**

Solvent:

A. 1-Butanol:water (84:16), 16 h.

B. 1-Butanol:water (84:16) + 0.25% p-toluenesulfonic acid, 16 h.

C. 1-Butanol:acetic acid:water (2:1:1), 16 h.

D. n-Butanol:water (84:16) + 2% piperidine.

E. 1-Butanol:water (4:96), 5 h.

F. 1-Butanol:water (4:96) + 0.25% p-toluenesulfonic acid, 5 h.

Detection:

R_f:

Solvent	$R_f^\star$ Lincomycin B
A	0.40–0.70
B	0.20–0.40
C	0.65
D	0.75
E	0.95
F	0.88

*Estimated from drawing.

Ref:

A.D. Argoudelis, M.E. Bergy and J.A. Fox, U.S. Patent 3,359,164; December 19, 1967.

TLC.

1. **Medium:**

Silica Gel G (Merck).

Solvent:

A. Methyl ethyl ketone:acetone:water (9.3:2.6:1).

B. Methyl propyl ketone:methyl ethyl ketone:water:methanol (2:2:1:1).

Detection:

Iodine vapor.

R_f:

Lincomycin   > U21,699   > U11,973.

Ref:

T.F. Brodasky and W.L. Lummis, Anti-microbial Agents and Chemotherapy, 1964 (1965) 18–23.

2. **Medium:**

Silica Gel.

Solvent:

Ethyl acetate:acetone:water (8:5:1).

Detection:

R_f:

	$R_f^\star$
Clindamycin	0.70
1'-Demethylclindamycin	0.17

*Estimated from drawing.

Ref:

A.D. Argoudelis, J.H. Coats, D.J. Mason and O.K. Sebek, J. Antibiotics, 22 (1969) 309–314.

3. **Medium:**

Silica Gel G.

Solvent:

Ethyl acetate:acetone:water (8:5:1).

Detection:

Bioautography vs. *Sarcina lutea*.

R_f:

	$R_f^\star$
Clindamycin	0.6
N-demethyl-N-hydroxymethyl-clindamycin (compound A)	0.4
Lincomycin	0.3
N-Demethylclindamycin	0.2

*Estimated from drawing.

Ref:

A.D. Argoudelis, J.H. Coats, B.J. Magerlein, J. Antibiotics, 25 (1972) 191–193.

GLC.

1. **Apparatus:**

Barber-Colman Model 500 with FID.

Column:

Glass, U-shaped, 6 ft × 3 mm I.D.; 5% SE-30 on Gas-Chrom-Q (80/100 mesh).

Temperature:

Column 257°; detector 280°; injector 280°.

Carrier gas:

N_2 at 20 p.s.i., 150 ml/min; H_2 at 32 p.s.i.; air 40 p.s.i.

Current:

2×10^{-8} f.s.d. (sens. 100 and atten. 2).

Silylating reagent:

Nine parts of hexamethyldisilane mixed with one part of trimethylchlorosilane. The mixture is cleared by filtration.

Lincomycin standard:

About 4 mg of lincomycin reference standard, accurately weighed and transferred to a centrifuge tube.

Internal standard:

A saturated soln. of tetraphenylcyclopentadienone prepared in cyclohexane, and cleared by filtration.

Derivatization:

A lincomycin standard is treated in the same manner as the samples. Each dry or dried sample is dissolved in 1 ml of pyridine, and 0.2 ml of the silylating reagent is added. The reaction mixtures are allowed to stand not less than 30 min. 1 ml of the internal standard soln. and 2 ml of water are added, and the mixture is shaken vigorously. The phases are separated by gravity or centrifugation.

Chromatography and calculations:

Five μl of the cyclohexane phase are injected into the gas chromatograph. The areas of each peak are measured by planimetry or by disc integration. The lincomycin content is determined by direct comparison of the ratio of the peak areas (lincomycin:internal standard) with that of the lincomycin reference standard treated in an identical manner. Lincomycin B content is determined as a fraction of the combined lincomycin plus lincomycin B.

Retention times of lincomycin and other compounds

	Retention time (min)	Relative retention time
Lincomycin	7.65	1.00
Lincomycin B	6.12	0.78
Lactose	4.11, 6.00	0.54, 0.78
Sucrose	4.35	0.57
Internal standard	11.10	1.45

Ref:

M. Margosis, J. Chromatogr., 37 (1968) 46–54.

LIPOXAMYCIN

PC.

1. **Paper:**

Whatman No. 1.

Solvent:

A. 1-Butanol:water (4:96) + 0.25% p-toluenesulfonic acid, 5 h.

B. 1-Butanol:water (84:16), 16 h.

C. 1-Butanol:water (84:16) + 0.25% p-toluenesulfonic acid, 16 h.

D. 1-Butanol:acetic acid:water (2:1:1), 16 h.

E. 2% Piperidine in 1-butanol:water (84:16), 16 h.

F. 1-Butanol:water (4:96), 5 h.

G. 1-Butanol:water (4:96) + 0.25% p-toluenesulfonic acid, 5 h.

Detection:

Bioautography vs. *Saccharomyces pastorianus*.

R_f:

Solvent	R_f
A	0.70
B	0.40–0.80
C	0.42–0.70
D	0.38, 0.78
E	0.20, 0.50
F	0.00, 0.50
G	0.38–0.65

Ref:

O.K. Sebek and H.A. Whaley, U.S. Patent 3,629,402; December 21, 1971. H.A. Whaley, O.K. Sebek and C. Lewis, Antimicrobial Agents and Chemotherapy, 1970 (1971) 455–461.

CCD.

1. **Solvent:**

Ethyl acetate:ethylene glycol monomethyl ether:water (2:1:1); 200 transfers of lipoxamycin-p-toluenesulfonic acid salt.

Distribution:

Lipoxamycin, free from coproduced antibiotic, was obtained from a pool of the contents of tubes 40 to 49.

Ref:

As PC (1).

LIVIDOMYCIN

PC.

1. **Paper:**
   Toyo No. 51.
   Solvent:
   n-Butanol satd. with water:p-toluenesulfonic
   acid:t-butanol (88:2:10), 40 h.
   Detection:
   As TLC (2).
   R_f:
   Lividomycin B moves 11.2 cm.
   Ref:
   T. Mori, Y. Kyotani, I. Watanabe and T. Oda,
   J. Antibiotics, 25 (1972) 149–150.

TLC.

1. **Medium:**
   A. Silica Gel D-5 (Camag).
   B. Aluminum Oxide G Type E (Merck).
   Solvent:
   Chloroform:methanol:17% ammonia
   (2:1:1), upper layer.
   Detection:
   R_f:

	R_f Medium	
	A	B
Lividomycin A	0.64	0.36
Lividomycin B	0.65	0.73

   Ref:
   T. Mori, T. Ichiyanagi, H. Kondo,
   K. Tokunaga and T. Oda, J. Antibiotics, 24
   (1971) 339–346.

2. **Medium:**
   A. Silica Gel D-5 (Camag).
   B. Aluminum Oxide G Type E (Merck).
   Solvent:
   A. Chloroform:methanol:17% ammonium
      hydroxide (2:1:1), upper layer.
   B. n-Butanol:acetic acid:water (1:1).
   C. Methanol:10% ammonium acetate (1:1).
   Detection:
   A. Ninhydrin.
   B. Bioautography.
   R_f:

Solvent	Medium	Lividomycin B R_f:
A	A	0.57
B		0.26
C		0.54
A	B	0.79

Ref:
As PC (1).

ELPHO.

1. **Medium:**
   Toyo No. 51.
   Buffer:
   Formic acid:acetic acid:water (22:75:900),
   pH 1.8.
   Conditions:
   3000 V (20 mA/10 cm).
   Detection:
   Ninhydrin.
   Mobility:

	R_m*
Lividomycin A	1.78
Lividomycin B	2.10

   *Relative mobility to alanine as 1.0.
   Ref:
   As TLC (1).

2. **Medium:**
   Paper, Toyo No. 51.
   Buffer:
   Formic acid:acetic acid:water (22:75:900),
   pH 1.8.
   Conditions:
   3000 V (1 mA/1 cm).
   Detection:
   As TLC (2).
   Mobility:
   R_m = 2.14 (Lividomycin B). R_m = relative
   mobility to alanine as 1.0.
   Ref:
   As PC (1).

GLC.

1. **Column:**
   0.3 × 100 cm tube, packed with 1.0% OV-1
   on Gas-Chrom Q (100–120 mesh).
   Gases:
   Carrier gas: N_2 at a flow rate of 30 ml/min.
   Temperatures:
   Oven temperature 265°C.
   Retention time:
   5.5 min.
   Ref:
   As PC (1).

LOMOFUNGIN

PC.

1. **Paper:**
   Solvent:
   - A. n-Butanol:water (84:16), 16 h.
   - B. n-Butanol:water (84:16) + 0.25% p-toluenesulfonic acid, 16 h.
   - C. n-Butanol:acetic acid:water (2:1:1), 16 h.
   - D. n-Butanol:water (84:16) + 2% piperidine, 16 h.
   - E. n-Butanol:water (4:96), 5 h.
   - F. n-Butanol:water (4:96) + 0.25% p-toluenesulfonic acid, 5 h.

   Detection:
   R_f:

Solvent	R_f*
A	0.00
B	0.10 and 0.20–0.30
C	0.79
D	0.00
E	0.30
F	0.10

   *Estimated from drawing.

   Ref:
   L.E. Johnson and A. Dietz, Appl. Microbiol., 17 (1969) 755–759.

TLC.

1. **Medium:**
   Silica Gel H_{254} (Merck). Solution of buffer salts (pH 6.7) composed of 0.2 M disodium phosphate and 0.2 M monopotassium phosphate. Air dry but not activate.

   Solvent:
   Methyl ethyl ketone:methanol (94:6).

   Detection:
   - A. Visible light.
   - B. Potassium permanganate-sodium meta-periodate spray.

   R_f:
   0.4

   Ref:
   M.E. Bergy, J. Antibiotics, 22 (1969) 126–128.

LYBANOMYCINE

PC.

1. **Paper:**
   Solvent:
   - A. Butanol:pyridine:water (6:4:3).

   - B. Butanol satd. with phosphate buffer M/15 at pH 3.
   - C. Same as B with buffer at pH 5.4.
   - D. Same as B with buffer at pH 7.0.
   - E. Same as B with buffer at pH 8.0.

   Detection:
   Bioautography vs. *Bacillus subtilis*.
   R_f:

Solvent	R_f Component A	B	C
A	0.65	0.78	0.40
B	0.60	0.85	—
C	0.55	0.75	—
D	0.90	0.90	—
E	0.50	0.75	0.30

   Ref:
   Belgium Patent No. 714,243; October 25, 1968.

LYDIMYCIN

PC.

1. **Paper:**
   Solvent:
   - A. 1-Butanol:water (86:16), 16 h.
   - B. 1-Butanol:water (84:16) + 0.25% p-toluenesulfonic acid, 16 h.
   - C. 1-Butanol:acetic acid:water (2:1:1), 16 h.
   - D. 2% Piperidine in 1-butanol:water (84:16), 16 h.
   - E. 1-Butanol:water (4:96), 5 h.
   - F. 1-Butanol:water (4:96) + 0.25% p-toluenesulfonic acid, 5 h.

   Detection:
   Bioautography vs. *Saccharomyces pastorianus*.
   R_f:

Solvent	R_f*
A	0.18
B	0.45
C	0.80
D	0.19
E	0.90
F	0.88

   *Estimated from drawing.

   Ref:
   M.E. Bergy, J.H. Coats and L.J. Hanka, U.S. Patent 3,395,220; February 23, 1965.

LYSOZYME

ELPHO.

1. **Medium:**
   Whatman No. 1 paper.
   Buffer:
   A. 0.05 M Veronal (pH 8.0 and 9.0) and glycine (pH 10.0) buffers were used.
   B. Trisethylenediaminetetraacetate buffer, pH 8.9.
   Conditions:
   A. A current of 4.5 ma and 90 V for 18 h at room temperature, for "A" buffer.
   B. A current of 6.5 ma for 16 h, for "B" buffer.
   Detection:
   After drying, the strips are stained with amide black 10B.
   Mobility:
   Ref:
   J. Hawiger, J. Bacteriol., 95 (1968) 376–384.

MACARBOMYCIN
PC.
1. **Paper:**
   Solvent:
   n-Butanol:pyridine:water (4:1:4).
   Detection:
   R_f:
   0.29 (major)
   0.47 and 0.56 (minor)
   Ref:
   H. Umezawa, K. Maeda, K. Nitta, M. Okanishi and S. Takahashi, U.S. Patent 3,564,090; February 16, 1971.

TLC.
1. **Medium:**
   Silica Gel GF$_{254}$ (E. Merck).
   Solvent:
   n-Propanol:2 N aq. ammonia (70:30).
   Detection:
   A. UV light at 253.6 nm.
   B. Spray with chlorosulfonic acid:acetic acid (1:2).
   C. Exposure to iodine vapor.
   R_f:
   0.25
   Ref:
   S. Takahashi, A. Okanishi, R. Utahara, K. Nitta, K. Maeda and H. Umezawa, J. Antibiotics, 23 (1970) 48–50.

MACROSIN
PC.
1. **Paper:**
   Solvent:
   A. Methyl ethyl ketone on pH 4 buffered paper.
   B. Methyl ethyl ketone.
   C. n-Butanol satd. with water on pH 4 buffered paper.
   D. n-Butanol satd. with water.
   E. Water with 7% sodium chloride and 2.5% methyl ethyl ketone.
   F. Ethyl acetate satd. with water on pH 4 buffered paper.
   Detection:
   R_f:

Solvent	R_f
A	0.45
B	0.66
C	0.92
D	0.80
E	0.74
F	0.39

   Ref:
   R.L. Hamill and W.M. Stark, J. Antibiotics, 17 (1964) 133–139.

MACROMOMYCIN
ELPHO.
1. **Medium:**
   Paper.
   Buffer:
   Barbital buffer (pH 8.6 μ = 0.05).
   Conditions:
   450 v., 4.5 h.
   Detection:
   Mobility:
   Moved 2.0 cm to cathode.
   Ref:
   H. Umezawa, T. Takeuchi, M. Hamada, M. Ishizuka, H. Chimura and K. Maeda, U.S. Patent 3,595,954; July 27, 1971.

MAGNAMYCIN
   cf. carbomycin
PC.
1. **Paper:**
   Solvent:
   A. Ethanol:hexane:water (90:10:0.15), 4 h, descending.

q B. Benzene:water:acetic acid (1:9:0.5), 4 h,
   ascending.
C. n-Butanol:water:acetic acid (4:5:1), 16 h,
   ascending.
D. Water satd. with n-butanol, 4 h, ascending.
Detection:
Bioautography vs. *M. pyogenes* var. *aureus*.
R_f:

Solvent	R_f
A	0.70
B	0.80
C	0.90
D	0.95

Ref:
J.F. Pagano, M.J. Weinstein and C.M. McKee,
Antibiotics and Chemotherapy, 3 (1953)
899–902.

TLC.

1. **Medium:**
   Solvent:
   A. Benzene:methanol (55:45).
   B. Butanol:acetic acid:water (3:1:1).
   Detection:
   R_f:

Solvent	R_f
A	0.75
B	0.49

Ref:
N. Nishimura, K. Kumagai, M. Ishida,
K. Saito, F. Kato and M. Asumi, J. Anti-
biotics, 18 (1965) 251–258.

MANNOSIDOSTREPTOMYCIN
See streptomycin

MARIDOMYCINS
TLC.

1. **Medium:**
   A. Spotfilm (Tokyokasei).
   B. Kieselgel G (Merck).
   Solvent:
   A. Benzene:acetone (3:2).
   B. Benzene:methanol (10:1).
   Detection:
   A. Conc. sulfuric acid.
   B. 5% Iodine in chloroform.
   C. 5% Phosphomolybic acid in ethanol.
   D. 5% Ceric sulfate in sodium sulfate.

R_f:

	R_f Solvent (Medium)		
	A (A)	A (B)	B (B)
Maridomycin I	0.48	0.68	0.71
Maridomycin II	0.42	0.63	0.66
Maridomycin III	0.37	0.57	0.61
Maridomycin IV	0.32	0.53	0.55
Maridomycin V	0.30	0.50	0.52
Maridomycin VI	0.43	0.43	0.48

Ref:
M. Muroi, M. Isawa, M. Asai, T. Kishi and
K. Mizuno, 183rd Scientific Mtg. of Japan
Antibiotic Res. Assn. May 26, 1972.

MEGALOMICINS
PC.

1. **Paper:**
   Solvent:
   A. 80% Methanol + 3% sodium chloride
      (1:1), descending. Paper buffered with
      0.95 M sodium sulfate + 0.05 M sodium
      bisulfate.
   B. Propanol:pyridine:acetic acid:water
      (6:4:1:3), ascending.
   C. Butanol:acetic acid:water (4:1:5),
      ascending.
   D. 80% Phenol, ascending.
   Detection:
   Bioautography vs. *Staphylococcus aureus*.
   R_f:

Solvent	R_f
A	0.90
B	0.93
C	0.78
D	0.86

Ref:
M.J. Weinstein, G.M. Luedemann,
G.H. Wagman and J.A. Marquez, U.S. Patent
3,632,750; January 4, 1972.

TLC.

1. **Medium:**
   Silica Gel G.
   Solvent:
   Chloroform:methanol (60:40).
   Detection:
   Bioautography vs. *Staphylococcus aureus*.

R_f:

	R_f
Megalomicin A	0.19
Megalomicin B	0.38
Megalomicin C_1	0.52
Megalomicin C_2	0.65

Ref:

M.J. Weinstein, G.H. Wagman, J.A. Marquez, E.M. Oden, R.T. Testa and J.A. Waitz, Antimicrobial Agents and Chemotherapy, 1968 (1969) 260–261. J.A. Marquez, A. Murawski and G.H. Wagman, J. Antibiotics, 22 (1969) 259–264.

2. **Medium**:

Solvent:

A. Chloroform:methanol:17% ammonia (2:1:1).

B. Butanol:acetic acid:water (3:1:1).

Detection:

A. Plates are sprayed with a mixture of conc. sulfuric acid:methanol (1:1) and developed by heating at 105°C for several min.

B. Bioautography vs. *Staphylococcus aureus*.

R_f:

Solvent	Color by sulfuric acid spray	R_f
A	Blue black	0.98
B	Red purple	0.13

Ref:

M.J. Weinstein, G.M. Luedemann, G.H. Wagman and J.A. Marquez, U.S. Patent 3,632,750; January 4, 1972. M.J. Weinstein, G.H. Wagman, J.A. Marquez, R.T. Testa, E.M. Oden and J.A. Waitz, J. Antibiotics, 22 (1969) 253–258.

MELINACIDINS

PC.

1. **Paper**:

Solvent:

A. 1-Butanol:water (84:16).

B. 1-Butanol:water (84:16) + 0.25% p-toluenesulfonic acid.

C. 1-Butanol:acetic acid:water (2:1:1).

D. 2% Piperidine in 1-butanol:water (84:16).

E. 1-Butanol:water (4:96).

F. 1-Butanol:water (4:96) + 0.25% p-toluenesulfonic acid.

G. 0.5 M phosphate buffer pH 7.0.

H. 0.075 N ammonium hydroxide satd. with methyl isobutyl ketone, lower phase.

I. Benzene:methanol:water (1:1:2).

Detection:

Bioautography vs. *Bacillus subtilis*.

R_f:

Solvent	R_f*
A	0.65–0.90
B	0.95
C	0.92
D	0.95
E	0.20–0.48
F	0.30; 0.50
G	0.05–0.22
H	0.10; 0.30
I	0.25; 0.60; 0.80

*Estimated from drawing.

Ref:

A.D. Argoudelis and F. Reusser, J. Antibiotics, 24 (1971) 383–389. Netherlands Patent No. 68,15117; April 29, 1969.

2. **Paper**:

Solvent:

A. 1-Butanol:water (84:16), 16 h.

B. 1-Butanol:water (84:16) + 0.25% p-toluenesulfonic acid, 16 h.

C. 1-Butanol:acetic acid:water (2:1:1), 16 h.

D. 2% Piperidine (v/v) in 1-butanol:water (84:16), 16 h.

E. 1-Butanol:water (4:96), 5 h.

F. 1-Butanol:water (4:96) + 0.25% p-toluenesulfonic acid, 5 h.

G. 0.5 M phosphate buffer, pH 7.0, 5 h.

H. 0.075 N ammonium hydroxide satd. with methyl isobutyl ketone, lower phase, 5 h.

I. Benzene:methanol:water (1:1:2), equilibrated 16 h, developed 5 h.

Detection:

Bioautography vs. *Bacillus subtilis*.

R_f:

Solvent	R_f*
A	0.60–0.80
B	0.80–0.90
C	0.88
D	0.95
E	0.20–0.45
F	0.30 and 0.50
G	0.10–0.20
H	0.10 and 0.30
I	0.25; 0.60; 0.80

*Estimated from drawing.

Ref:

A.D. Argoudelis, J.H. Coats and F. Reusser,
U.S. Patent 3,639,581; February 1, 1972.

3. **Paper:**
Solvent:

Benzene:methanol:water (1:1:2).

Detection:

Bioautography vs. *Bacillus subtilis.*

R_f:

	R_f*
Melinacidin II	0.9
Melinacidin IV	0.8
Melinacidin III	0.7

*Estimated from drawing.

Ref:

A.D. Argoudelis, J. Antibiotics, 25 (1972)
171–178.

TLC.

1. **Medium:**
Silica Gel G.

Solvent:

Toluene:ethyl acetate mixtures (50:50
or 60:40).

Detection:

A. Bioautography vs. *Bacillus subtilis.*

B. Periodate–permanganate spray reagent.

R_f:

	R_f
Melinacidin II	0.40
Melinacidin III	0.25
Melinacidin IV	0.20

Ref:

As PC (3).

CCD.

1. **Solvent:**

Cyclohexane:ethyl acetate:95% ethanol:
water (1:1:1:1), 1000 transfers.

Distribution:

Tubes 260–300 contained melinacidin IV.

Ref:

As PC (3).

METHYMYCIN
CCD.

1. **Solvent:**

10 ml volumes of mutually satd. ether and
M/2 potassium phosphate buffer, pH 6.8,
24 transfers.

Distribution:

Peak tubes No. 15 and 16. K = 1.85.

Ref:

M.N. Donin, J. Pagano, J.D. Dutcher and
C.M. McKee, Antibiotics Annual, 1953–
1954, 179–185.

MIAMYCIN
CCD.

1. **Solvent:**

Ethyl acetate:0.1 M phosphate buffer, pH 6.9,
120 transfers.

Distribution:

The peak concentration was found around
tube 40.

Ref:

H. Schmitz, M. Misiek, B. Heinemann,
J. Lein and I.R. Hooper, Antibiot. and
Chemotherap., 7 (1957) 37–39.

MICROMONOSPORA CHALCEA ANTIBIOTIC
PC.

1. **Paper:**
Solvent:

Benzene:hexane:acetone (20:5:6).

Detection:

R_f:

7 Biologically active components.

Ref:

G.F. Gause, M.G. Brazhnikova, U.A. Shorin,
T.S. Moksimova, O.L. Olkhovatova,
M.K. Kudinova, I.A. Vishnyakova,
N.S. Pezner and S.P. Shapovalova,
Antibiotiki, 15 (1970) 483–486.

TLC.

1. **Medium:**
Silicic Acid.

Solvent:

Benzene:acetone (5:1).

Detection:

R_f:

As PC (1).

Ref:

As PC (1).

MICROMONOSPORIN
PC.

1. **Paper:**

As everninomicin PC (1).

Solvent:

As everninomicin PC (1).

Detection:

As everninomicin PC (1).

R_f:

1.0

Ref:

As everninomicin PC (1).

MICROPOLYSPORINS

PC.

1. **Paper:**

Solvent:

A. Butanol satd. with water.

B. Methanol.

C. Butanol satd. with water and 2% piperidine.

D. Butanol:pyridine:water (1:0.6:1).

E. Butanol:acetic acid:water (2:1:1).

F. Butanol satd. with water and 2% p-toluenesulfonic acid.

Detection:

Bioautography vs. *Sarcina lutea*.

R_f:

Solvent	Component	R_f
A	Micropolysporin A	0.35–0.41
	Micropolysporin B	0.07–0.13
B	Micropolysporin A	0.82
C	Micropolysporin A	0.40
D	Micropolysporin A	0.67; 0.84
E	Micropolysporin A	0.83
F	Micropolysporin A	0.60

Ref:

N.O. Blinov, E.A. Babkova and L.V. Kalakutskii, Antibiotiki, 11 (1966) 587–590.

MINIATOMICINS

PC.

1. **Paper:**

Solvent:

A. Water.

B. 0.1% Aq. ammonium chloride.

C. 0.5% Aq. ammonium chloride.

D. 1.0% Aq. ammonium chloride.

E. 2.0% Aq. ammonium chloride.

F. 3.0% Aq. ammonium chloride.

G. 5.0% Aq. ammonium chloride.

H. 10.0% Aq. ammonium chloride.

I. 20.0% Aq. ammonium chloride.

J. Satd. ammonium chloride.

K. Water satd. n-butanol.

L. 75% Phenol.

M. n-Butanol:methanol:water:methyl

N. orange (40 ml:10 ml:20 ml:1.5 g). n-Butanol:methanol:water (40:10:20).

O. Benzene:methanol (80:20).

P. Water.

Q. pH 8 buffer.

R. Satd. soln. picric acid.

S. 96% Methanol.

T. Acetone.

U. Water satd. soln. ethyl acetate.

V. Water satd. n-butanol.

W. Water satd. ethyl ether.

X. Chloroform.

Y. Benzene.

Z. Petroleum ether.

Detection:

Bioautography.

R_f:

Solvent	R_f^* Miniatomicin M_2	M_3
A	0.00–0.2	0.00–0.32
B	0.00–0.3	0.00–0.50
C	0.00–0.4	0.08–0.70
D	0.00–0.45	0.08–0.73
E	0.00–0.47	0.15–0.79
F	0.00–0.55	0.18–0.83
G	0.00–0.60	0.25–0.90
H	0.00–0.55	0.15–0.87
I	0.00–0.43	0.07–0.84
J	0.00–0.32	0.00–0.59
K	0.45–1.00	0.00–0.80
L	0.00–0.35	0.45–0.90
M	0.80–1.00	0.70–1.00
N	0.75–1.00	0.52–0.90
O	0.60–1.00	0.47–0.90
P	0.05, 0.90	0.60–0.97
Q	0.00–0.20	0.00–0.48
R	0.05	0.08
S	—	—
T	0.25–0.50	0.00–0.2 0.35–0.8
U	0.05	0.00–0.60
V	0.05 0.10–0.25	0.08
W	0.47–1.00	0.03–0.41 0.85

X	0.05	0.10
Y	0.05	0.10
	0.1−0.25	
Z	0.05	0.10
AA	0.05	0.10

*Estimated from drawing.

Ref:

M.F. de Albuquerque, F.D. de Andrade Lyra, O.G. de Lima, L.L. de Oliverira, J.S. de Barros Coelho, G.M. Maciel and M. da Salete Barros Cavalcanti, Recife, 6 (1966) 35−51.

ELPHO.

1. **Medium:**
   Paper.
   Buffer:
   A. pH 5.4 phosphate buffer.
   B. pH 8.0 phosphate buffer.
   Conditions:
   A. For buffer A, 6.04 V/cm, 6 h.
   B. For buffer B, 6.6 V/cm, 6 h.
   Detection:
   Mobility:
   Miniatomicin M_2.
      A. Moves slightly to cathode.
      B. Moves slightly to cathode.
   Miniatomicin M_3.
      A. Moves toward anode.
      B. Moves slightly toward anode.
   Ref:
   As PC (1).

MINIMYCIN

TLC.

1. **Medium:**
   Silica Gel.
   Solvent:
   A. Wet butanol.
   B. Butanol:acetic acid:water (4:1:2).
   C. Ethanol:water (4:1).
   D. Chloroform:methanol:17% ammonium hydroxide (2:1:1, upper phase).
   E. Propanol:pyridine:acetic acid:water (15:10:3:12).
   Detection:
   R_f:

Solvent	R_f
A	0.42
B	0.57
C	0.75

D	0.88
E	0.85

Ref:

Y. Kusakabe, J. Nagatsu, M. Shibuya, O. Kawaguchi, C. Hirose and S. Shirato, J. Antibiotics, 25 (1972) 44−47.

MITOCHROMINS

PC.

1. **Paper:**
   Solvent:
   Benzene:chloroform:acetic acid:water (2:2:1:1), vs. wet paper.
   Detection:
   Bioassay.
   R_f:

Compound	R_f
Mitochromin A	0.6
Mitochromin B	0.5
Mitochromin C	0.3
Mitochromin D	0.05

   Ref:
   W. Liu, W.P. Cullen and K.V. Rao, J. Antibiotics, 22 (1969) 608−611.

2. **Paper:**
   Whatman No. 4 impregnated with acetone: water (7:3).
   Solvent:
   Benzene:chloroform:acetic acid:water (2:2:1:1).
   Detection:
   R_f:

	R_f
Mitochromin A	0.35
Mitochromin B	0.25

   Ref:
   French Patent No. 2,024,316; October 29, 1969.

TLC.

1. **Medium:**
   Silica Gel.
   Solvent:
   Chloroform:methanol (9:1) with 1% formic acid.
   Detection:
   R_f:
   0.2−0.3
   Ref:
   As PC (1).

MOENOMYCINS

PC.

1. Paper:
Solvent:
n-Butanol:pyridine:water (4:1:4).
Detection:
R_f:
0.29, 0.38, 0.64, 0.47 (minor)
Ref:
H. Umezawa, K. Maeda, K. Nitta, M. Okanishi
and S. Takahashi, U.S. Patent 3,564,090;
February 16, 1971.

2. Paper:
Solvent:
A. n-Butanol:triethyl amine:methyl isobutyl
ketone:water (14:1:1:5).
B. Benzene:glacial acetic acid:water (2:2:1).
C. n-Butanol:glacial acetic acid:water
(4:1:5).
D. tert. butanol:glacial acetic acid:water
(60:6:34).
E. Butanol satd. with water.
F. Sec. butanol:glacial acetic acid:water
(4:1:1).
Detection:
R_f:

Solvent	R_f
A	0.05
B	0
C	0.88
D	0.70
E	0
F	0.05

Ref:
U. Schacht, R. Tschesche and I. Duphorn,
U.S. Patent 3,660,569; May 2, 1972.

TLC.

1. Medium:
Silica Gel GF (Merck).
Solvent:
Isopropanol:2N ammonia (70:30).
Detection:
Spray with chlorosulfonic acid:acetic acid
(1:2) and heat for 10 min at 100°C; appear
as red-violet spots.
R_f:

	R_f
Moenomycin A	0.5

Moenomycin B_1 0.4
Moenomycin B_2 0.3
Moenomycin C   0.6
Ref:
G. Huber, U. Schacht, H.L. Weidenmüller,
J. Schmidt-Thome, J. Duphorn and
R. Tschesche, Antimicrobial Agents and
Chemotherapy, 1965 (1966) 737—742.

2. Medium:
Silica Gel GF.
Solvent:
A. Chloroform:ethanol:water (40:70:20).
B. Isopropanol:water:borate buffer pH 9.0
(70:25:5).
Detection:
R_f:

	R_f Moenomycin				
Solvent	D	E	F	G	H
A	0.20	0.25	0.14	0.22	0.14
B	0.48	0.67	0.47	0.65	0.35

Ref:
Derwent Farmdoc No. 31774 (1966).

3. Medium:
Silica Gel GF_{254} (E. Merck).
Solvent:
n-Propanol:2N aq. ammonia (70:30).
Detection:
A. UV light at 253.6 nm.
B. Spray with chlorosulfonic acid:acetic acid
(1:2).
C. Exposure to iodine vapor.
R_f:
0.25, 0.33, 0.41, 0.47
Ref:
As PC (1).

4. Medium:
Silica Gel.
Solvent:
A. Isopropanol:2N ammonia (70:30).
B. Isopropanol:water:borate buffer, pH 9.0
(70:25:5).
C. Ethanol:water (4:1).
Detection:
R_f:

	R_f Moenomycin		
Solvent	A	B	C
A	0.45	0.36	0.53
B	0.38	0.55	0.38
C	0.70	0.44	0.77

Ref:

As PC (1).

ELPHO.

1. **Medium:**

Paper.

Buffer:

pH 1.9 or 7.8.

Conditions:

Detection:

Mobility:

Migrates to anode at pH 7.8 only.

Ref:

As PC (1).

MONAMYCINS

TLC.

1. **Medium:**

Kieselgel G (E. Merck). Activate before use by heating at 120°C for 1 h.

Solvent:

Chloroform:methanol (20:1).

Detection:

A. Spray with a soln. of iodine (2 g/100 ml of methanol:water, 50:1).

B. Scrape sections (0.5 by 2 cm) and apply the Kieselgel to small wells (7-mm diameter) in the agar medium of an assay plate seeded with *Staphylococcus aureus*.

R_f:

0.4–0.6

Ref:

M.J. Hall and C.H. Hassall, Appl. Microbiol., 19 (1970) 109–112.

2. **Medium:**

Kieselgel G (Merck).

Solvent:

Benzene:methanol:acetic acid (10:2:1).

Detection:

A. 0.1% soln. of ninhydrin in acetone, heat at 100°C for 5 min.

B. 5% soln. of p-dimethylaminobenzaldehyde in hydrochloric acid:methanol (5:100) (Ehrlich's reagent).

C. 5% Aq. potassium permanganate.

D. Exposure to iodine vapor.

R_f:

	R_f
Monamycin A	0.31
Monamycin B_1	0.38
Monamycin B_2	0.38
Monamycin B_3	0.38
Monamycin C	0.35
Monamycin D_1	0.43
Monamycin D_2	0.43
Monamycin E	0.38
Monamycin F	0.45
Monamycin G_1	0.55
Monamycin G_2	0.55
Monamycin G_3	0.57
Monamycin H_1	0.57
Monamycin H_2	0.60
Monamycin I	0.60

Ref:

K. Bevan, J.S. Davies, C.H. Hassall, R.B. Morton and D.A.S. Phillips, J. Chem. Soc., (C) (1971) 514–522.

3. **Medium:**

Solvent:

A. Butanol satd. with water.

B. Butanol:glacial acetic acid:water (4:1:5).

C. Butanol satd. with water + 2% p-toluene-sulfonic acid.

D. Butanol satd. with water + 2% piperidine.

E. Butanol:pyridine:water (6:4:3).

F. 80% Ethanol + 1.5% sodium chloride; Whatman No. 4 paper impregnated with 0.95 M sodium sulfate + 0.05 M sodium hydrosulfate.

G. Butanol:ethanol:water (1:1:2).

H. Butanol:butyl acetate:glacial acetic acid: water (10:3:1.3:14.3), supernatant phase.

Detection:

Bioautography vs. *Staphylococcus aureus* or *Bacillus subtilis*.

R_f:

	R_f Component	
Solvent	A	B
A	0.00	0.00
B	0.49	0.63
C	0.34	0.58
D	0.05	0.15

E	0.32	0.32
F	0.47	0.47
G	0.74	0.74
H	2.7*	7.6*

*Distance in cm from origin after 16 h.

CCD.
1. Solvent:
n-Butanol:benzyl alcohol:0.001N hydrochloric acid:satd. aq. sodium chloride (10:5:15:3).
Distribution:
25°C.

| Component A | K = 0.372 |
| Component B | K = 0.175 |

Ref:
As PC (1).

MONAZOMYCIN
PC.
1. Paper:
Solvent:
A. Water satd. butanol.
B. Butanol:acetic acid:water (4:2:1).
C. Ethanol:acetic acid:water (33:5:62).
D. Butanol:acetic acid:water (2:2:4).
Detection:
R_f:

Solvent	R_f
A	0.23
B	0.77
C	0.93
D	0.95

Ref:
K. Akasaki, K. Karasawa, M. Watanabe, H. Yonehara and H. Umezawa, J. Antibiotics, 16 (1963) 127–131.

MONENSIN
PC.
1. Paper:
Whatman No. 1.
Solvent:
Water:methanol:acetic acid:benzene (72.0:24.5:3.0:0.5).
Detection:
Bioautography vs. *Bacillus subtilis* ATCC 6633.
R_f:

	R_f*
Monensin A	0.50
Monensin B	0.90
Monensin C	0.35

*Estimated from drawing.

Ref:
M.E. Haney, Jr. and M.M. Hoehn, Antimicrobial Agents and Chemotherapy, 1967 (1968) 349–352.

TLC.
1. Medium:
Silica Gel.
Solvent:
Ethyl acetate.
Detection:
Spray the dried plates with 3% vanillin in 1.5% ethanolic sulfuric acid and then heat the plates at 100°C for 5 min to develop a bright red color.
R_f:

	R_f*
Monensin A	0.4
Monensin B	0.5
Monensin C	0.2
Monensin D	0.3

*Estimated from drawing.

Ref:
As PC (1).

MYCOBACILLIN
PC.
1. Paper:
Whatman No. 1.
Solvent:
A. Water satd. phenol.
B. Water satd. butanol.
C. n-Butanol:acetic acid:water (4:1:1).
D. n-Butanol:pyridine:water (2:1:4).
E. Pyridine:water (3:2).
F. Ammonium chloride in water (3.0%).
Detection:
Bioautography vs. *Aspergillus niger*.
R_f:

Solvent	R_f
A	0.92
B	0.83
C	0.93
D	0.92
E	0.92
F	0.10

Ref:

S.K. Majumdar and S.K. Bose, Arch.
Biochem. Biophys., 90 (1960) 154–158.

ELPHO.
1. **Medium:**

Whatman No. 3 MM paper previously soaked
in a buffer soln.

Buffer:

A. Veronal buffer, pH 8.6, μ 0.05.
B. Acetate buffer, pH 4.8, μ 0.1.

Conditions:

220 V, 9 mA, 5.5 h.

Detection:

A. Blue color with 20% sodium carbonate
and phenol reagent of Folin and Ciocalteu.
B. Bioautography vs. *Aspergillus niger.*

Mobility:

Migrates to anode 3 cm at pH 8.6 and
0.0–1.0 cm at pH 4.8.

Ref:

As PC (1).

MYCOBACTOCIDINS
PC.
1. **Paper:**

Whatman No. 1.

Solvent:

0.067M phosphate buffer pH 7.

Detection:

Stain with Amido Black 10B.

R_f:

Fraction B separated into 2 areas.
Fraction D has only 1 area.

Ref:

G.B. Fregnan and D.W. Smith, J. Bacteriol.,
83 (1962) 1069–1076.

MYCOPHENOLIC ACID
PC.
1. **Paper:**

Whatman No. 1.

Solvent:

n-Butanol satd. with water + 2% p-toluenesulfonic acid and 2% piperidine.

Detection:

Bioautography vs. vaccinia virus-infected
BSC-1 monkey kidney cells.

R_f:

0.6

Ref:

R.H. Williams, L.D. Boeck, J.C. Cline,
D.C. DeLong, K. Gerzon, R.S. Gordee,
M. Gorman, R.E. Holmes, S.H. Larsen,
D.H. Lively, T.R. Matthews, J.D. Nelson,
G.A. Poore, W.M. Stark and M.J. Sweeney,
Antimicrobial Agents and Chemotherapy,
1968 (1969) 229–233.

TLC.
1. **Medium:**

Silica Gel.

Solvent:

Amyl acetate:n-propanol:acetic acid:water
(4:3:2:1).

Detection:

Spray with a soln. of 1% ferric chloride in
methanol.

R_f:

0.65

Ref:

As PC (1).

MYCORHODIN
CCD.
1. **Solvent:**

A. Methanol:water:chloroform:carbon
tetrachloride (3:1:1.5:4), 200 transfers.
B. Methanol:methyl isobutyl ketone:water
(1:1:1), 100 transfers.

Distribution:

Mycorhodin A: Peak in tube 65.
Mycorhodin B: Peak in tube 86.

Ref:

M. Misiek, A. Gourevitch, B. Heinemann,
M.J. Cron, D.F. Whitehead, H. Schmitz,
I.R. Hooper and J. Lein, Antibiot. and
Chemotherap., 9 (1959) 280–285.

MYCOTRIENIN
CCD.
1. **Solvent:**

Chloroform:ligroin:water:methanol (2:1:1:2).

Distribution:

K = 0.56

Ref:

C. Coronelli, R.C. Pasqualucci, J.E. Thiemann
and G. Tamoni, J. Antibiotics, 20 (1967)
329–333.

NAEMATOLIN

TLC.

1. **Medium:**
    Kieselgel GF.
    Solvent:
    A. Cyclohexane:chloroform:ethanol (2:8:1).
    B. Benzene:methanol (9:1).
    C. n-Hexane:acetone (4:1).
    D. Benzene:acetone (4:1).
    E. Ether.
    F. n-Hexane:ethyl acetate (4:1).
    G. Chloroform:methanol (4:1).
    H. n-Hexane:ether (1:4).
    I. Ether:ethyl acetate (1:1).
    Detection:
    R_f:

Solvent	R_f
A	0.47
B	0.25
C	0.19
D	0.35
E	0.71
F	0.05
G	0.91
H	0.50
I	0.91

Ref:
Y. Ito, H. Kurita, T. Yamaguchi, T. Okuda and M. Sato, 156th Scientific Meeting of Japan Antibiotics Res. Assn, July 21, 1967.

NEBRAMYCIN

PC.

1. **Paper:**
    Whatman No. 1.
    Solvent:
    Water satd. n-butanol:p-toluenesulfonic acid: t-butanol (88:2:10), 40 h.
    Detection:
    Bioautography.
    R_f:

Component	R_f[*]
Factor 2	0.35
Factor 3	0.35
Factor 4	0.50
Factor 5	0.58
Factor 6	0.75

[*]Estimated from drawing.

Ref:
W.M. Stark, M.M. Hoehn and N.G. Knox, Antimicrobial Agents and Chemotherapy, 1967 (1968) 314–323.

2. **Paper:**
    As PC (1).
    Solvent:
    A. Water satd. n-butanol containing 2% p-toluenesulfonic acid, 40 h.
    B. 80% Ethanol + 1.5% sodium chloride, paper buffered with 0.95M sulfate-bisulfate, 40 h.
    C. Propanol:pyridine:acetic acid:water (15:10:3:12), 40 h.
    D. Water satd. with methyl isobutyl ketone + 1% p-toluenesulfonic acid, 6 h.
    E. Propanol:water (1:1); paper buffered with 0.75M phosphate, pH 1.0, 24 h.
    F. n-Butanol satd. with water, 18 h.
    G. Water satd. n-butanol containing 2% p-toluenesulfonic acid and 2% piperidine, 18 h.
    Detection:
    R_f:

Component	R_E[*] Solvent						
	A	B	C	D	E	F	G
Factor 1	0.20	—	—	—	—	—	—
Factor 1'	0.27	—	—	—	—	—	—
Factor 2	0.40	0.17	0.32	—	—	—	—
Factor 3	0.40	0.34	0.41	—	—	—	—
Factor 4	0.49	0.20	0.32	—	—	—	—
Factor 5	0.55	0.22	0.35	—	—	—	—
Factor 6	0.71	0.31	0.38	—	—	—	—
Nebramycin complex	—	—	—	0.65	0.32	0.00	0.00

[*]R_E = ratio of distance traversed by the antibiotic with respect to the end of the tape.

Ref:

R.Q. Thompson and E.A. Presti, Antimicrobial Agents and Chemotherapy, 1967 (1968) 332—340; Belgian Patent 697,319; October 20, 1967.

3. **Paper:**

Solvent:

Water satd. n-butanol:p-toluenesulfonic acid:t-butanol (88:2:10).

Detection:

Bioautography vs. *Bacillus subtilis*.

R_f:

Component	R_f*
Factor 2	0.35
Factor 3	0.35
Factor 4	0.45
Factor 5	0.60
Factor 6	0.80

*Estimated from drawing.

Ref:

W.M. Stark, N.G. Knox and R.M. Wilgus, Folia Microbiologica, 16 (1971) 206—217.

TLC.

1. **Medium:**

Silica Gel F_{254} (E. Merck).

Solvent:

Chloroform:methanol:ammonium hydroxide (1:3:2).

Detection:

A. As PC (3).

B. Spray as follows:

  1. With 5 ml of 5% sodium hypochlorite in 95 ml water.

  2. With 3A ethanol.

  3. With benzidine (100 mg) + potassium iodide (100 mg) in 100 ml water + 2 ml of glacial acetic acid.

Ref:

As PC (3).

NEGAMYCIN

ELPHO.

1. **Medium:**

Buffer:

Formic acid:acetic acid:water (25:75:900).

Conditions:

3,500 V for 15 min.

Detection:

Mobility:

Moved 12 cm to cathode.

Ref:

M. Hamada, T. Takeuchi, S. Kondo, Y. Ikeda, H. Naganawa, K. Maeda, Y. Okami and H. Umezawa, J. Antibiotics, 23 (1970) 170—171.

NEOCARZINOSTATIN

ELPHO.

1. **Medium:**

Buffer:

Barbital buffer (pH 8.6; μ = 0.05).

Conditions:

450 V, 4.5 h.

Detection:

Mobility:

Moves to cathode 5.6 cm.

Ref:

H. Umezawa, T. Takeuchi, M. Hamada, M. Ishizuka, H. Chimura and K. Maeda, U.S. Patent 3,595,954; July 27, 1971.

NEOMYCINS

PC.

1. **Paper:**

Solvent:

n-Butanol:acetic acid:water (50:25:25), 16 h, descending.

Detection:

A. Ninhydrin.

B. Bioautography vs. *Bacillus subtilis*.

R_f:

Neomycin 0.0

Neamine   0.05—0.10

Ref:

B.E. Leach and C.M. Teeters, J. Am. Chem. Soc., 73 (1951) 2794—2797.

2. **Paper:**

Whatman No. 1.

Solvent:

Butanol:pyridine:water (6:4:3).

Detection:

Reagents.

a. Sodium hypochlorite. Add 1 part of "Clorox" (5.25% sodium hypochlorite in water) to 20 parts of water.

b. Ethanol, 95%.

c. Starch-iodide reagent. Mix equal volumes

of a 1% soluble starch soln. and a 1% potassium iodide soln.

The developed paper chromatogram is sprayed with a. When dry, it is sprayed with b; finally after b has evaporated, the chromatogram is sprayed with c. The acetylated neomycins show up as deep blue spots against a colorless background.

R_f:

Component	R_f
N-acetyl neomycin B	0.29
N-acetyl neomycin C	0.19

Ref:

S.C. Pan and J.D. Dutcher, Anal. Chem., 28 (1956) 836–838.

3. **Paper:**

Toyo Roshi No. 50.

Solvent:

0.4% Aq. ammonium chloride and 20% methanol-water.

Detection:

Bioautography vs. *Bacillus subtilis*.

R_f:

Neomycin methanesulfonate, 1.0.

Ref:

H. Umezawa, M. Murase and S. Yamazaki, J. Antibiotics, 12 (1959) 341–342.

4. **Paper:**

Solvent:

n-Propanol:glacial acetic acid:water (9:1:10), descending.

Detection:

R_f:

	R_f
Neomycin B	0.26
Neomycin C	0.30
Neamine	0.43

Ref:

K.L. Rinehart, Jr., A.D. Argoudelis, W.A. Goss, A. Sohler and C.P. Schaffner, J. Am. Chem. Soc., 82 (1960) 3938–3946.

5. **Paper:**

Whatman No. 4. (Quantitative Radioisotopic Method.)

Solvent:

1-Butanol:water:piperidine (84:16:2), descending 48 h.

Detection:

Carbon C^{14} N-acetyl derivatives are located by passing the chromatogram through an automatic scanner and quantitated by liquid scintillation counting.

R_f:

	R_f
N-acetyl neomycin B	0.43
N-acetyl neomycin C	0.24
Neamine	0.68

Ref:

D.G. Kaiser, Anal. Chem., 35 (1963) 552–554.

6. **Paper:**

Solvent:

1-Butanol:pyridine:water (3:2:2), descending, 18–20 h.

Detection:

As PC (2).

R_f:

N-acetate reference	R_f	N-acetate to be correlated	R_{rel}
Neomycin B	0.44		
		Neomycin C	0.75
		Neamine	0.93

Ref:

H. Maehr and C.P. Schaffner, Anal. Chem., 36 (1964) 104–108.

7. **Paper:**

Toyo No. 50.

Solvent:

n-Butanol:pyridine:water:acetic acid (6:4:3:1), descending.

Detection:

Ninhydrin; 0.25% in pyridine.

R_f:

Neamine: R_f paromomine   0.47

Ref:

K. Tatsuta, E. Kitazawa and S. Umezawa, Bull. Chem. Soc. Japan, 40 (1967) 2371–2375.

8. **Paper:**

A. Whatman No. 1.

B. Whatman No. 4.

Solvent:

A. 1-Butanol:water:piperidine (84:16:2), descending, 34°C, 24 h.

B. 1-Butanol:water:piperidine (6:3:4).

C. Isoamyl alcohol:water:pyridine (1:0.8:1), ascending, 28°C.

Detection:

As PC (2).

R_f:

	Paper	R_{rel}[*] values in Solvent		
		A	B	C
N-acetyl neomycin B	B	0.69	1.11	1.09
N-acetyl neomycin C	A	0.35	0.73	0.84
N-acetyl neamine	A	1.00	1.00	1.00

[*]R_{rel} Migration of the substance relative to N-acetyl neamine.

Ref:

M.K. Majumdar and S.K. Majumdar, Anal. Chem., 39 (1967) 215–217.

9. **Paper:**

Solvent:

1-Butanol:pyridine:water (6:4:3).

Detection:

As PC (2).

R_f:

Modified neomycins	R_f
N-acetyl hybrimycin A_1	0.32
N-acetyl hybrimycin A_2	0.19
N-acetyl hybrimycin B_1	0.37
N-acetyl hybrimycin B_2	0.19
N-acetyl neomycin B	0.41
N-acetyl neomycin C	0.30

Ref:

W.T. Shier, K.L. Rinehart, Jr. and D. Gottlieb, Biochem., 63 (1969) 198–204.

10. **Paper:**

Whatman No. 1.

Solvent:

Methyl ethyl ketone:tert. butanol:methanol: 6.5N ammonium hydroxide (16:3:1:6), descending, 24–36 h.

Detection:

Sprayed with ninhydrin reagent; 0.25 g of ninhydrin, 10 ml of methanol, 47 ml of butanol, 3 ml of water, and 50 ml of pyridine and finally heated at 80 to 90°C for 30 min. For quantitation, spots were cut and extracted for 30 min with 3 ml of 75% methanol, and the absorbances of the soln. were measured spectrophotometrically at 570 nm with a 1 cm cell. The amount of neomycin was determined by reference to standard curves.

R_f:

	R_{rel}[*]
Neamine	1.00
Neomycin B	0.54
Neomycin C	0.30

[*]Migration of the substance relative to neamine.

Ref:

M.K. Majumdar and S.K. Majumdar, Appl. Microbiol., 17 (1969) 763–764.

11. **Paper:**

Solvent:

Butanol:water:acetic acid:pyridine:sodium chloride (30:12:7:2:0.1).

Detection:

A. Ponceau S.

B. Ninhydrin.

R_f:

Useful for separation of neomycin from polymyxin B and bacitracin.

Ref:

J.P. Carr, R.J. Stretton, J.W. Watson, Final Year Study Proj. Theses, 10 (1969) 17–18 (Eng.). Pharm. Anal., 73 (1970) 247.

TLC.

1. **Medium:**

Carbon. Thirty g of Nuchar (C-190-N) vegetable carbon black and 1.5 g of calcium sulfate-1/2 water were slurried with 220 ml of distilled water adjusted to pH 2 with sulfuric acid. The carbon prepared with distilled water was applied to the glass plates immediately; however, the acidified carbon must stand a minimum of 16 h prior to preparation of the plates. The carbon was applied with a film thickness of 3×10^{-2} cm and air dried.

Solvent:

A. Water.

B. 0.5N sulfuric acid.

Detection:

Bioautography vs. *Bacillus pumilus* after neutralizing by exposure to ammonia 5 min.

R_f:

	Acid Carbon Solvent		Untreated Carbon Solvent	
	A	B	A	B
Neomycin A	0.60	0.61	0.00	0.51
Neomycin B	0.10	0.21	0.00	0.24
Neomycin C	0.10	0.43	0.00	0.45

Ref:

T.F. Brodasky, Anal. Chem., 35 (1963) 343—345.

2. **Medium**:

Silica Gel.

Solvent:

3% Ammonia:acetone (160:40), 1 h.

Detection:

Ninhydrin.

R_f:

Neomycin B   0.33

Neomycin C   0.33

Ref:

R. Foppiano and B.B. Brown, J. Pharm. Sci., 54 (1965) 206—208.

3. **Medium**:

Kieselgel G (Merck); activate at 110°C for 45 min.

Solvent:

A. n-Butanol:glacial acetic acid:water: pyridine (30:22:38:6).

B. n-Butanol:water:pyridine:glacial acetic acid:ethanol (60:10:6:15:5).

Detection:

Ninhydrin spray reagent followed by heating at 105°C for 5 min.

R_f:

Solvent	R_f
A	0.14
B	0.05

Ref:

R.J. Stretton, J.P. Carr and J. Watson-Walker, J. Chromatogr., 45 (1969) 155—158.

4. **Medium**:

Silica Gel.

Solvent:

Butanol:water:pyridine:acetic acid:95% ethanol (60:10:6:15:5).

Detection:

A. Ponceau S stain.

B. Ninhydrin.

R_f:

Useful for separation of neomycin from polymyxin B and bacitracin.

Ref:

As PC (11).

ELPHO.

1. **Medium**:

A. Cellulose acetate (Oxoid) strips of 2.5 × 20 cm.

B. Whatman No. 1.

Buffer:

A. Glacial acetic acid:formic acid:water (60:30:910).

B. Pyridine:glacial acetic acid:water (75:2.5:922.5), pH 6.6.

Conditions:

Paper, 700 V for 40 min; cellulose acetate strips, 400 V, for 60 min.

Detection:

A. Ninhydrin.

B. Stain with Ponceau S reagent for 10 min and remove excess stain by soaking for 15 min in 5% acetic acid. Quantitative estimations of the antibiotics present in the electrophoresis strips are made by eluting the Ponceau S stained material with 2 ml of 0.1 N sodium hydroxide and estimating the color produced at 510 nm. Alternatively two strips were run in parallel, the presence of the antibiotics located on one and the corresponding section removed from the other and the antibiotic eluted from this with 2 ml of pH 5.0 acetate buffer. To this soln. 1 ml of quantitative ninhydrin reagent was added and the color was developed by heating at 98°C for 10 min. The color produced was estimated at 570 nm and by comparison with calibration curves of the pure antibiotic the amount in each sample could be determined.

Mobility:

Medium	Neomycin
A	11.2 towards the cathode
B	17.7 towards the cathode

Ref:

As PC (11), and TLC (3).

GLC.

1. **Apparatus**:

F and M Model 400 with F.I.D.

Column:

A glass column, 3 mm × 1830 mm (6 ft) and packed with 0.75% OV-1 on GAS-CHROM Q, 100—120 mesh (Applied Science

Laboratory, Inc., State College, Pa.) was used.

Temperature:

Column, 330°C; oven, 290°C; temperature programming: 10°C/min from 150 to 310°C.

Gases:

Gas flow rates of hydrogen 20 ml/min, air 550 ml/min, and carrier gas (helium) 40 ml/min.

Internal standard:

Prepare a pyridine soln. containing approximately 3 mg/ml of trilaurin (Superco Inc., St. Bellefonte, Pa.). TRI-SIL Z (Pierce Chemical) may be substituted for pyridine for better stability of silylated neomycin.

Reference standard:

Use USP lot I neomycin Reference Standard at 767 μg neomycin base per mg anhydrous neomycin sulfate. Weigh approximately 6 mg neomycin powder into a one-dram vial and dissolve with one ml water. Place this vial in an appropriate apparatus and freeze-dry. The resulting freeze dried sample dissolves more readily during silylation.

Sample:

As Reference standard.

Derivative:

Silylation Procedure. Add 1.0 ml of the internal standard soln. and 80 μl of N-trimethylsilyldiethylamine (Pierce Chemical) to each vial containing the freeze dried sample. Heat the vial in a 75°C oil bath for 40 min. Silylated neomycins thus prepared are extremely sensitive to moisture and better stability may be obtained when the sample is prepared in a 1.5 ml serum vial with a 13 mm natural red rubber closure.

Calculations:

$[R_1/R_2] \times [Wr/Ws] \times F = \mu g$ neomycin per mg of sample.

Where:

$R_1 = \dfrac{\text{Area of the neomycin sample peak}}{\text{Area of the internal standard peak}}$

$R_2 = \dfrac{\text{Area of the neomycin standard peak}}{\text{Area of the internal standard peak}}$

Wr : Weight of neomycin reference standard in mg.

Ws : Weight of neomycin sample in mg.

F : Assigned value of neomycin reference standard expressed in μg of anhydrous neomycin base per mg of reference standard.

A mixture of silylated neamine, neobiosamine, and neomycins B and C were chromatographed using temperature programming. Neamine and neobiosamine were clearly separated from each other and from neomycins B and C.

Ref:

K. Tsuji and J.H. Robertson, Anal. Chem., 41 (1969) 1332—1335. Cf: K. Tsuji, J.H. Robertson, R. Baas and D.J. McInnis, Appl. Microbiol., 18 (1969) 396—398.

2. **Apparatus:**

An F and M model 402 gas chromatograph with flame-ionization detector was used.

Column:

Glass, 3 mm i.d. × 61 cm (2 ft) packed with 3% OV-1 on Gas Chrom Q, 100—120 mesh is used. To precondition the column before packing, fill the empty column with a 50% soln. of dimethyldichlorosilane in hexane and allow to stand for 5 min. Empty the column and wash with 50 ml of hexane followed by 50 ml of chloroform. Dry the column with a stream of dry air. Pack the column to within 8—9 mm of each end, and fill the remaining portions of the column with a small piece of silylated glass wool.

Temperature:

Oven temperature, 290°C; detector temperature, 310°C; and flash heater, 290°C.

Gases:

The gas flow rates are: hydrogen, 50 ml/min; air, 600 ml/min; and helium, 70 ml/min. The chart speed is 0.64 cm (0.25 in)/min. min.

Internal standard:

Add 50 μl N-trimethylsilyldiethylamine and 2 mg trilaurin/ml.

Reference standard:

Prepare a water soln. containing 5.0 mg/ml of neomycin sulfate, USP Lot I Reference Standard. Before using, dry the neomycin sulfate standard at 60° in a vacuum oven (< 5 mm, Hg) for 3 h.

Derivatives:

Add 1 ml of internal standard-silylation mixture to each vial, using 1 ml tuberculin syringe. Heat the vials in a 75° oil bath for 35 min, swirling occasionally.

Calculations:

Measure each peak area. Add one-third of the area of neomycin C to the area of neomycin B, and determine the peak area ratio of neomycin to trilaurin. The biopotency is determined by comparing area ratios between sample and standard soln.

Retention times:

Estimated from curve.

Neomycin B   9.5 min.

Neomycin C   11–12 min.

Ref:

B. Van Giessen and K. Tsuji, J. Pharm. Sci., 60 (1971) 1068–1070.

NEOPLURAMYCIN

TLC.

1. **Medium:**

Silica Gel G (E. Merck).

Solvent:

A. Acetone.

B. Acetone:ethanol (4:1).

C. Acetone:ethanol (1:1).

D. Acetone:ethanol (1:4).

E. Acetone:methanol (4:1).

F. Acetone:methanol (9:1).

G. Methanol.

H. Chloroform.

I. Chloroform:methanol (9:1).

J. Ethanol:28% ammonia:water (8:1:1).

K. n-Butanol:acetic acid:water (4:1:2).

Detection:

R_f:

Solvent	R_f
A	0.05
B	0.03–0.09
C	0.06–0.18
D	0.00–0.10
E	0.05–0.10
F	0.00–0.10
G	0.05–0.20
H	0.00
I	0.00–0.05
J	0.80–0.90
K	0.25–0.30

Ref:

S. Kondo, T. Wakashiro, M. Hamada, K. Maeda, T. Takeuchi and H. Umezawa, J. Antibiotics, 23 (1970) 354–359.

NETROPSIN

PC.

1. **Paper:**

Solvent:

Butanol:acetic acid:water (2:1:1).

Detection:

R_f:

0.39

Ref:

As kikumycin PC (1).

NEUTRAMYCIN

PC.

1. **Paper:**

Solvent:

A. Dibutyl ether:diethyl ketone:0.2M acetic acid (3:2:4).

B. Cyclohexane:sec.-butanol:0.4% ammonium hydroxide (4:1:4).

C. n-Heptane:diethyl ketone:tetrahydrofuran (8:3:3:8).

Detection:

Bioautography vs. *Bacillus cereus*, *Corynebacterium xerosis* or *Staphylococcus aureus*.

R_f:

Solvent	R_f
A	0.50
B	0.18
C	0.40

Ref:

D.V. Lefemine, F. Barbatschi, M. Dann, S.O. Thomas, M.P. Kunstmann, L.A. Mitscher and N. Bohones, Antimicrobial Agents and Chemotherapy, 1963 (1964) 41–44.

NIDDAMYCIN

PC.

1. **Paper:**

Circular.

Solvent:

A. Sec.-butanol:acetic acid:water (4:1:1).

B. Pyridine:n-butanol:water (4:6:3).

C. Sec. butanol:triethanolamine:methyl isobutyl ketone:water (14:1:1:5).

D. Cyclohexane:tetrahydrofuran (1:2), paper impregnated with formamide.

E. Toluene, paper impregnated with
   propylene glycol.
F. 3% Aq. ammonium chloride.
G. 0.01N ammonium hydroxide satd. with
   methyl isobutyl ketone.
Detection:
A. Bioautography vs. *Staphylococcus aureus*
   209P.
B. UV fluorescence.
C. Spray with 15% phosphoric acid and heat
   5 min at 105°C to give a dark brown
   color.
R_f:

Solvent	R_f
A	1.00
B	1.00
C	1.00
D	0.45
E	0.70
F	1.00
G	0.90

Ref:
G. Huber, K.H. Wallhäuser, L. Fries,
A. Steigler and H.-L. Weidenmüller, Arztl.
Forschung, 12 (1962) 1191–1195.

TLC.
1. **Medium:**
   Silica Gel.
   Solvent:
   Isopropyl ether:methanol (8:2).
   Detection:
   As PC (1), C.
   R_f:
   0.8
   Ref:
   As PC (1).

ELPHO.
1. **Medium:**
   Paper.
   Buffer:
   Buffers at pH 1.9 and 7.8.
   Conditions:
   Detection:
   Mobility:
   Moved toward cathode.
   Ref:
   As PC (1).

NIFIMYCIN
PC.
1. **Paper:**
   Solvent:
   A. Butanol satd. with water.
   B. Butanol satd. with water + 2% piperidine.
   Detection:
   A. UV absorption.
   B. Ninhydrin.
   C. Bioautography vs. *Candida albicans*.
   D. Bioautography vs. *Bacillus subtilis*.
   R_f:
   Solvent A: 0.27, 0.65 (vs. *Candida albicans*).
   Solvent B: 2 spots active against *Candida
   albicans*; additional zone ca. R_f 0.9 active vs.
   Bacillus subtilis only.
   Ref:
   E.I. Khlebarova, N.O. Blinov, Farmatsiya
   (Sofia), 19 (1969) 1–6; Chem. Abstr., 72
   (1970) 296.

NOGALAMYCIN
PC.
1. **Paper:**
   Solvent:
   A. 1-Butanol:water (84:16), 16 h.
   B. 1-Butanol:water (84:16) + 0.25%
      p-toluenesulfonic acid, 16 h.
   C. 1-Butanol:acetic acid:water (2:1:1), 16 h.
   D. 2% Piperidine in n-butanol:water (84:16),
      16 h.
   E. 1-Butanol:water (4:96), 5 h.
   F. 1-Butanol:water (4:96) + 0.25% p-toluene-
      sulfonic acid, 5 h.
   Detection:
   R_f:

Solvent	R_f
A	0.80
B	0.60
C	0.82
D	0.70
E	0.18
F	0.62

Ref:
B.K. Bhuyan and A. Dietz, Antimicrobial
Agents and Chemotherapy, 1965 (1966)
836–844.

NOGALAROL; NOGALARENE
TLC.
1. **Medium:**
   Silica Gel.
   Solvent:
   Chloroform:methanol:water (78:20:2).
   Detection:
   R_f:

	R_f
Nogalarol	0.16
Nogalarene	0.37

   Ref:
   P.F. Wiley and E.L. Caron, Jr., U.S. Patent 3,501,569; March 17, 1970.

NOVOBIOCIN
PC.
1. **Paper:**
   The lower part of the paper was dipped in a mixture of 1:5 capryl alcohol:methanol up to the point of application of the sample and blotted.
   Solvent:
   0.1 M phosphate buffer pH 8.2 equilibrated with capryl alcohol.
   Detection:
   R_f:

Novobiocin	0.25
Dihydronovobiocin	0.61

   Ref:
   E.J. Wolf and R. Nescot, Antibiotics Annual, 1956–1957, 1035–1039.

2. **Paper:**
   Solvent:
   Benzene:hexane:methyl ethyl ketone:ethanol (45:39:13:3).
   Detection:
   Spectrophotometric procedure.
   R_f:

	R_f	
	Descending	Ascending
Novobiocin	0.22	0.08
Isonovobiocin	0.33	0.13
Descarbamyl novobiocin	0.47	0.20

   Ref:
   V.B. Korchagin, V.V. Stepushkina and Z.E. Voinova, Antibiotiki, 11 (1966) 107–112.

3. **Paper:**
   Whatman No. 4 or 20 dipped in ethylene glycol containing 2% of 85% lactic acid as stationary phase.
   Solvent:
   Isopropyl ether satd. with ethylene glycol, descending, 16 h at 28°C and dried.
   Detection:
   UV absorbance at 324 nm.
   R_f:
   Novobiocin acid > decarbamylnovobiocin > isonovobiocin > O-demethyldecarbamylnovobiocin > O-demethylnovobiocin (No R_f given).
   Ref:
   L.A. Kominek, Antimicrobial Agents and Chemotherapy, 1 (1972) 123–134.

NYSTATIN
PC.
1. **Paper:**
   As chromin, PC (1).
   Solvent:
   As chromin, PC (1).
   Detection:
   As chromin, PC (1).
   R_f:
   0.40
   Ref:
   As chromin, PC (1).

2. **Paper:**
   Whatman No. 1.
   Solvent:
   Water satd. n-butanol, descending.
   Detection:
   A. Bioautography vs. *Saccharomyces carlsbergensis* K-20.
   B. 2,3,5-triphenyltetrazolium chloride in glucose.
   R_f:
   0.22
   Ref:
   J. Burns and D.F. Holtman, Antibiotics and Chemotherapy, 9 (1959) 398–405.

TLC.
1. **Medium:**
   Silica Gel G (Merck), activate 30 min at 105°C.

Solvent:
>   A. n-Butanol:acetic acid:water (4:1:2).
>   B. Butanol:pyridine:water (2:1:2).

Detection:
>   0.02 N potassium permanganate.

R_f:

Solvent	R_f
A	0.45
B	0.73–0.75

Ref:
>   P.-A. Nussbaumer, Pharm. Acta Helv., 43
>   (1968) 462–464.

OCHRAMYCIN

PC.

1. **Paper:**
>   Whatman No. 1.

>   Solvent:
>   >   A. Methanol:water:ammonium hydroxide
>   >   (20:4:1).
>   >   B. Propan-2-ol:water (6:4).
>   >   C. Butanol:pyridine:water (6:4:3).
>   >   D. Butanol:acetic acid:water (4:1:5).
>   >   E. Butanol satd. with phosphate buffer
>   >   M/15 at pH 4.1.
>   >   F. As E but pH 5.4.
>   >   G. As E but pH 6.0.
>   >   H. As E but pH 7.0.
>   >   I. As E but pH 8.0.

>   Detection:

> R_f:

Solvent	R_f
A	0.70
B	0.90
C	0.73
D	0.73
E	0.12
F	0.32
G	0.22
H	0.67
I	0.26

Ref:
>   G. Cassinelli, A. Grein, P. Orezzi,
>   P. Pennella and A. Sanfilippo, Archiv
>   Mikrobiologie, 55 (1967) 358–368.

TLC.

1. **Medium:**
>   A. Kieselgel G.
>   B. Alumina G.

>   Solvent:
>   >   A. Ethanol:butanol:0.1 N hydrochloric acid
>   >   (1:1:1).

>   B. Butanol:acetic acid:water (4:1:5).
>   C. Ethanol:water:ammonia (8:1:1).
>   D. Butanol:acetic acid:water (4:1:5).
>   E. Propanol:ethyl acetate:water:25%
>   ammonium hydroxide (6:1:3:1).

Detection:

R_f:

Medium	Solvent	R_f
A	A	0.60
	B	0.30
	C	0.10
B	D	0.80
	E	0.70

Ref:
>   As PC (1).

OLEANDOMYCINS

PC.

1. **Paper:**
>   Solvent:
>   >   A. Benzene:cyclohexane (1:1); formamide
>   >   treated papers.
>   >   B. Benzene; formamide treated papers.
>   >   C. Benzene:chloroform (3:1); formamide
>   >   treated papers.
>   >   D. Benzene:chloroform (1:1); formamide
>   >   treated papers.

>   Detection:

> R_f:

Solvent	R_f
A	0.00
B	0.02
C	0.32
D	0.63

>   Ref:
>   >   K. Murai, B.A. Sobin, W.D. Celmer and
>   >   F.W. Tanner, Antibiotics and Chemotherapy,
>   >   9 (1959) 485–490.

2. **Paper:**
>   Whatman No. 4 impregnated with 50%
>   methanolic formamide.

>   Solvent:
>   >   A. Benzene:cyclohexane (1:1).
>   >   B. Benzene:cyclohexane (2:1).
>   >   C. Benzene:chloroform (3:1).
>   >   D. Benzene:chloroform (1:1).
>   All systems satd. with formamide.

>   Detection:
>   >   Bioautography vs. *Bacillus subtilis* ATCC
>   >   6633.

> R_f:

| | R_f Solvent | | | |
	A	B	C	D
Oleandomycin base	0.02	0.05	0.05	0.30
3-monoacetyloleandomycin	0.05	0.10	0.15	0.50
2-monoacetyloleandomycin	0.10	0.25	0.40	0.70
2,3-diacetyloleandomycin	0.20	0.35	0.70	0.95
1-monoacetyloleandomycin	0.30	0.50	0.95	0.95
1,3-diacetyloleandomycin	0.40	0.65	0.95	0.95
1,2-diacetyloleandomycin	0.80	0.90	0.95	0.95
triacetyloleandomycin	0.95	0.95	0.95	0.95

Ref:

T.M. Lees, P.J. DeMuria and W.H. Boegemann, J. Chromatogr., 5 (1961) 126–130.

TLC.

1. **Medium:**

Silica.

Solvent:

Chloroform:methanol:toluene (80:17:23).

Detection:

Dragendorff Reagent.

R_f:

	R_f
Triacetyloleandomycin	0.7
Diacetyloleandomycin	0.5
Monoacetyloleandomycin	0.2

Ref:

P. Gantes, J.-C. Garinot, J. Barat and J.P. Juhasz, Annales Pharm. Franc., 23 (1965) 137–140.

2. **Medium:**

Silica Gel:Plaster of Paris:Water (6:0.3:15).

Solvent:

Butanol:acetic acid:water (3:1:1).

Detection:

A. Visualized by spraying with sulfuric acid and heat at 100° for 5 min.

B. Bioautography vs. *Bacillus subtilis*.

R_f:

0.53

Ref:

M.V. Kalinina and E.I. Surikova, Antibiotiki, 13 (1968) 112–114.

CCD.

1. **Solvent:**

Benzene:cyclohexane:95% ethanol:water (5:5:8:2).

Distribution:

Coefficient = 0.25.

Ref:

As carbomycin PC (2).

OLEFICIN

PC.

1. **Paper:**

Solvent:

Propanol:ethyl acetate:0.25 N ammonium hydroxide (6:1:4).

Detection:

Bioautography vs. *Bacillus subtilis*.

R_f:

0.84

Ref:

J. Gyimesi, I. Ott, I. Horvath, I. Koczka and K. Magyar, J. Antibiotics, 24 (1971) 277–282.

TLC.

1. **Medium:**

Kieselgel G.

Solvent:

A. As PC (1), A.

B. Butanol:acetic acid:water (4:1:5).

C. Ethanol:water:ammonium hydroxide (8:1:1).

D. Benzene:ethyl acetate (1:1).

Detection:

R_f:

Solvent	R_f
A	0.60
B	0.79
C	0.62
D	0.10

Ref:

As PC (1).

CCD.
1. **Solvent:**
    Pyridine:ethyl acetate:water (3.5:6.5:8.3),
    100 transfers.
   Distribution:
    Peak in tube 59.
   Ref:
    As PC (1).

OLIGOMYCIN

PC.
1. **Paper:**
    Eaton-Dikeman No. 613.
   Solvent:
    Water:ethanol:acetic acid (70:24:6), 18—20
    h at 30°.
   Detection:
    Bioautography vs. *Glomerella cingulata*.
   R_f:

Component	R_f
A moves 22 cm	0.70
B moves 29 cm	0.85
C moves 13 cm	0.60

   Ref:
    S. Masamune, J.M. Sehgal, E.E. van Tamelen,
    F.M. Strong and W.H. Peterson, J. Amer.
    Chem. Soc., 80 (1958) 6092—6095;
    M.H. Larson and W.H. Peterson, Appl.
    Microbiol., 8 (1960) 182—189; E.W. Marty,
    Jr. and E. McCoy, Antibiotics and
    Chemotherapy, 9 (1959) 286—293.

OLIVOMYCIN

PC.
1. **Paper:**
    Circular.
   Solvent:
    A. Benzene:acetic acid:water (20:25:5).
    B. Benzene:butanol:water (18:2:20).
    C. Chloroform:carbon tetrachloride (satd.
        with water):methanol (5:4:1).
    D. Di-isoamyl ether (satd. with water):
        butanol (20:10).
   Detection:
    Bioautography vs. *Staphylococcus aureus*
    209P.
R_f:
    Olivomycin (greatest R_f) can be separated
    from aburamycin, NSCA-649 and LA-7017.
   Ref:
    E.V. Kruglyak, V.N. Borisova,
    M.G. Brazhnikova, Antibiotiki, 8 (1963)
    1064—1067.

OOSPORA VIRESCENS (Link) Wallr.
ANTIBIOTIC GLYCOSIDES

TLC.
1. **Medium:**
    Kieselgel H (Fluka). Activate at 110°C.
   Solvent:
    A. Chloroform:methanol (85:15).
    B. Chloroform:methanol:acetic acid
        (80:15:5).
   Detection:
    50% sulfuric acid; heat 110°C approximately
    5 min.
   R_f:

	R_f Solvent	
Component	A	B
A	0.16	
B	0.34	
C	0.52	
D	0.65	
E	0.36	
F		
G		0.32
H	0.42	0.18

   Ref:
    German "Offenlegungsschrift" 2100918,
    July 15, 1971.

ORYZOXYMYCIN

PC.
1. **Paper:**
    Toyo No. 51.
   Solvent:
    A. 80% ethanol.
    B. n-Butanol:acetic acid:water (4:1:2).
   Detection:
   R_f:

Solvent	R_f
A	0.66
B	0.13

   Ref:
    T. Hashimoto, S. Kondo, T. Takita,
    M. Hamada, T. Takeuchi, Y. Okami and
    H. Umezawa, J. Antibiotics, 21 (1968)
    653—658.

TLC.
1. **Medium:**
    Kieselgel G (Merck).

Solvent:

   A. Methanol.

   B. n-Butanol:acetic acid:water (4:2:1).

   C. n-Propanol:acetic acid:pyridine:water (50:6:20:24).

   D. Methanol:ethyl acetate (1:1).

Detection:

   A. Bioautography vs. *Xanthomonas oryzae*.

   B. Color with 0.5% potassium permanganate.

R_f:

Solvent	R_f
A	0.42
B	0.32
C	0.64
D	0.07

Ref:

   As PC (1).

ELPHO.

1. **Medium:**

   Paper.

   Buffer:

   Formic acid:acetic acid:water (25:75:900).

   Conditions:

   3,300 V/42 cm, 65 mA/20 cm, 15 min.

   Detection:

   Mobility:

   Moves 7 cm to cathode.

   Ref:

   As PC (1).

OSSAMYCIN

TLC.

1. **Medium:**

   A. Silica Gel.

   B. Cellulose Powder.

   Solvent:

   A. Benzene:methanol:water (100:110:10).

   B. Benzene:methanol:Skellysolve B:water (25:150:25:15).

   Detection:

   R_f:

Solvent	R_f
A	0.66
B	0.43

Ref:

   H. Schmitz, S.D. Jibinski, I.R. Hooper, K.E. Crook, Jr., K.E. Price and J. Lein, J. Antibiotics, 18 (1965) 82–88.

CCD.

1. **Solvent:**

   Skellysolve:benzene:ethanol:water (2:3:4:1), 100 transfers.

   Distribution:

   Peak in tube 71.

   Ref:

   As TLC (1).

OUDEMANSIELLA MUCIDA **ANTIBIOTIC**

TLC.

1. **Medium:**

   Aluminum oxide.

   Solvent:

   Petroleum ether:ether:acetic acid (9:10:1).

   Detection:

   Bioautography vs. *Saccharomyces cerevisiae*.

   R_f:

   0.5 (estimated from figure).

   Ref:

   Belgian patent no. 704076; published March 20, 1968.

OXYTETRACYCLINE

   See tetracyclines

OXYTOCIN

PC.

1. **Paper:**

   Whatman No. 1.

   Solvent:

   Butanol:acetic acid:water (4:1:5).

   Detection:

   R_f:

	R_f
4-glycine-oxytocin	0.58
3-glycine-oxytocin	0.36
2-glycine-oxytocin	0.38

   Ref:

   S. Drabarek, J. Am. Chem. Soc., 86 (1964) 4477.

PAECILOMYCEROL

TLC.

1. **Medium:**

   Silica Gel.

   Solvent:

   A. Benzene:acetone (2:1).

   B. Chloroform:methanol (7:1).

   C. Ethyl acetate.

Detection:

R_f:

Solvent	R_f*
A	0.50
B	0.25
C	0.50

*Estimated from drawing.

Ref:

A. Kato, K. Ando, T. Kimura, G. Tamura and K. Arima, J. Antibiotics, 22 (1969) 419–422.

PAROMOMYCIN

TLC.

1. **Medium:**

    Mixture of Kieselgel G and Aluminum Oxide.

    Solvent:

    n-Propanol:ethyl acetate:water:25% ammonium hydroxide (50:10:30:10).

    Detection:

    Ninhydrin.

    R_f:

    $$R_{glucosamine} = \frac{\text{distance spot moved}}{\text{distance glucosamine moved}} = 0.31$$

    Ref:

    V.R. Huttenrauch and I. Schulze, Pharm. Zentralblatt, 104 (1965) 85–87.

GLC.

Procedure for GLC as kanamycin GLC (1).

Separation of Paromomycin I and II:

Paromomycin II is retained longer on the OV-1 column than paromomycin I.

Ref:

As kanamycin GLC (1).

PATHOCIDIN

PC.

1. **Paper:**

    Solvent:

    A. Acetone:water (3:7).

    B. Acetone:water (1:1).

    C. Acetone:water (8:2).

    D. Pyridine:water (2:1).

    E. Methanol:pH 9 phosphate buffer (4:1).

    F. Butanol satd. with water.

    G. Butanol:acetic acid:water (4:1:2).

    H. pH 9 phosphate buffer.

    Detection:

    A. Fluorescence under UV light.

B. Bioautography vs. *Penicillium chrysogenum*.

R_f:

Solvent	R_f
A	0.70
B	0.52
C	0.10
D	0.70
E	0.38
F	0.00
G	0.00

Ref:

K. Anzai, J. Nagatsu and S. Suzuki, J. Antibiotics, 14 (1961) 340–342.

PATULIN

TLC.

1. **Medium:**

    Solvent:

    A. Ethanol:water (4:1).

    B. Toluene:ethyl acetate:90% formic acid (6:3:1).

    C. Benzene:methanol:acetic acid (24:2:1).

    D. Benzene:propionic acid:water (2:2:1).

    E. Chloroform.

    F. Chloroform:methanol (1:1).

    G. Methanol.

    Detection:

    Spray with O-dianisidin in acetic acid.

    R_f:

Solvent	R_f
A	0.71
B	0.37
C	0.13
D	0.64
E	0.04
F	0.71
G	0.66

Ref:

J. Reiss, Chromatographia, 4 (1971) 576–577.

PELIOMYCIN

TLC.

1. **Medium:**

    Silica Gel.

    Solvent:

    Ligroin:ethyl acetate (1:1).

    Detection:

    A. 0.3% Aq. potassium permanganate.

    B. Exposure to iodine vapor.

R_f:
Ref:

H. Schmitz, S.B. Deak, K.E. Crook, Jr.
and I.R. Hooper, Antimicrobial Agents and
Chemotherapy, 1963 (1964) 89—94.

CCD.

1. **Solvent:**

    A. Chloroform:carbon tetrachloride:
       methanol:water (2:2:3:1), 100 transfers.
    B. Skellysolve B:benzene:80% ethanol
       (2:3:5), 100 transfers.

    Distribution:

    A. Peak in tube 27.
    B. Peak in tube 37.

    Ref:

    As TLC (1).

PENICILLINS

PC.

1. **Paper:** (Quantitative Radioactive Method)
   Whatman No. 1, pH 6.2 buffered strips.

    Solvent:

    Ether.

    Detection:

    The developed strips are left in contact
    with X-ray film in a cassette for several days
    and the film is then developed.

    A. With these radio-autographs as guides, the
       corresponding paper strips are cut into
       squares or, where necessary, rectangles,
       in such a way as to avoid having parts of
       different penicillin zones on the same
       square. The squares are then fitted into
       planchettes and measured radiometrically
       in a thin end-window Geiger-Müller
       counter. From the total counts for each
       penicillin species, the proportions by
       weight (more strictly, the molar
       proportions) can readily be calculated.
    B. Alternatively, again using the radio-
       autographs as a guide, a strip is cut into
       sections each containing the whole of one
       penicillin species. Each section is then
       extracted by boiling for a few minutes
       with very dilute phosphate buffer. An
       aliquot of each extract is evaporated
       down on a planchette and the radio-
       activity measured.

    R_f:

Ref:

E.L. Smith and D. Allison, Analyst, 77
(1952) 29—33.

2. **Paper:**
   Whatman No. 4.

    Solvent:

    Water-satd. diethyl ether. The wet ether is
    kept at the temperature of development for
    several hours before use. Layers of water and
    ether are kept at the bottom of each tank
    and, for the purpose of maintaining the
    equilibrium, unbuffered filter papers are
    suspended from the top of the tank, close to
    the walls and dipping into the water layer.

    Detection:

    A. Bioautography vs. *Bacillus subtilis* 288.
    B. Methylene blue prints. Flood the surface
       with a 1.0% aq. soln. of methylene blue
       (containing 1.0% phenol to kill the test
       organism), wash off the surplus stain
       after a minute or so, blot with Whatman
       No. 1 filter paper by quickly smoothing
       a sheet over the surface, leave the paper
       in contact with the surface until the dye
       has been taken up sufficiently to give a
       clear print.

    R_f:

Compound	R_f*
Penicillin G	0.85
Penicillin V	0.7
Penicillin K	0.15

    *Estimated from drawing.

    Ref:

    J. Stephens and A. Grainger, J. Pharm.
    Pharmacol., 7 (1955) 702—705.

3. **Paper:**
   Whatman No. 1.

    Solvent:

    Butanol:ethanol:water (40:10:50), upper
    layer.

    Detection:

    The reaction with phenyl acetyl chloride in
    the presence of sodium bicarbonate is
    readily adapted to the detection of 6-amino-
    penicillanic acid on paper chromatograms,
    which are sprayed with the appropriate
    reagents before plating on agar seeded with
    a sensitive bacterium in the usual way. This

conversion of 6-amino-penicillanic acid to benzylpenicillin on paper strips also provides a convenient method of assay, being similar to the well known paper disc method.

R_f:

Penicillin G > 6-amino-penicillanic acid.

Ref:

F.R. Batchelor, F.P. Doyle, J.H.C. Nayler and G.N. Rolinson, Nature, 183 (1959) 257–258.

4. **Paper:**

Solvent:

Butanol:ethanol:water (40:10:50), upper layer.

Detection:

Bioautography vs. *Bacillus subtilis*.

R_f:

Penicillin K,FH$_2$ > F,G > penicillin 4 > penicillin 3 > penicillin 2 > penicillin 1.

Ref:

A. Ballio, E.B. Chain and F.D. Di Accadia, Nature, 183 (1959) 180–181.

5. **Paper:**

Whatman No. 1.

Solvent:

A. n-Butanol:ethanol:water (40:10:50), 5°C.
B. 70% Aq. n-propanol.

Detection:

R_f:

	Solvent	R_f
4-carboxy-n-butyl-penicillin	A	0.00
	B	0.35
Benzylpenicillin	B	0.75

Ref:

A. Ballio, E.B. Chain, F.D. Di Accadia, M.F. Mastropietro-Cancellieri, G. Morpurgo, G. Serlupi-Crescenzi and G. Sermonti, Nature, 185 (1960) 97–99.

6. **Paper:**

Whatman No. 1.

Solvent:

Butanol:acetic acid:water (4:1:5), 4 h.

Detection:

A. Spray with 0.5 N sodium hydroxide then, after an interval of 10–15 min to allow partial drying, it is further sprayed with a reagent composed of a mixture of 1% aq.

starch, glacial acetic acid and 0.1 N iodine in 4% potassium iodide soln. (50:3:1). Decolorization of the iodine reagent by the hydrolysed penicillins is fairly rapid, yielding maximum contrast after 5–10 min.

B. The reagent contains a mixture of SchenLabs (SchenLabs Pharmaceuticals Inc., New York) purified *Bacillus cereus* penicillinase (10,000 units/ml), 1% starch, 0.1 N iodine and pH 7 M sodium phosphate buffer, in the ratio 5:50:1:1. The rate of decolorization of the spray by the penicillin substrate is found to be dependent on the penicillinase conc. and, with this mixture, development is complete at room temperature (ca. 22°) in 10–15 min after hydrolysis of the β-lactam ring with alkali or penicillinase. The resulting penicilloic acid rapidly consumes nine equivalents of iodine. Under suitable conditions it is found that both penicillins and the related products cephalosporin C and cephalosporin N are readily detected as white zones against a dark blue background, with a sensitivity of 1–2 μgm.

R_f:

Cephalosporin C > Cephalosporin N > 6-aminopenicillanic acid.

Ref:

R. Thomas, Nature, 191 (1961) 1161–1163.

7. **Paper:**

Toyo No. 50; immerse in 2% liquid paraffin in ether and dry in air.

Solvent:

Butyl acetate, 2 h.

Detection:

Bioautography.

R_f:

Compound	R_f
Penicillin F	0.22
Penicillin G	0.48
Penicillin K	0.14
Penicillin V	0.36
Penicillin X	0.59

Ref:

T. Watanabe, S. Endo and Y. Iida, J. Antibiotics, 15 (1962) 112.

8. **Paper:**
   Solvent:
   A. Petroleum ether.
   B. Carbon tetrachloride.
   C. Methanol.
   D. Isooctanol.
   E. Propyl ether.
   F. Octyl ether.
   G. Water satd. with butanol.
   H. Water.
   I. 3% Aq. soln. of ammonium chloride.
   Solvents which are not miscible with water
   are preliminarily satd. with it.
   Detection:
   Chromatograms are first processed in alkali
   and then in iodine-starch reagent. Penicillin
   and related substances isomerize into
   penicilloic acids which are detected through
   the decoloration of the iodine-starch reagent.
   R_f:

Solvent	R_f Benzyl penicillin methyl ether	Phenoxy methyl-penicillin methyl ether
A	0.18	0.19
B	0.76	0.80
C	0.83	0.76
D	0.86	0.86
E	0.77	0.77
F	0.53	0.53
G	0.75	0.63
H	0.90	0.64
I	0.81	0.67

   Ref:
   A.S. Khokhlov and I.N. Blinova, Antibiotiki,
   15 (1962) 35–39.

9. **Paper:**
   Whatman No. 1 paper buffered with a soln. of
   10% citric acid monohydrate adjusted with
   aq. satd. sodium hydroxide to pH 5.7 and
   dried at room temperature.
   Solvent:
   Water satd. diethyl ether.
   Detection:
   Bioautography vs. *Sarcina lutea*.
   R_f:

Penicillin derived from	R_{bp}*
Methionine	0.54
Ethionine	0.94
S-methylcysteine	0.39
S-ethylcysteine	0.88

   *R_{bp} = mobility relative to benzyl penicillin (= 1.00).
   Ref:
   E. Albu and R. Thomas, Biochem. J., 87
   (1963) 648–652.

10. **Paper:**
    Whatman No. 1.
    Solvent:
    Butanol:acetic acid:water (4:1:5),
    descending, 16 h.
    Detection:
    Dry and dip in 0.2% ninhydrin in acetone
    containing 1% pyridine and heat at 80° for
    10 min.
    R_f:

Compound	R_f
Penicillin G	0.80
6-amino-penicillanic acid	0.53

    Ref:
    J.M.T. Hamilton-Miller, Biochem., 87 (1963)
    209–214.

11. **Paper:**
    Whatman No. 1 buffered with 1/15 M
    phosphate, pH 4.5.
    Solvent:
    Butanol:ether:water:acetone (7:2:2.5:2),
    4 h.
    Detection:
    Air dry, expose to ammonia vapor 30 min;
    spray with 0.02 N iodine soln.
    R_f:
    Useful for chromatography of 6-amino-
    penicillanic acid.
    Ref:
    B. Vassileva, Comptes rendus de l'Academie
    bulgare des Sciences, 16 (1963) 369–372.

12. **Paper:**
    Whatman No. 1.
    Solvent:
    n-Butanol:2% aq. oxalic acid (2:1), upper
    layer. Spot paper, allow to dry and then
    expose the strip to ammonia fumes in a
    closed container for 10 min. Remove and
    air dry. Place in the developing tank so that
    about 1/4 in. of the bottom of the strip is
    immersed in the mobile phase. Allow to

develop to the 15 cm mark, remove, and air dry.

Detection:

Place the strip in ammonia vapor for 10 min, remove, air dry, and spray once lightly with 0.02 M iodine soln. White spots on an iodine-colored background indicate the presence of phenethicillin.

R_f:

Phenethicillin, approximately 0.55.

Ref:

W   Cox and B.E. Greenwell, J. Pharm. Sci., 5   965) 1076–1077.

13. Paper:

Solvent:

A. 2-Butanol:formic acid:water (75:15:10).
B. 1-Propanol:water (60:40).
C. 1-Propanol:water (70:30).
D. 1-Propanol:ethanol:water (30:40:30).
E. 1-Propanol:ethanol:water (50:20:30).
F. 1-Propanol:ethanol:water (50:30:20).
G. 1-Butanol:1-propanol:water (25:40:35).
H. 1-Butanol:1-propanol:water (20:50:30).
I. 1-Butanol:1-propanol:water (25:50:25).

Detection:

Dip paper in a soln. of silver nitrate in acetone (1 ml satd. soln. silver nitrate added drop wise to 100 ml acetone until a precipitate begins to form). Air dry. Dip in a soln. of 2.5 ml of 50% sodium hydroxide in methanol to maximum color and wash briefly in water. Decolorize the background by dipping in 6 N ammonium hydroxide and wash in running water.

R_f:

	R_f	
Solvent	Penicillin V	6-amino-penicillanic acid
A	0.92	0.52
B	0.81	0.66
C	0.70	0.42
D	0.80	0.65
E	0.71	0.59
F	0.65	0.43
G	0.60	0.43
	0.60	0.43
I	0.55	0.38

Ref:

M. Rohr, Mikrochim. Acta, 4 (1965) 705–707.

14. Paper:

Whatman No. 1.

Solvent:

A. n-Butanol:pyridine:water (1:1:1).
B. n-Butanol:ethanol:water (4:1:5).

Detection:

Bioautography vs. *Bacillus subtilis* after activation by phenylacetylation if required.

R_f:

	Solvent	R_f
Methylpenicillin	A	0.58
Penicillin X	A	0.3
6-amino-penicillanic acid	A	0.48
Penicillin	A	0.75
Penicillin	B	0.4–0.5

Ref:

M. Cole, Appl. Microbiol., 14 (1966) 98–104.

15. Paper:

Whatman No. 1.

Solvent:

n-Butanol:ethanol:water (4:1:5), upper phase.

Detection:

Bioautography vs. *Bacillus subtilis.*

R_f:

α-azidobenzylpenicillin > ampicillin.

Ref:

E. Hansson, L. Magni and S. Wahlqvist, Antimicrobial Agents and Chemotherapy, 1967 (1968) 568–572.

16. Paper:

Papers impregnated with phthalate buffers, pH 4 or 5.

Solvent:

Both phases of isopropyl ether:isopropanol: water (70:30:100).

Detection:

A. Iodine-sodium azide reagent in combination with starch soln. produces white spots on a blue-gray background, but they are labile and have to be photographed.

B. Positive spots are produced by an alkaline silver reagent (0.1 M silver nitrate, 1 M ammonia, 1 M sodium hydroxide), but the chromatograms have to be treated with sodium thiosulfate and rinsed well with water.

R$_f$:

Penicillins	R$_f$ pH 5.0	pH 4.0
Ampicillin	0.00	0.00
Methicillin	0.04	0.12
Benzyl penicillin	0.23	0.65
Phenoxymethyl penicillin	0.33	
Oxacillin	0.50	
Phenoxylethyl penicillin	0.55	
Cloxacillin	0.56	
Phenoxypropyl penicillin	0.80	

Ref:

H. Hellberg, J. A.O.A.C., 51 (1968) 552—557.

17. **Paper:**

Whatman No. 1.

Solvent:

A. Butanol:ethanol:water (4:1:5), upper phase.

B. Water satd. ether, pH 6.2.

Detection:

A. Bioautography vs. *Bacillus subtilis* ATCC 6633.

B. 6-amino-penicillanic acid is detected by phenylacetylation of one of a pair of chromatograms before bioautography.

R$_f$:

Reaction mixture of 6-amino-penicillin acid + carboxylic acid	R$_f$ A	Migration (cm) B
n-Butyric	0.36	3.0
n-Valeric	0.46	8.0
n-Hexanoic	0.49	15.5
3-Hexanoic	0.46	13.0
n-Heptanoic	0.54	12—15.5
n-Octanoic	0.56	11.0
Pimelic	—	5.0
γ-Amino-n-valeric	—	4.8
ϵ-Aminocaproic	—	4.5
α-Hydroxyisocaproic	—	4.2
Butylthioacetic	0.53	10.0
Phenylacetic	0.47	6.5
N-phenylglycine	0.37	3.0
α-Ketophenylacetic	0.37	2.5
DL-α-hydroxyphenylacetic	0.40	3.4
DL-α-ethylphenylacetic	0.43	—
DL-α-methoxyphenylacetic	0.41	3.5—6.5
p-Hydroxyphenylacetic	0.29	0.5
p-Aminophenylacetic	0.21	0.0
m-Aminophenylacetic	0.22	0.0
p-Methoxyphenylacetic	0.39	4.2

Reaction mixture of 6-amino-penicillin acid + carboxylic acid	R$_f$ A	Migration B
3,4-Dichlorophenylacetic	0.57	6.4
3,4-Dihydroxyphenylacetic	0.24	0.0
p-Hydroxy-α-hydroxyphenylacetic	0.32	0.0
α-Methyl-α-hydroxyphenylacetic	0.46	6.9
Homogentisic acid lactone	0.31	0.0
Phenoxyacetic	—	7.0
p-Chlorophenoxyacetic	—	6.5
2-Thienylacetic	0.40	5.3
1-Naphthylacetic	0.48	6.0
2-Naphthylacetic	0.52	7.4

Reaction mixture of 6-amino-penicillin acid + amide		
Valeramide	0.49	7.5
Hexanamide	0.55	13.5
Heptanamide	0.58	15.5
Phenylacetamide	0.5	7.2
Phenylacetic acid control (pH 5)	0.5	7.5
p-Aminophenylacetamide	0.23	0.0
DL-mandelamide	0.48	4.5
DL-α-aminophenylacetamide	0.25	0.0
DL-α-phenoxypropionamide	0.58	16.0

Reaction mixture of 6-amino-penicillanic acid + N-acyl derivatives of glycine		
Valerylglycine	0.51	7.5
Hexanoylglycine	0.55	14.0
Heptanoylglycine	0.58	10.5
Octanoylglycine	0.62	25.0
Benzoylglycine	0.00	0.0
Phenylacetylglycine	0.50	8.0
Phenoxyacetylglycine	0.50	12.0
DL-α-phenoxypropionylglycine	0.54	14.5
DL-α-hydroxyphenylacetylglycine	0.45	5.0
D-α-aminophenylacetylglycine	0.03	0.0
	0.24	
Phenylacetic acid control (pH 5.0)	0.50	8.0
Phenylacetamide control (pH 7.0)	0.50	8.5

Ref:

M. Cole, Biochem. J., 115 (1969) 747—756.

18. **Paper:**

Whatman No. 1.

Solvent:

A. Butanol:ethanol:water (4:1:5), upper phase.

B. Butanol:pyridine:water (1:1:1).

C. Butanol:acetic acid:water (12:3:5).

Detection:

As PC (17).

R$_f$:

	R$_f$ Solvent		
	A	B	C
Benzylpenicillin amide	0.9	–·	—
Benzylpenicillin methyl ester	0.95	—	—
Benzylpenicillin cyanomethyl ester	—	—	0.92
Benzylpenicillin acetoxymethyl ester	0.92	—	—
Benzylpenicillin diethylaminoethyl ester HI	0.78	—	—
Benzylpenicillin phenacyl ester	0.92	—	—
Benzylpenicillin acetonyl ester	—	—	0.94
Benzylpenicillin thiomethyl ester (contaminated with some benzylpenicillin)	0.94	—	—
Benzylpenicilloic acid	—	0.51	—
N-Phenylacetyl-cyclic-DL-cysteinyl-D-valine	—	0.7	—
2-Furylmethylpenicillin methyl ester	0.89	—	—
n-Propoxymethylpenicillin cyanomethyl ester	—	—	0.85
2-Thienylmethylcephalosporin	0.32	—	—
	—	0.71	—
	—	—	0.75
2-Thienylmethylcephalosporin pyridine	0.26	—	—
	—	0.63	—
	—	—	0.45

Ref:

M. Cole, Biochem. J., 115 (1969) 733–739.

TLC.

1. **Medium:**

Silica Gel; activate 30 min at 110°C.

Solvent:

Benzene:isopentyl acetate:carbon tetra-
chloride:acetic acid:water (20:39:35:6:0.5).

Detection:

Spray with 40% sulfuric acid.

R$_f$:

Separates phenethicillin and phenoxymethyl
penicillin.

Ref:

P.J. Weiss, B. Taliaferro, R. Huckins and
R. Chastonay, J. A.O.A.C., 50 (1967)
1294–1297.

2. **Medium:**

A. Silica Gel G.
B. Silica Gel G adjusted to pH 6.1 with
McIlvaines buffer.

Solvent:

Nitromethane:toluene:butanol:pyridine:
acetic acid (60:30:15:9:6).

Detection:

R$_f$:

Useful for separation of semisynthetic
penicillins.

Ref:

F. Saccani, Boll. Chim. Farm., 106(9) (1967)
625–628; also Chem. Abstr., 68 (1968)
2375.

3. **Medium:**

Silica Gel H.

Solvent:

Acetic acid:acetone (5:95).

Detection:

Bioautography vs. *Bacillus subtilis*.

R$_f$:

Useful for detection of α-azidobenzyl
penicillin and a metabolite; also for
ampicillin.

Ref:

As PC (15).

4. **Medium:**
   A. Cellulose MN 300.
   B. Silica Gel G.

   Solvent:
   A. 0.1 M sodium chloride soln.
   B. 0.3 M citric acid soln. satd with n-butanol.
   C. Isoamyl acetate:methanol:formic acid: water (65:20:5:10).
   D. Acetone:acetic acid (95:5).

   Detection:
   A. 10% Ferric chloride:5% aq. potassium ferricyanide (20:10 ml) are mixed with 20% sulphuric acid (70 ml) and used on the day of preparation.
   B. Ninhydrin.
   C. 50% Aq. sulphuric acid.

   R_f:

	R_f Solvent			
	Medium A		Medium B	
	A	B	C	D
Benzylpenicillin Na	0.90	0.90	0.61	0.58
Ampicillin Na	0.97	0.98	0.12	0.15
Cloxacillin Na	0.65	0.38	0.64	0.77
Dicloxacillin Na	0.47	0.22	0.65	0.77
Nafcillin Na	0.47	0.22	0.64	0.77
Oxacillin	0.74	0.49	0.65	0.63
Phenethicillin K	0.84	0.73	0.66	0.77
Phenoxymethylpenicillin K	0.82	0.76	0.52	0.75
Methicillin Na	0.93	0.93	0.52	0.59
Hetacillin K	0.96	0.98	0.30	0.64

   Ref:
   I.J. McGilveray and R.D. Strickland, J. Pharm. Sci., 56 (1967) 78.

5. **Medium:**
   Solvent:
   Butanol:ethyl ether:butyl acetate:water (14:4.5:4.5:1).

   Detection:
   Bioautography.

   R_f:
   Useful for chromatography of 6-(α-amino-acylamido) penicillanic acids.

   Ref:
   J. Cieslak, B. Wasilewa, D. Roslik, Acta, Pol. Pharm. 25(2) (1968) 515—516; Chem. Abstr., 69 (1968) 8121.

6. **Medium:**
   Kieselguhr G (Merck) buffered to pH 5.3. Prepare slurry with a mixture of 100 ml 0.05 M potassium hydrogen phthalate and 32 ml 0.1 M sodium hydroxide. Dry the plates 1 h at 105°C.

   Solvent:
   Carbon tetrachloride:isopropanol:water (6.5:3.5:0.4). Pour the solvent, after clarification, on the bottom of the tank and moisten the paper lining. Use the tank preferably 10—48 h after preparation. Develop 30—40 min.

   Detection:
   Iodine-azide soln: Dissolve 1 g sodium azide in a mixture of 10 ml 0.1 M iodine soln. and 90 ml water. Starch soln: 0.5% soln. of soluble starch. Dry in air and spray well with starch soln. Finally dry with warm air and spray with iodine-azide reagent; repeat this alternate drying and spraying with iodine-azide until the white spots are distinct (2—3 times).

   R_f:
   Useful for separation of semi-synthetic penicillins.

   Ref:
   As PC (16).

7. **Medium:**
   Eastman Chromagram Sheet No. 6061.
   Solvent:
   Ethyl acetate:acetic acid:water (8:1:1).

Detection:

Bioautography vs. *Bacillus subtilis* ATCC 6633.

R_f:

Separation of ampicillin and cloxacillin. The inhibition zone near the origin is due to ampicillin; zone near the front is cloxacillin.

Ref:

T. Murakawa, Y. Wakai, M. Nishida, R. Fujii, M. Konno, K. Okada, S. Goto and S. Kuwahara, J. Antibiotics, 23 (1970) 250−251.

8. **Medium:**

Silica Gel.

Solvent:

Butyl acetate:butanol:acetic acid:methanol: phosphate buffer pH 5.8 (80:15:40:5:24).

Detection:

R_f:

Benzylpenicilloic acid > benzylpenicillanic acid > benzylpenicillin > benzylpenicillic acid.

Ref:

E.E. Imozemtzeva, D.M. Trachtenberg and E.N. Navoilneva, Khim. Farm. Zh., 4 (1970) 26−30.

9. **Medium:**

Solvent:

A. Isopropanol:acetone:water (1:1:1).

B. n-Butanol:ethanol:isopropanol:acetone: water (4:1:2:2:2).

C. Isopropanol:acetone:n-butanol:water (4:2:4:2).

D. n-Butanol:ethanol:acetone:water (4:1:4:1).

E. n-Butanol:ethanol:water (4:1:5).

F. n-Butanol:ethanol:isopropanol:acetone: water (4:1:1:1:1).

Detection:

R_f:

Solvent	R_f 6-amino-penicillanic acid	Benzyl penicillin
A	0.76	0.87
B	0.44	0.63
C	0.53	0.71
D	0.37	0.58
E	0.20	0.45
F	0.28	0.50

Ref:

J. Mikolajczyk, J. Kazimierczak and J. Cieslak, Chemia Analityczna, 16 (1971) 877−882.

10. **Medium:**

Silica Gel.

Solvent:

Acetone:acetic acid (95:5), followed by methanol:butanol:formamide:heptane (46:16:11:5).

Detection:

The separated compounds are detected by spraying with 0.01N iodine soln. containing 20 mg sodium azide per 100 ml, followed by spraying with 1% aq. starch soln. The spots appear as white zones on a bluish violet background.

R_f:

	R_s*
Phenoxymethylpenicillic acid	0.25
Phenoxymethylpenicilloic acid	0.33
Phenoxymethylpenilloic acid	0.73
Phenoxymethylpenicillin	1.00
Phenoxymethylpenicillanic acid	1.15

*R_s = mobility relative to phenoxymethyl-penicillin (= 1.00).

Ref:

V.B. Korchagin, L.I. Serova, S.P. Dement'eva, I.N. Navol'neva, I.I. Inozemtseva, D.M. Trakhtenberg, N.I. Kotova, Antibiotiki, 16 (1971) 8−11; Chem. Abs., 74 (1971) 218, No. 79535n.

ELPHO.

1. **Medium:**

Paper:

Buffer:

0.1 M phosphate buffer, pH 6.8.

Conditions:

25 V/cm.

Detection:

Mobility:

Benzylpenicillin, 10.5 cm/h.

4-carboxy-n-butyl-penicillin, 20 cm/h.

Ref:

As PC (5).

2. **Medium:**

Agarose plates (1% agarose).

Buffer:

Potassium phosphate, pH 7.0; ionic strength = 0.02.

Conditions:

2 V/mm^{-1}, 18 mA, 30 min.

Detection:

A. Bioautography vs. *Bacillus subtilis*. 6-amino-penicillanic acid is converted into benzylpenicillin before the addition of the seeded agar layer. This is achieved by placing a series of filter papers, impregnated with either a 5% aq. soln. of sodium hydrogen carbonate or with a 5% soln. of phenylacetyl chloride in acetone on the gel surface for 5 min each and finally repeating the 5% aq. sodium hydrogen carbonate soln.

B. The penicilloic acids are detected by placing the gel in iodine vapor from a few crystals of iodine contained in a chromatographic tank. The acids were visible as dark blue spots on a blue background. Penicillins are detected by this method after they have been hydrolyzed *in situ* to the corresponding penicilloic acids. The plate is immersed in 0.5 N hydrochloric acid for 5 min to hydrolyse the penicillins (alkali treatment at this stage interferes with the iodine reaction). The gel surface is thoroughly freed from liquid by wiping with paper tissues and the plate exposed to iodine vapor. The penicilloic acids already present in the gel are unaffected by the hydrolytic procedure and both the penicilloic acids and the hydrolysed penicillins are visible as dark blue spots.

Mobility:

6-amino-penicillanic acid, ampicillin and carbenicillin are readily distinguished; separation of the other penicillins tested is only marginal.

Ref:

A.H. Thomas and R.A. Broadbridge, Analyst, 95 (1970) 459–462.

GLC.

1. **Column:**

1.5 m $\times$ 4 mm column of stationary phase on acid-washed silanized Gas-Chrom P 60–80 mesh.

Temperature:

Column, 230°C; detector, 240°C; flash heater, 300°C.

Carrier gas:

N_2 75 ml/min.

Retention times:

(Est. from graph): Penicillin G, 7.3 min; penicillin V, 8.7 min (as methyl esters).

Ref:

S. Kawai and S. Hashiba, Japan Analyst, 13 (1964) 1223–1226.

2. **Apparatus:**

Argon Chromatograph (Pye Instruments, Cambridge, England) modified to permit the injection of a sample directly on the top of the column through a silicone rubber septum.

Column:

130 cm $\times$ 4 mm internal diameter borosilicate glass tubing, filled with acid-washed, silanized Gas-Chrom P, 100–120 mesh, coated with stationary phase at the percentage indicated in table.

Temperature:

Column, 300°C; detector, 250°C.

Carrier gas:

Argon, inlet pressure, 1 kg/cm^2.

Detector voltage:

800–1000 V.

Reagent solvent:

Acetone.

Derivative:

Different penicillanic acids are transformed into their methyl esters by reaction with an ethereal soln. of diazomethane.

Relative retention time:

Methyl ester of	Relative retention time				
	QF-1 80%	QF-1 0.75%	SE-30 0.4%	SE-52 0.4%	SE-52 0.4%
Penicillanic acid	0.59	—	—	—	—
6-chloropenicillanic acid	0.81	—	—	—	—
6-bromopenicillanic acid	1.04	—	—	—	—
Benzoylglycine	1.00	—	—	—	—
Benzylpenicillin	—	1.00	1.00	1.00	1.00
Phenoxymethylpenicillin	—	1.17	1.24	1.35	1.18
α-phenoxyethylpenicillin side-chain:					
D-isomer	—	0.864	1.07	1.08	—
L-isomer	—	0.913	1.14	1.20	—
3,4-Dichloro-α-methoxybenzyl side chain:					
L-isomer	—	—	—	—	2.69
D-isomer	—	—	—	—	3.14
6-tritylaminopenicillanic acid	—	2.72	—	—	6.05

Ref:

E. Evrard, M. Claesen and H. Vanderhaeghe, Nature, 201 (1964) 1124–1125.

3. **Apparatus:**

A Varian Aerograph Model 2100 gas chromatograph equipped with F.I.D.

Column:

A 4-mm i.d. × 660 mm glass U-tube column is packed with 2% OV-17 (Applied Science Laboratories, State College, Pa.) on 80–100 mesh Supelcoport (Supelco, Inc., Bellefonte, Pa.).

Temperature:

Column oven temperatures of 245 and 275°C are used; injector and detector temperatures are maintained at 275°C.

Gases:

Helium, 165–215 ml/min; hydrogen, 85 ml/min; air, 260 ml/min.

Internal standard-silylating reagent:

A 50% soln. of HMDS in pyridine containing 0.375 mg/ml of 5-α-cholestane or 5-α-cholestan-3-one.

Reference standard:

Penicillin reference standards are dissolved in water at a conc. of 20 mg/ml. To 2.0 ml of the standard soln., 8.0 ml of chloroform and 2.0 ml of pH 2.2 buffer are added. The mixture is immediately taken vigorously for 1 min and centrifuged. A 2.0 ml aliquot of the organic phase is transferred to an 8.2 ml serum vial for silylation.

Silylation procedure:

To each vial is added 2.0 ml of internal standard-silylating reagent. The vials are sealed, mixed, and allowed to stand at room temperature with occasional shaking.

Relative retention time:

Compound	Relative retention time
5-α-Cholestan-3-one	1.00 (2.0 min)[*]
Methicillin	1.51
Oxacillin	1.58
Cloxacillin	2.16
Dicloxacillin	2.83
5-α-Cholestane	1.00 (2.3 min)[**]
Penicillin G	1.65
D-Phenethicillin	1.60
L-Phenethicillin	1.71
Penicillin V	2.05

[*] 275°C at 215 ml/min.
[**] 245°C at 165 ml/min.

Ref:

C. Hishta, D.L. Mays and M. Garofalo, Anal. Chem., 43 (1971) 1530–1535.

ADDITIONAL PENICILLIN REFERENCES

R.R. Goodall and A.A. Levi. A microchromatographic method for the detection and approximate determination of the different penicillins in a mixture. *Nature*, 158 (1946) 675–676.

W. Awe, F. Neuwald and G.A. Ulex. Die Anwendung der Jod-Azid-Reaktion im Papierchromatogramm. *Naturwissen.*, 41 (1954) 528.

L.N. Astanina and L.M. Yakobson. Paper chromatographic separation of penicillin metabolites. *Lab. Delo.*, 11 (1967) 666-9 (Russ.); *Chem. Abstr.*, 68 (1968) 4638.

D.M. Trakhtenberg, I.I. Inozemtseva, G.S. Rozenfeld, Z.F. Kamokina and L.I. Ermakova, Counter-current distribution and chromatography of benzylpenicillin salts. *Antibiotiki*, 13(8) (1968) 696–691; *Chem. Abstr.*, 69 (1968) 7518.

P.A. Nussbaumer. Application de la chromatographie en couche mince à l'analyse de quelques penicillines usuelles. *Pharm. Acta Helv.*, 38 (1963) 245–251.

V. Betina. "pH chromatography" of Antibiotics VI. Separation of mixtures of natural penicillins. *Chemicke Zvesti*, 18 (1964) 209–213.

G.L. Biagi, A.M. Barbaro and M.C. Guerra. The influence of pH in buffered reversed-phase thin-layer chromatography of penicillins and cephalosporins. *J. Chromatogr.*, 51 (1970) 548–552.

G.L. Biagi, A.M. Barbaro, M.F. Gamba and M.C. Guerra. Partition data of penicillins determined by means of reversed-phase thin-layer chromatography. *J. Chromatogr.*, 41 (1969) 371–379.

V. Bettina. A Paper chromatography method for the determination of suitable pH values for the extraction of antibiotics. *Nature*, 182 (1958) 796–797.

PERIMYCIN
PC.
1. **Paper:**
   Solvent:
   Pyridine:1-butanol:water (4:6:5).
   Detection:
   Bioautography vs. *Candida albicans* 204.
   R_f:
   0.80
   Ref:
   E. Borowski, C.P. Schaffner, H. Lechevalier and B.S. Schwartz, Antimicrobial Agents Annual, 1960, 532–538.

CCD.
1. **Solvent:**
   A. Pyridine:ethyl acetate:water (3.5:6.5:8.3), 200 transfers.
   B. Chloroform:methanol:borate buffer (2:2:1).
   Distribution:
   Solvent A: K = 2.2.
   Solvent B; K = 0.1.
   Ref:
   As PC (1).

PETRIN
PC.
1. **Paper:**
   Solvent:
   Chloroform:n-butanol:water (46:4:50).

Detection:
Activity vs. *Haemophilus pertussis*.
R_f:
Separation of petrin into three fractions:
(1) antibiotic; (2) haemolytic; (3) fluorescent.
Ref:
A.I. Tiffin, Nature, 181 (1958) 907–908.

PHENAZINES and PHENOXAZINONES
PC.
1. **Paper:**
   A. Whatman No. 1, previously washed with 2.8% ammonium hydroxide.
   B. Schleicher and Schuell No. 2497 (fully acetylated).
   Solvent:
   A. Acetic acid:chloroform (1:10).
   B. Toluene:ethanol:water (4:17:1).
   C. Ethanol:water (1:1).
   D. Butanol:acetic acid:water (4:1:1).
   E. Butanol:acetic acid:water (4:1:5), upper layer.
   F. Toluene vs. Whatman No. 1 paper dipped in acetone:dimethyl sulfoxide (3:1) and dried 15 min in air.
   G. 15% Acetone.
   H. 50% Methanol.
   I. Methanol:10% hydrochloric acid (1:1).
   Detection:
   R_f:

	Paper	Solvent	R
1,6-phenazinediol-5,10 dioxide (iodinin)	B	B	0
	–	D	0
		C	n (
1,6-phenazinediol	B	B	0
		D	0
		F	0
2-aminophenoxazin-3-one	A	E	0
		G	0
		H	0
		I	0
2-acetamidophenoxazine-3-one	A	E	0
		F	0
	B	B	0
		D	0

Ref:
N.N. Gerber and M.P. Lechevalier, Biochem., 3 (1964) 598–602.

TLC.

1. **Medium:**

     Silica Gel.

   Solvent:

     As PC (1), A.

   Detection:

   R_f:

Compound	R_f
1,6-Phenazinediol-5,10 dioxide (iodinin)	0.80
2-Aminophenoxazin-3-one	0.30
2-Acetomidophenoxazine-3-one	0.60

   Ref:

     As PC (1).

PHENOMYCIN

ELPHO.

1. **Medium:**

     Cellulose acetate film.

   Buffer:

     pH 7.0 buffer (0.01 M phosphate and 0.1 M sodium chloride).

   Conditions:

     10 mA/4 cm, 1 h.

   Detection:

     Purple-red spot by treatment with Ponceau 3R.

   Mobility:

     Moves 2.3 cm to cathode.

   Ref:

     S. Nakamura, T. Yajima, M. Hamada, T. Nishimura, M. Ishizuka, T. Takeuchi, N. Tanaka and H. Umezawa, J. Antibiotics, 20 (1967) 210−216.

PHLEOMYCINS

PC.

1. **Paper:**

   Solvent:

     A. 0.5% Ammonium chloride.
     B. 1.0% Ammonium chloride.

   Detection:

   R_f:

	R_f Solvent	
	A	B
Phleomycin C	0.73	0.79
Phleomycin D	−	0.88
Phleomycin D_1	0.81	0.88
Phleomycin D_2	0.76	0.88
Phleomycin E	0.84	0.88
Phleomycin F	0.78	0.76
Phleomycin G	0.81	0.86
Phleomycin H	0.73	0.87
Phleomycin I	0.83	0.88
Phleomycin J	−	0.81
Phleomycin K	−	0.88

   Ref:

     T. Ikekawa, F. Iwami, H. Hiranaka and H. Umezawa, J. Antibiotics, 17 (1954) 194−199.

2. **Paper:**

   Solvent:

     10% Ammonium chloride.

   Detection:

     Sakaguchi reaction.

   R_f:

     All phleomycins showed R_f below 0.80 and gave positive Sakaguchi reaction.

   Ref:

     H. Umezawa, Y. Suhara, T. Takita and K. Maeda, J. Antibiotics, 19 (1966) 210−215.

TLC.

1. **Medium:**

   Solvent:

     10% Ammonium acetate:methanol (1:1).

   Detection:

   R_f:

	R_f
Phleomycin C	0.72
Phleomycin D_1	0.65
Phleomycin D_2	0.64
Phleomycin E	0.56
Phleomycin F	0.50
Phleomycin G	0.48
Phleomycin H	0.42
Phleomycin I	0.38
Phleomycin J	0.35
Phleomycin K	0.23

   Ref:

     As PC (1).

ELPHO.

1. **Medium:**

     Paper.

   Buffer:

     Formic acid:acetic acid:water (25:75:900).

Conditions:
  3,300 V and 25 mA for 20 min.
Detection:
Mobility:

	R_f*
Phleomycin C	0.75
Phleomycin D_1	0.94
Phleomycin D_2	0.98
Phleomycin E	1.08
Phleomycin F	1.12
Phleomycin G	0.86
Phleomycin H	0.88
Phleomycin I	0.89

  *L-alanine as the standard (= 1.00).
Ref:
  As PC (1).

PHOSPHONOMYCIN

PC.
1. **Paper:**
  Solvent:
    A. n-Propanol:2N methylamine (7:3).
    B. n-Propanol:2N isopropylamine (7:3).
    C. n-Butanol:acetic acid:water (3:1:1).
    D. n-Butanol:acetic acid:water (4:1:1).
    E. Isopropanol conc. ammonia:water
       (7:1:2).
    F. Methanol:water:triethylamine (80:20:5).
  Detection:
    A. Bioautography vs. *Proteus vulgaris*
       MB-838.
    B. Reagent containing 3% perchloric acid
       and 1% ammonium molybdate in 0.01 N
       hydrochloric acid readily reveals an
       intense blue zone after heating for 5 min
       at 85°.
    C. Spray with 0.1% ferric chloride in 80% aq.
       ethanol. After drying, the antibiotic is
       revealed as a white or light buff colored
       zone on a pinkish background by spraying
       with a 1% soln. of sulfosalicylic acid in
       80% ethanol.
  R_f:

Solvent	R_f
A	0.19
B	0.26
C	—*
D	0.26
E	—*
F	—*

  *See TLC (2).

Ref:
  H. Shafer, W.J.A. Vandenheuvel, R. Ormond,
  F.A. Kuehl and F.J. Wolf, J. Chromatog.,
  52 (1970) 111–117.

2. **Paper:**
  Whatman No. 3 M.
  Solvent:
    A. Isopropanol:0.01 M phosphate buffer
       pH 6.0 (7:3).
    B. Methanol:2% sodium chloride (7.5:2.5).
  Detection:
  Bioautography vs. *Proteus vulgaris* or *Erwinia
  atroseptica*.
  R_f:

Solvent	R_f
A	0.25
B	0.74

  Ref:
  E.O. Stapley, D. Hendlin, J.M. Mata,
  M. Jackson, H. Wallick, S. Hernandez,
  S. Mochales, S.A. Currie and R.M. Miller,
  Antimicrobial Agents and Chemotherapy,
  1969 (1970) 284–290.

TLC.
1. **Medium:**
  Silica Gel G.
  Solvent:
    A. Methanol:isopropanol:water (7:3).
    B. Methanol:water (1:1).
    C. Ethanol:water:conc. ammonia (25:3:4).
    D. Aq. ammonia and diethylamine.
  Detection:
  Bioautography.
  R_f:

Solvent	R_f
A	0.0
B	0.0
C	slight mobility
D	1.0

  Ref:
  L. Chaiet, T.W. Miller, R.T. Goegelman,
  A.J. Kempf and W.J. Wolf, J. Antibiotics, 23
  (1970) 336–347.

2. **Medium:**
    A. Cellulose.
    B. Silica Gel G.

Solvent:

    A. As PC (1), C.

    B. As PC (1), D.

    C. As PC (1), E.

    D. As PC (1), F.

Detection:

    As PC (1).

R_f:

Medium	Solvent	R_f
A	B	0.26
	C	0.18
B	A	0.33
	D	0.75

Ref:

    As PC (1).

ELPHO.

1. **Medium:**

    Schleicher and Schuell SS-598.

    Buffer:

    Refrigerated unit, 0.165 M pH 7.0 phosphate buffer, 2.5 h.

    Conditions:

    600 V.

    Detection:

    As PC (1).

    Mobility:

    Moves to anode 12.7 cm.

    Ref:

    As PC (1).

PICROMYCIN

PC.

1. **Paper:**

    Whatman No. 1. Saturate with 0.3 M phosphate buffer (pH 3.0) and air dry.

    Solvent:

    1-Hexanol satd. with water, developed 24 h; solvent runs off strips.

    Detection:

    Bioautography vs. *Corynebacterium xerosis*.

R_f:

    Picromycin moved 15 in. (38.1 cm) from origin.

Ref:

    S.E. DeVoe, H.B. Renfroe and W.K. Hausmann, Antimicrobial Agents and Chemotherapy, 1963 (1964) 125–129.

PILOSOMYCINS

PC.

1. **Paper:**

    Whatman No. 1, except F (below).

    Solvent:

    A. Butanol satd. with water.

    B. Butanol:glacial acetic acid:water (4:1:5), upper phase.

    C. Butanol satd. with water + 2% p-toluenesulfonic acid.

    D. Butanol satd. with water + 2% piperidine.

    E. Butanol:pyridine:water (6:4:3).

    F. 80% ethanol + 1.5% sodium chloride; Whatman No. 4 paper impregnated with 0.95 M sodium sulfate + 0.05 M sodium hydrosulfate.

    G. Butanol:ethanol:water (1:1:2).

    H. Butanol:butyl acetate:glacial acetic acid: water (10:3:1.3:14.3), upper phase, developed 16 h.

Detection:

    Bioautography vs. *Staphylococcus aureus* or *Bacillus subtilis*.

R_f:

Solvent	R_f Pilosomycin A	Pilosomycin B
A	0.00	0.00
B	0.49	0.63
C	0.34	0.58
D	0.05	0.15
E	0.32	0.32
F	0.47	0.47
G	0.74	0.74
H	2.7*	7.6*

*Distance from origin in cm after 16 h.

Ref:

    E. Gaeumann, H. Bickel and E. Visher; U.S. Patent 3,033,760; May 8, 1962.

ELPHO.

1. **Medium:**

    Paper.

    Buffer:

    0.1 M acetate buffer, pH 4.6.

    Conditions:

    Detection:

    Mobility:

    Pilosomycin migrates toward cathode.

    Ref:

    As PC (1).

PIMARICIN
PC.
1. **Paper:**
   Whatman No. 1.
   Solvent:
   A. Butanol:ethanol:water (5:1:4).
   B. Propanol:water (7:3).
   C. As B, but (8:2).
   Detection:
   Bioautography vs. *Saccharomyces cerevisiae.*
   R_f:

Solvent	R_f
A	0.25
B	0.15
C	0.45

   Ref:
   A.P. Struyk, I. Hoette, G. Drost,
   J.M. Waisvisz, T. van Eek and J.C. Hooger-
   heide, Antibiotics Annual, 1957–1958,
   878–885.

PIOMYCIN
PC.
1. **Paper:**
   Toyo No. 51.
   Solvent:
   A. Butanol:acetic acid:water (4:1:2).
   B. 75% phenol.
   Detection:
   A. Bioautography vs. *Piricularia oryzae.*
   B. Ninhydrin.
   C. UV lamp.
   R_f:

Solvent	R_f
A	0.17
B	0.36

   Ref:
   M. Matsuoka, N. Hattori and T. Ishiyama,
   paper presented at Japan Antibiotics
   Research Association March 22, 1968;
   Netherlands Patent 67,13997, published
   April 16, 1968.

TLC.
1. **Medium:**
   Silica Gel G.
   Solvent:
   A. Butanol:acetic acid:water (4:1:2).
   B. Butanol:ethanol:0.1 N hydrochloric acid
   (1:1:9).
   C. Propanol:pyridine:acetic acid:water
   (15:10:3:12).
   D. Chloroform:methanol:17% ammonium
   hydroxide (2:1:1).
   E. Ethanol:water (4:1).
   Detection:
   A. Ninhydrin.
   B. Potassium permanganate.
   C. UV lamp.
   R_f:

Solvent	R_f
A	0.22
B	0.35
C	0.88
D	0.82
E	0.50

   Ref:
   As PC (1).

2. **Medium:**
   As TLC (1).
   Solvent:
   As TLC (1) A–E.
   Detection:
   As TLC (1) A–C.
   R_f:

Solvent	R_f
A	0.21
B	0.45
C	0.86
D	0.87
E	0.74

   Ref:
   As PC (1), reference 2.

ELPHO.
1. **Medium:**
   Paper, Toyo No. 51.
   Buffer:
   Formic acid:acetic acid:water (25:75:900),
   pH 2.0.
   Conditions:
   Temperature, 0°C; 3000 V/40 cm; 30 mA;
   20 min.
   Detection:
   Mobility:
   Piomycin moves 1.8 cm toward cathode.
   Ref:
   As PC (1), reference 2.

PLICACETIN

PC.

1. **Paper:**
   Solvent:
   As amicetin, PC (2).
   Detection:
   As amicetin, PC (2).
   R_f:
   0.86
   Ref:
   As amicetin, PC (2).

PLURALLIN

TLC.

1. **Medium:**
   Alumina.
   Solvent:
   n-Butanol:ethanol:water (4:1:2).
   Detection:
   Bioautography vs. *Corynebacterium xerosis*.
   R_f:
   0.0 (plurallin); 0.5–0.7
   Ref:
   H. Umezawa, H. Ogawara, K. Maeda,
   K. Nitta, Y. Okami and T. Takeuchi,
   U.S. Pat. No. 3,655,877; April 11, 1972.

POLYANGIUM CELLULOSUM var. fulvum ANTIBIOTIC

PC.

1. **Paper:**
   Whatman No. 1.
   Solvent:
   A. Water.
   B. Water satd. n-butanol.
   C. Water satd. ethyl acetate.
   Detection:
   Bioautography vs. *Microsporum canis*.
   R_f:

Solvent	R_f
A	0.74
B	0.93
C	0.71

   Ref:
   S.M. Ringel, S. Roemer and A.L. Gutt,
   U.S. Patent 3,651,216; March 21, 1972.

TLC.

1. **Medium:**
   A. Cellulose Eastman Sheet 6065.

B. Silica Gel Eastman Sheet 6060.
C. Silica Gel G Plates.
Solvent:
   A. Butanol.
   B. 95% Ethanol.
   C. n-Propanol:ethyl acetate:water (7:2:1).
   D. Methanol:ethanol (1:1).
   E. Water:methanol:ethanol (2:3:5).
   F. Water:ethanol (5:95).
   G. Methanol:ethyl acetate (1:1).
   H. Ammonium hydroxide:water:isopropanol (5:15:85).
   I. Water:ethanol (1:4).
Detection:
   As PC (1).
R_f:

Medium	Solvent	Complex	R_f Component A	B	C
A	A	0.23			
A	B	0.65			
A	C	0.70			
B	B		0.69	0.38	0.00
B	C		0.50	0.28	0.00
C	D		0.05	0.30	0.50
C	E		0.50	0.75	0.82
C	F		0.10	0.85	0.35
C	G		0.02	0.33	0.18
C	H			0.57	0.61
C	I				0.75

Ref:
As PC (1).

CCD.

1. **Solvent:**
   Water satd. n-butanol:butanol satd. water (1:1), 30 transfers.
   Distribution:
   Component A in tubes 16–29.
   Ref:
   As PC (1).

POLYETHERIN A

TLC.

1. **Medium:**
   A. Silica Gel G.
   B. Aluminum oxide.
   Solvent:
   A. Chloroform:methanol (9:1).
   B. Benzene:ethyl acetate:methanol (6:4:1).

C. Ethyl acetate:tetrachloroethane:water (3:1:3).

Detection:

Sulfuric acid.

R_f:

Medium	Solvent	R_f
A	A	0.44–0.60
A	B	0.40–0.46
B	C	0.33–0.48

Ref:

S. Shoji, S. Kozuki, S. Matsutani, T. Kubota, H. Nishimura, M. Mayama, K. Motokawa, Y. Tanaka, N. Shimaoka and H. Otsuka, J. Antibiotics, 21 (1968) 402–409.

TLC.

1. **Medium:**

Silica Gel.

Solvent:

Methanol:chloroform:water (2:2:1).

Detection:

As PC (1).

R_f:

Component A	0.5	(est.)
Component B	0.7	(est.)

Ref:

As PC (1).

POLYFUNGINS

PC.

1. **Paper:**

Solvent:

Water satd. butanol.

Detection:

Bioautography vs. *Saccharomyces cerevisiae.*

R_f:

Component A	0.12–0.38	(est.)
Component B	0.39–0.61	(est.)

Ref:

German "Offenlegungsschrift" 2,044,004, April 1, 1970.

POLYKETO ACIDOMYCIN (PKAM)

PC.

1. **Paper:**

Solvent:

A. Distilled water.

B. 3% Ammonium chloride soln.

C. Chloroform.

D. Ethyl acetate:water (1:1).

E. Acetone.

F. Methanol.

G. Ethanol.

H. n-Butanol:water (1:1).

I. n-Butanol:acetic acid:water (4:1:5).

J. Petroleum ether:water (1:1).

K. Diethyl ether:water (1:1).

Detection:

A. Bioautography vs. *Bacillus subtilis.*

B. Potassium permanganate spray.

C. Ninhydrin.

R_f:

Solvent	R_f*
A	0.80
B	0.75
C	0.85
D	0.82
E	0.90
F	0.85
G	0.80
H	0.70
I	0.65
J	0.05
K	0.55

*Estimated from drawing.

Ref:

I.R. Shimi, G.M. Inam and Y.M. Shehata, J. Antibiotics, 20 (1967) 204–209.

POLYMYXINS

PC.

1. **Paper:**

Whatman No. 1 pretreated with 0.2 M glycine: HCl at pH 2.5.

Solvent:

Butanol, 6–18 h.

Detection:

Bioautography vs. *Brucella bronchiseptica.*

R_f:

Polymyxin A	0.18
Polymyxin B	0.56
Polymyxin D	0.38
Polymyxin E	0.54

Ref:

H.A. Nash and A.R. Smashey, Arch. Biochem. Biophys., 30 (1951) 237.

2. **Paper:**

Whatman No. 1.

Solvent:

Butanol:water:isopropylamine (125:60:4).

Detection:

R_f:

Polymyxin B	0.43
Polymyxin D	0.23

Ref:

A.G. Mistulta, Antibiotics and Chemotherapy, 6 (1956) 196–198

3. **Paper:**

A. Whatman No. 1.
B. Whatman No. 2.
C. Whatman No. 4.
D. Whatman No. 20.

Solvent:

A. 1-Butanol:acetic acid:water (120:30:50).
B. As A, but (4:1:5), upper phase.
C. As B, but lower phase.
D. 1-Butanol:pyridine:acetic acid:water (30:20:6:24).
E. 1-Butanol:acetic acid:1% aq. sodium chloride (120:30:50).
F. 1-Butanol:acetic acid:5% aq. sodium chloride (120:30:50).
G. 1-Butanol:pyridine:acetic acid:1% aq. sodium chloride (30:20:6:24).

Detection:

R_f:

Ref:

S. Wilkinson and L.A. Lowe, J. Chem. Soc., (1964) 4107.

4. **Paper:**

Whatman No. 1.

Solvent:

A. n-Butanol:acetic acid:water (4:1:5).
B. n-Butanol:pyridine:acetic acid:water (30:20:6:24).
C. n-Butanol:acetic acid:water (12:3:5).

Detection:

R_f:

	R_f Solvent		
Component	A	B	C
Polymyxin A_1	0.33	0.58	0.39
Polymyxin A_2	0.33	0.58	0.39
Polymyxin B_1	0.48	0.73	0.54
Polymyxin B_2	0.48	0.73	0.54
Polymyxin E_1	0.46	0.77	0.51
Polymyxin E_2	0.46	0.77	0.51

Ref:

S. Wilkinson, Antimicrobial Agents and Chemotherapy, 1966 (1967) 651–654.

5. **Paper:**

Solvent:

A. n-Butanol:acetic acid:water (4:1:5).
B. n-Butanol:pyridine:acetic acid:water (15:10:3:12).

		R_f		
Solvent	Paper	Polymyxin A	Polymyxin B	Polymyxin E
A	A	0.39	0.54	0.51
	B	0.29	0.42	0.40
	C	–	0.52	0.51
	D	0.15	0.31	0.30
B	A	–	0.50	0.46
	C	–	0.46	0.45
	D	–	–	0.20
C	A	0.92	0.86	0.90
D	A	0.58	0.73	0.77
	C	–	0.73	0.72
	D	–	–	0.64
E	A	–	0.42	0.42
F	A	–	0.37	0.37
	C	–	0.46	0.46
G	A	–	0.24	0.24

C. t-Butanol:acetic acid:water (74:3:25).

D. t-Butanol:methyl ethyl ketone:formic acid:water (8:6:3:3).

Detection:

Ninhydrin.

R_f:

Solvent	R_f Polymyxin B
A	0.23
B	0.76
C	0.54
D	0.60

Ref:

M.J. Daniels, Biochim. Biophys. Acta, 156 (1968) 119–127.

TLC.

1. **Medium:**

Kieselgel G (Merck).

Solvent:

Acetone:water:acetic acid:2 N ammonium hydroxide (15:5:1:2).

Detection:

A. Ninhydrin.

B. Bioautography vs. *Bordetella bronchiseptica.*

R_f:

Polymyxin B	0.45
Polymyxin D	0.51
Polymyxin E	0.45
Polymyxin M	0.36
Polymyxin E-methanesulfonate	0.95

Ref:

M. Igloy and A. Mizsei, J. Chromatogr., 28 (1967) 458–461; ibid., 34 (1968) 546–547.

2. **Medium:**

Silica Gel.

Solvent:

n-Butanol:acetic acid:water (4:1:3) and 1/20 vol. of pyridine; upper layer.

Detection:

R_f:

Polymyxin A	0.34
Polymyxin B	0.48

Ref:

Y. Kimura, E. Murai, M. Fujisawa, T. Tatsuki and F. Nobue, J. Antibiotics, 22 (1969) 449–450.

3. **Medium:**

As gramicidin, TLC (1) A and B.

Solvent:

As gramicidin, TLC (1) A–K.

Detection:

As gramicidin, TLC (1).

R_f:

Medium	Solvent	R_f Polymyxin E	Polymyxin B
A	A	0.21	0.23
	B	0.35	0.36
	C	0.21	0.23
	D	0.07	0.08
	E	0.43	0.44
	F	0.32	0.33
	G	0.00	0.00
	H	0.00	0.00
	I	0.78	0.80
	J	0.00	0.00
B	C	0.38	0.38
	K	0.68	0.69

Ref:

As gramicidin, TLC (1).

4. **Medium:**

Silica Gel G.

Solvent:

As PC (1), A.

Detection:

R_f:

Component	R_f
Polymyxin A_1	0.47
Polymyxin A_2	0.47
Polymyxin B_1	0.57
Polymyxin B_2	0.57
Polymyxin E_1	0.57
Polymyxin E_2	0.57

Ref:

As PC (1).

CCD.

For separation of polymyxin P components.

1. **Solvent:**

n-Butanol:sec.-butanol:0.1 N hydrochloric acid (6:30:40), 2100 transfers.

Distribution:

P_1 K = 0.056

P_2 K = 0.041

Ref:

As TLC (2).

POLYOXINS

PC.

1. Paper:

Solvent:

n-Butanol:acetic acid:water (4:1:2).

Detection:

R_f:

At least four active components seen:
Following R_f values given (main components).

Polyoxin A   0.23
Polyoxin B   0.13

Ref:

K. Isono, J. Nagatsu, Y. Kawashima and
S. Suzuki, Agr. Biol. Chem., 29 (1965)
848–854.

2. Paper:

Toyo No. 51.

Solvent:

A. As PC (1).
B. 75% Phenol.

Detection:

R_f:

Polyoxin	R_f Solvent A	Solvent B
A	0.21	0.53
B	0.10	0.18
D	0.10	0.08
E	0.13	0.12
F	0.21	0.38
G	0.12	0.30
H	0.27	0.66

Ref:

Derwent Farmdoc no. 29960, South Africa;
published April 10, 1967.

3. Paper:

As PC (2), ascending.

Solvent:

A. As PC (1).
B. Butanol:pyridine:water (4:1:2).
C. As PC (2) B.

Detection:

A. UV light.
B. Ninhydrin.
C. Biological activity.

R_f:

Polyoxin	R_f Solvent A	Solvent B	Solvent C
A	0.19	0.07	0.53
B	0.07	0.03	0.18
C	0.09	0.03	0.27
D	0.07	0.01	0.06*
E	0.08	0.01	0.09*
F	0.18	0.03	0.38
G	0.09	0.03	0.30
H	0.25	0.12	0.66
I	0.23	0.08	0.61

*Tailing was observed.

Ref:

K. Isono, J. Nagatsu, K. Kobinata, K. Sasaki
and S. Suzuki, Agr. Biol. Chem., 31 (1967)
190–199.

4. Paper:

As PC (2).

Solvent:

As PC (1).

Detection:

R_f:

Polyoxin J   0.08
Polyoxin K   0.22
Polyoxin L   0.08

Ref:

Netherlands Patent 68,09186; published
December 31, 1968.

5. Paper:

As piomycin PC (1).

Solvent:

As piomycin PC (1) A and B.

Detection:

As piomycin PC (1) A–C.

R_f:

	R_f Polyoxin			
Solvent	A	B	G	H
A	0.19	0.07	0.09	0.25
B	0.63	0.16	0.30	0.66

Ref:

As piomycin PC (1), reference 2.

TLC.

1. Medium:

Silica Gel G.

Solvent:

A. As PC (1).

B. Butanol:ethanol:0.1 N hydrochloric acid (1:1:1).

C. Butanol:pyridine:water (15:10:3).

D. Chloroform:methanol:17% ammonia (2:1:1).

E. Ethanol:water (4:1).

Detection:

A. Permanganate spray.

B. As PC (3) A.

C. As PC (3) C.

R_f:

Polyoxin	R_f Solvent				
	A	B	C	D	E
A	0.15	0.39	0.66	0.85	0.32
B	0.11	0.23	0.56	0.83	0.23
C	0.12	0.33	0.59	0.83	0.23
D	0.08	0.07	0.25	0.03	0.00
E	0.08	0.07	0.29	0.04	0.00
F	0.16	0.16	0.47	0.06	0.00
G	0.12	0.36	0.59	0.84	0.30
H	0.20	0.44	0.67	0.85	0.39
I	0.18	0.41	0.66	0.85	0.35

Ref:

As PC (3).

2. **Medium:**

Silica Gel G.

Solvent:

As piomycin TLC (1) C, E.

Detection:

As piomycin TLC (1) A–C.

R_f:

Solvent	R_f Polyoxin			
	A	B	G	H
C	0.66	0.56	0.59	0.67
E	0.28	0.23	0.28	0.32

Ref:

As piomycin TLC (1).

PORFIROMYCIN

PC.

1. **Paper:**

Solvent:

A. 1-Butanol:water (84:16).

B. As A + 0.25% p-toluenesulfonic acid.

C. 1-Butanol:acetic acid:water (2:1:1).

D. As A + 2% piperidine.

E. Methanol:benzene:water (1:1:2).

F. Water satd. ethyl acetate.

Detection:

A. Bioautography vs. *Sarcina lutea.*

B. UV at 360 nm.

R_f:

Solvent	R_f
A	0.60–0.75
B	0.55–0.72
C	no zone
D	0.58–0.75
E	0.10–0.22
F	0.55–0.80

Ref:

German Patent 1,122,671; patented January 25, 1962.

PRIMYCIN

PC.

1. **Paper:**

Schleicher and Schull 2043/b.

Solvent:

Butanol:acetic acid:water (4:1:5).

Detection:

A. Bioautography vs. *Bacillus subtilis.*

B. N-bromo-succinimide modification of Sakaguchi color test.

R_f:

0.56–0.61

Ref:

I. Szilagyi, T. Valyi-Nagy and T. Keresztes, Nature, 205 (1965) 1225–1227.

PROACTINOMYCINS

CCD.

1. **Solvent:**

Ether: m/2 potassium phosphate buffer, pH 6.8; 24 transfers.

Distribution:

Antibiotic	Peak tubes
Proactinomycin A	4
Proactinomycin B	8–9
Proactinomycin C	20

Ref:

R.Q. Marston, Brit. J. Exptl. Pathol., 30 (1949) 398–407.

PROCEOMYCIN
PC.
1. **Paper:**
   Solvent:
   A. Wet butanol.
   B. Aq. 3% ammonium chloride.
   C. 75% Phenol.
   D. 50% Acetone.
   E. Butanol:methanol:water (4:1:2) + 1.5% methyl orange.
   F. Butanol:methanol:water (4:1:2).
   G. Benzene:methanol (4:1).
   H. Water.
   All solvents developed ascending.
   Detection:
   R_f:

Solvent	R_f
A	0.95
B	0.10
C	0.95
D	0.90
E	0.90
F	0.90
G	0.65
H	0.25

Ref:

H. Tsukiura, M. Okanishi, H. Koshiyama, T. Ohmori, T. Miyaki and H. Kawaguchi, J. Antibiotics, 17 (1964) 223–229.

PROTICIN
TLC.
1. **Medium:**
   Silica Gel F_{254} (E. Merck, Darmstadt).
   Solvent:
   Chloroform:methanol (3:2).
   Detection:
   Staining was done with a mixture of chlorosulfonic acid and glacial acid by heating to 110°C.

R_f:
   0.38
Ref:
   L. Vertesy, J. Antibiotics, 25 (1972) 4–10.

PROTOMYCIN
PC.
1. **Paper:**
   Solvent:
   A. Ether.*
   B. Benzene.*
   C. Chloroform.*
   D. Methyl isobutyl ketone.*
   E. Petroleum ether.*
   F. Cyclohexane.*
   G. 3% Aq. ammonium chloride.
   *Water satd.
   All solvents developed ascending.
   Detection:
   R_f:

Solvent	R_f
A	0.85
B	0.35
C	0.75
D	0.78
E	0.00
F	0.00
G	0.86

Ref:

R. Sugawara, J. Antibiotics, 16 (1963) 115–120.

CCD.
1. **Solvent:**
   Benzene:methanol:0.001 N hydrochloric acid (10:2:8), 30 transfers.
   Detection:
   UV at 232 nm.
   Distribution:
   K = 0.9
   Ref:
   As PC (1).

PRUMYCIN
TLC.
1. **Medium:**
   Silicic acid (Kieselgel G, Merck).
   Solvent:
   A. Propanol:pyridine:acetic acid:water (15:10:3:12).

B. Butanol:acetic acid:water (3:1:2).

Detection:

R$_f$:

Solvent	R$_f$
A	0.68
B	0.21

Ref:

T. Hata, S. Omura, M. Katagiri, K. Atsumi,
J. Awaya, S. Higashikawa, K. Yasui,
H. Terada and S. Kuyama, J. Antibiotics, 24
(1971) 900—901.

PRUNACETIN

ELPHO.

1. **Medium:**

Starch block.

Buffer:

5 mM phosphate, pH 8.5, $\mu = 0.045$.

Conditions:

Detection;

Color (purple band).

Mobility:

Migrates toward anode.

Ref:

T. Arai, S. Kushikata, K. Takamiya,
F. Yanagisawa and T. Koyama, J. Antibiotics,
20 (1967) 334—343.

PSEUDOMONAS ANTIFUNGAL SUBSTANCE

PC.

1. **Paper:**

Solvent:

A. n-Butanol:acetic acid:water (4:1:5).

B. Isopropanol:ammonium hydroxide:water
(20:1:2).

C. Water:satd. phenol.

D. n-Butanol:pyridine:water (1:1:1).

E. n-Amyl alcohol satd. with 3% ammonium
hydroxide.

F. Benzene:acetic acid:water (2:2:1).

G. Hydrous acetone (50%).

H. n-Butanol:satd. water.

I. Ethyl acetate:pyridine:water (2:1:2).

J. n-Propanol:2.5% sodium chloride:acetic
acid (10:8:1).

K. Methanol:0.1 N hydrochloric acid (3:1).

L. Methanol:water (3:1).

M. Ammonium chloride (3%).

N. Water.

Detection:

A. Bioautography.

B. Visible yellow zone color.

R$_f$:

Solvent	R$_f$
A	1.00
B	0.99
C	0.96
D	0.98
E	0.97
F	0.95
G	0.98
H	0.00
I	1.00
J	0.99
K	0.83
L	0.80
M	0.02
N	0.00

Ref:

W.A. Ayers and G.C. Papavizas, Appl.
Microbiol., 11 (1963) 533—538.

PSICOFURANINE

PC.

1. **Paper:**

Whatman No. 1.

Solvent:

A. n-Butanol:water (84:16).

B. As A + 0.25% p-toluenesulfonic acid.

C. n-Butanol:acetic acid:water (2:1:1).

D. As A, but 2 ml piperidine added to
98 ml solvent mixture.

E. Water:n-butanol (96:4).

F. As E + 0.25% p-toluenesulfonic acid.

All solvents developed descending.

Detection:

UV at 262 nm.

R$_f$:

Solvent	R$_f$*
A	0.15
B	0.15
C	0.45
D	0.15
E	0.65
F	0.55

*Estimated from drawing.

Ref:

W.T. Sokoloski, N.J. Eilers and T.E. Eble,
Antibiotics and Chemotherapy, 9 (1959)
435—438.

2. Quantitative procedure.
   Paper:
   Schleicher and Schuell 589 (blue ribbon special). 0.5 × 22.5 inch strips. Satd. soln. containing 1 mg psicofuranine per ml water applied to strips at doses of 1, 2, 4, 5, 6, 8, 10 or 20 μl/strip. Each test soln. applied to 3 strips using 3 different doses estimated to contain 1—20 μg antibiotic.
   Solvent:
   As PC (1) D, developed without equilibration, 40 h.
   Detection:
   UV scan at 262 nm with recording scanning spectrophotometer. O.D. proportional to quantity of antibiotic.
   Ref:
   As PC (1).

CCD.
1. **Solvent:**
   1-Butanol:water.
   Distribution:
   K = 0.28—0.35
   Ref:
   T.E. Eble, H. Hoeksema, G.A. Boyack and G.M. Savage, Antibiotics and Chemotherapy, 9 (1959) 418—420.

PYRACRIMYCIN A
PC.
1. **Paper:**
   Whatman No. 1.
   Solvent:
   A. Water satd. n-butanol.
   B. Water satd. n-butanol + 2% p-toluene-sulfonic acid.
   C. Water satd. n-butanol + 2% conc. ammonia.
   D. n-Butanol satd. water.
   E. Ammonium chloride (20% soln. in water).
   F. n-Butanol:methanol:water (40:10:20) containing 0.75 g methyl orange.
   G. n-Butanol:methanol:water (40:10:30).
   H. Water:acetone (1:1).
   I. Water satd. ethyl acetate.
   Detection:
   Bioautography vs. *Staphylococcus aureus*.
   R_f:

Solvent	R_f
A	0.60
B	0.29
C	0.53
D	0.14
E	0.71
F	0.65
G	0.71
H	0.52
I	0.00

Ref:
C. Coronelli, G. Tamoni, G. Beretta and G.C. Lancini, J. Antibiotics, 24 (1971) 491—496.

TLC.
1. **Medium:**
   Silica Gel HF/UV$_{254}$.
   Solvent:
   Chloroform:methanol (9:1).
   Detection:
   UV absorption.
   R_f:
   0.22
   Ref:
   As PC (1).

PYRIDOMYCIN
TLC.
1. **Medium:**
   Eastman chromatogram sheet type K301R2.
   Solvent:
   1-Butanol:acetic acid:water (3:1:1).
   Detection:
   A. Bioautography vs. *Mycobacterium* 607.
   B. UV light.
   C. Spray sheet with 3% ferric chloride.
   R_f:
   0.25
   Ref:
   H. Ogawara, K. Maeda and H. Umezawa, Biochem., 7 (1968) 3296—3302.

PYRROLE ANTIBIOTIC from marine bacterium
TLC.
1. **Medium:**
   Silica Gel G.
   Solvent:
   Chloroform.

Detection:

A. Iodine vapor.

B. Conc. sulfuric acid.

R_f:

0.50

Ref:

P.R. Burkholder, R.M. Pfister and F.H. Leitz, Appl. Microbiol., 14 (1966) 649–653.

PYRROLNITRIN

PC.

1. **Paper:**

Solvent:

A. 50% acetone.

B. 1% ammonium chloride.

C. n-Butanol:methanol:water (4:1:2).

D. n-Butanol:methanol:water satd. with methyl orange (4:1:2).

E. n-Butanol:acetic acid:water (2:1:1).

F. Benzene:methanol (8:2).

G. n-Butanol satd. with water.

H. Water.

Detection:

R_f:

Solvent	R_f*
A	0.90
B	0.00
C	0.95
D	0.90
E	0.90
F	0.85
G	0.90
H	0.00

*Estimated from drawing.

Ref:

K. Arima, H. Imanaka, M. Jousaka, A. Fukuda and G. Tamura, J. Antibiotics, 18 (1965) 201–204.

TLC.

1. **Medium:**

Solvent:

A. Chloroform.

B. Benzene.

C. Benzene:n-hexane (1:1).

Detection:

R_f:

Solvent	R_f*
A	0.70
B	0.60
C	0.25

*Estimated from drawing.

Ref:

As PC (1).

2. **Medium:**

Solvent:

Benzene.

Detection:

Purplish green spot with sulfuric acid spray.

R_f:

0.75

Ref:

D.H. Lively, M. Gorman, M.E. Haney and J.A. Mabe, Antimicrobial Agents and Chemotherapy, 1966 (1967) 462–469.

3. **Medium:**

Silica Gel G.

Solvent:

Benzene:Skellysolve F (3:7).

Detection:

R_f:

Component A	0.31
Component B	0.37 (fluorpyrrolnitrin)

Ref:

M. Gorman, M.E. Haney, Jr., D.H. Lively and J.D. Davenport, U.S. Patent 3,590,051; June 29, 1971.

GLC.

1. Pyrrolnitrin and derivatives.

Apparatus:

F and M model 402 gas chromatograph.

Column:

Glass, U-shaped, 120 cm × 0.3 cm I.D.

A. Packed with 3.8 UCC-W98 [silicone gum rubber (methyl vinyl)] coated on 80–100 mesh Diatoport S.

B. 3% OV-1 coated on 100–200 mesh Gas Chrome Q.

Temperatures:

A. 230°C for flash heater, 180°C for column oven, 210°C for flame detector.

B. 240°C for flash heater, 200°C for column oven, 210°C for flame detector.

C. 240°C for flash heater, 180°C for column oven, 200°C for flame detector.

Carrier gas:

Helium, 70 ml/min.

Solvent:

Ethyl acetate.

Chromatography:

Injection, 1 μg.

Relative retention times:

Compound	System (Packing-temperatures)		
	A-A	A-B	B-C
Aminopyrrolnitrin	0.52	0.75	0.76
Isopyrrolnitrin		0.86	
Pyrrolnitrin	1.00	1.00	1.00
2-Chloropyrrolnitrin	1.50	1.38	1.47
Oxypyrrolnitrin		1.68	
3'-Methyl-3'-dechloropyrrolnitrin	0.66		
4'-Fluoropyrrolnitrin	0.86		
3'-Fluoro-3'-dechloropyrrolnitrin	0.50		
4'-Trifluoromethyl-3'-dechloro-aminopyrrolnitrin	0.23		

Ref:

R.L. Hamill, H.R. Sullivan and M. Gorman, Appl. Microbiol., 18 (1969) 310–312.

2. **Apparatus:**

F and M model 402 gas chromatograph.

Column:

4 ft × 0.25 in. glass column of 3.8% UC-W 98 on diatoport-S.

Temperatures:

Inlet temperature, 240°C; column temperature, 200°C.

Detection:

The eluate from the column is split (1:1) and passed through a flame ionization detection (220°C) and an electron capture detector (210°C). The resulting signals are recorded separately.

Solvent:

Compounds are run at a conc. of 1 mg/ml in ethyl acetate. Samples of 1 μ-liter are injected.

Chromatography:

Substances are eluted in the following order: amino derivative, isopyrrolnitrin, pyrrolnitrin, 2-chloropyrrolnitrin and oxypyrrolnitrin.

Ref:

R. Hamill, R. Elander, J. Mabe and M. Gorman, Antimicrobial Agents and Chemotherapy, 1967 (1968) 388–396.

QUINOMYCINS

PC.

1. **Paper:**

Solvent:

n-Butyl ether:s-tetrachloroethane:10% o-cresotinate (2:1:3).

Detection:

Bioautography vs. *Bacillus subtilis*.

R_f:

Quinomycin A   0.13
Quinomycin C   0.59

Ref:

T. Yoshida and K. Katagiri, J. Antibiotics, 14 (1961) 330–334.

TLC.

1. Circular TLC.

Medium:

Aluminum oxide GF$_{254}$ (Merck).

Solvent:

Ethyl acetate:tetrachloroethane:water (3:1:3), lower phase.

Detection:

R_f:

1. Quinomycin C > B$_o$ > A.
2. Quinomycin C > E > B > D > A.

Ref:

H. Otsuka and J.-I. Shoji, J. Antibiotics, 19 (1966) 128–131.

2. **Medium:**

Silica Gel G (Merck).

Solvent:

Methyl ethyl ketone.

Detection:

UV light.

R$_f$:

Quinomycin A	0.34	(UV absorbing).
NX Quinomycin A	0.52	(fluorescent).
QN Quinomycin A	0.70	(fluorescent).

Ref:

T. Yoshida, Y. Kimura and K. Katagiri,
J. Antibiotics, 21 (1968) 465—467.

RABELOMYCIN
TLC.
1. **Medium:**
   Silica Gel.
   Solvent:
   A. Chloroform:methanol:piperidine
   (94:5:1).
   B. Benzene:methanol (9:1).
   Detection:
   R$_f$:

Solvent	R$_f$
A	0.4
B	0.5

Ref:

W.C. Liu, W.L. Parker, D.S. Slusarchyk,
G.L. Greenwood, S.F. Graham and
E. Meyers, J. Antibiotics, 23 (1970)
437—441.

RACEMOMYCIN
PC.
1. **Paper:**
   Toyo-Roshi No. 51, UH-type; circular
   development.
   Solvent:
   n-Butanol:pyridine:acetic acid:water:tert.-
   butanol (15:10:3:12:4).
   Detection:
   A. Bioautography vs. *Bacillus subtilis.*
   B. Ninhydrin.
   R$_f$:

Racemomycin A	0.33
Racemomycin B	0.18
Racemomycin C	0.24
Racemomycin D	0.11

Ref:

H. Taniyama, Y. Sawada and T. Kitagawa,
J. Chromatogr., 56 (1971) 360—362.

RAMNACIN
PC.
1. **Paper:**

Solvent:
n-Butanol:acetic acid:water (4:1:5).
Detection:
Bioautography.
R$_f$:
0.92
Ref:

K. Ahmad and M.F. Islam, Nature, 176
(1955) 646—647.

RELOMYCIN
PC.
1. **Paper:**
   Whatman No. 1; 0.5 in. wide strips.
   Solvent:
   Isopropyl ether:methyl isobutyl ketone:2%
   aq. ammonium carbonate (2:1:2).
   Detection:
   Bioautography vs. *Bacillus subtilis* at pH 7.9.
   R$_f$:
   0.24
   Ref:

H.A. Whaley, E.L. Patterson, A.C. Dornbush,
E.J. Backus and N. Bohonus, Antimicrobial
Agents and Chemotherapy, 1963 (1964)
45—48.

RESISTAPHYLLIN
TLC.
1. **Medium:**
   Silica Gel.
   Solvent:
   A. Ethyl acetate.
   B. Ethyl acetate:benzene (1:1).
   C. Ethyl acetate:methanol (10:1).
   D. Chloroform.
   E. Acetone.
   Detection:
   Bioautography vs. *Bacillus subtilis.*
   R$_f$:

Solvent	R$_f$
A	0.45
B	0.00
C	0.90
D	0.00
E	1.00

Ref:

S. Aizawa, J. Nagatus, M. Shibuya,
H. Sugawara, C. Hirose and S. Shirato,
172nd Meeting Japan Antibiotics Assn.
April 4, 1970.

RHODOMYCINS
PC.
1. **Paper:**
   Circular paper chromatography.
   Solvent:
   Butanol:M/15 phosphate buffer pH 5.8.
   Detection:
   Color.
   R_f:
   Rhodomycin B > iso-rhodomycin B >
   rhodomycin A > iso-rhodomycin A.
   Ref:
   H. Brockmann and P. Patt, Chem. Ber., 88
   (1955) 1455–1468.

RIFAMYCINS
PC.
1. **Paper:**
   Whatman No. 1. Paper dipped in aq. buffered
   phase and dried.
   Solvent:
   A. n-Amyl alcohol:n-butanol (9:1) satd.
      with phosphate buffer, pH 8.6.
   B. As A, but 0.1% sodium ascorbate added.
   Detection:
   Bioautography vs. *Sarcina lutea*, pH 5.9.
   R_f:

Rifamycin	R_f Solvent A	Solvent B
B	0.25, 0.73	0.40
O	0.25, 0.73	0.40
S	0.73	0.87
SV	0.73	0.87

   Ref:
   P. Sensi, C. Coronelli and B.J.R. Nicolaus,
   J. Chromatogr., 5 (1961) 519–525.

2. **Paper:**
   As PC (1).
   Solvent:
   A. Phosphate buffer, pH 7.3 containing 0.1%
      sodium ascorbate satd. with n-amyl
      alcohol:n-butanol (9:1).
   B. n-Butanol satd. with phosphate buffer,
      pH 7.3 containing 0.1% sodium ascorbate.
   C. Phosphate buffer, pH 8.6 containing 0.1%
      sodium ascorbate satd. with n-butanol.
   Detection:
   As PC (1).
   R_f:

Rifamycin	R_f Solvent A	B	C
B	0.67	0.75	0.86
SV	0.51	0.95	0.67

   Ref:
   As PC (1).

3. **Paper:**
   Whatman No. 1.
   Solvent:
   Water containing 3% ammonium chloride
   + 1% ascorbic acid.
   Detection:
   Bioautography vs. *Sarcina lutea*.
   R_f:

Rifamycin	$R_f^\star$
A	0.05
B	0.25
C	0.45
D	0.60
E	0.75

   $\star$Estimated from drawing.
   Ref:
   P. Sensi, A.M. Greco and R. Ballotta,
   Antibiotics Annual (1959–1960) 262–270.

4. **Paper:**
   Whatman No. 1.
   Solvent:
   A. Water containing 3% ammonium chloride
      + 1% ascorbic acid.
   B. Butanol satd. with water.
   C. Water satd. with butanol.
   D. Butanol:acetic acid:water (4:1:5).
   E. Butanol:acetic acid:ethanol:water
      (25:3:25:47).
   F. Acetone:water (1:1).
   G. Chloroform:cyclohexane:water (8:1:2).
   Detection:
   As PC (3).
   R_f:
   Rifamycin B

Solvent	R_f
A	0.25
B	0.87
C	0.87
D	0.95
E	0.85
F	0.88
G	0.92

Ref:

As PC (3).

5. Centrifugal circular chromatography.
   Paper:
   As PC (1).
   Solvent:
   As PC (1) A. Solvent flow aimed 2 cm from center of paper rotating at 1500 r.p.m.; about 4 min.
   Detection:
   As PC (1).
   R_f:
   Rifamycin B can be separated from rifamycin SV.
   Ref:
   As PC (1).

6. **Paper:**
   Reversed phase paper partition chromatography. Paper impregnated with sec.-octyl alcohol.
   Solvent:
   M/15 phosphate buffer pH 8.6 with or without addition of sodium ascorbate.
   Detection:
   Color.
   R_f:

Rifamycin	Color	R_f
S	violet	0.04
O	yellow	0.08
SV	brown	0.50
B	yellow	0.80

   Ref:
   S. Sferruzza and R. Rangone, Il Farmaco, Ed. Pr. 19 (1964) 486–490.

TLC.
1. **Medium:**
   Silica Gel G. Plates dried at 105–110°C for 30 min and cooled in a desiccator.
   Solvent:
   Acetone.
   Detection:
   Color. Rifamycins B, O and SV are yellow; rifamycin S is red-violet.
   R_f:
   Rifamycin SV > O = S > B. Mixture of O and S can be detected by color difference.
   Ref:
   As PC (1).

2. **Medium:**
   Silica Gel G.
   Solvent:
   Chloroform:ethanol (2:1).
   Detection:
   Color (yellow-orange spot).
   R_f:
   Rifampicin [3-(4-methyl-piperazinyl-iminomethyl)rifamycin SV].
   Ref:
   N. Maggi, C.R. Pasqualucci, R. Ballotta and P. Sensi, Chemotherapia, 11 (1966) 285–292.

3. **Medium:**
   Silica Gel.
   Solvent:
   Chloroform:acetone (6:4).
   Detection:
   R_f:
   0.51
   Ref:
   H. Bickel and B. Fechtig, U.S. Pat. No. 3,644,337; February 22, 1972.

4. **Medium:**
   Eastman Chromagram Sheet No. 6060.
   Solvent:
   Chloroform:ethanol:0.1 N hydrochloric acid (84:15.9:0.1).
   Detection:
   The components are identified by their individual colors.
   R_f:
   0.55
   Ref:
   O.T. Kolos and L.L. Eidus, J. Chromatogr., 68 (1972) 294–295.

CCD.
1. **Solvent:**
   Methanol:0.01 N hydrochloric acid:benzene: petroleum ether (10:5:15:5), 100 transfers.
   Distribution:

Rifamycin	Tube No.
E	1–10
D	40–55
C	60–75
A	90–100

   Ref:
   As PC (3).

0165

RIMOCIDIN
PC.
1. Paper:
Whatman No. 1.
Solvent:
Water satd. n-butanol, descending, 18 h.
Detection:
Bioautography vs. *Saccharomyces carlsbergensis.*
R_f:
0.38
Ref:
J. Burns and D.F. Holtman, Antibiotics and Chemotherapy, 9 (1959) 398–405.

2. Paper:
As chromin, PC (1).
Solvent:
As chromin, PC (1).
Detection:
As chromin, PC (1).
R_f:
0.55
Ref:
As chromin, PC (1).

RISTOCETIN
PC.
1. Paper:
Eaton-Dikeman No. 613.
Solvent:
A. n-Butanol satd. with water:equilibrate 3 h, descending 16–17 h.
B. As A + 2% p-toluenesulfonic acid, 16–17 h.
C. As B + 2% piperidine, 16–17 h.
D. Methyl isobutyl ketone satd. with water; no equilibration, 3 h.
E. As D + 2% p-toluenesulfonic acid, 3 h.
F. As D + 2% piperidine (v/v), 3 h.
G. Water satd. with methyl isobutyl ketone: no equilibration, 3 h.
H. As G + 1% p-toluenesulfonic acid, 3 h.
I. As G + 1% piperidine (v/v), 3 h.
J. Water:methanol:acetone, 3:1 (3:1). Adjust to pH 10.5 with ammonium hydroxide than back to pH 7.5 with phosphoric acid; no equilibration, 3 h.
K. Methanol:water (80:20) + 1.5% sodium chloride. Paper buffered with soln. containing 0.95 M sodium sulfate +

0.05 M sodium bisulfate; equilibration 3 h; develop 16–17 h.
L. Amyl acetate satd. with 0.1 M potassium phosphate buffer, pH 6.15; equilibration 3 h; develop 16–17 h.
M. n-Butanol:methanol:water (40:10:20). Add excess methyl orange (ca. 1.5 g) and let stand at 28°C. Separate from insolubles; equilibration 3 h; develop 16–17 h.
All solvents run ascending except (A).
Detection:
Bioautography vs. *Bacillus subtilis.*
R_f:

Solvent	R_f
A	0.00
B	0.05
C	0.00
D	0.00
E	0.00
F	0.00
G	0.05
H	0.68
I	0.90
J	0.25
K	0.40
L	0.00
M	0.44

Ref:
J.E. Philip and J.R. Schenck, U.S. Patent 2,990,329; June 27, 1961.

2. Paper:
Whatman No. 1.
Solvent:
A. Pyridine:s-collidine:sec.-butanol:water (2:2:1:1).
B. As PC (1) K.
Both solvents run descending.
Detection:
Bioautography vs. *Bacillus subtilis* or *Corynebacterium xerosis.*
R_f:

Solvent	R_f	
A	0.85	
B	Ristocetin A	0.40
	Ristocetin B	0.15

Ref:
M.P. Kunstmann, L.A. Mitscher, J.N. Porter, A.J. Shay and M.A. Darken, Antimicrobial Agents and Chemotherapy, 1968 (1969) 242–245.

RORIDINES
TLC.
1. **Medium:**
    As verrucarines, TLC (1), A, B.
    Solvent:
    As verrucarines, TLC (1), A, B.
    Detection:
    As verrucarines, TLC (1), A, B.
    R_f:

	R_f (Medium-solvent)		
	(A-A)	(B-A)	(B-B)
Roridine A	0.70	0.18	0.21
Roridine B	0.55	0.26	0.49
Roridine C	–	–	0.41

Ref:
    As verrucarines, TLC (1).

2. **Medium:**
    As verrucarines, TLC (2).
    Solvent:
    As verrucarines, TLC (2), A, B, C.
    Detection:
    As verrucarines, TLC (2).
    R_f:

	R_f Solvent		
	A	B	C
Roridine E	0.40	0.35	0.24
Roridine D	0.35	0.29	0.18
Roridine A	0.21	0.20	0.14

Ref:
    As verrucarines, TLC (2).

RUBIDIN
PC.
1. **Paper:**
    Solvent:
    A. Dioxane:water (1:1).
    B. Ethanol:water (1:1).
    C. Water.
    D. Dioxane:water:benzene (12:2:3).
    E. n-Butanol:M/15 phosphate buffer, pH 5.8 (circular chromatography).
    Detection:
    R_f:

Solvent	R_f
A	0.80
B	0.78
C	0.63
D	1.00
E	1.00

Ref:
    A.K. Banerjie, G.P. Sen and P. Nandi, Antibiotics Annual (1955–1956) 640–647.

Color	
Iodine	UV
yellow brown	dark
dark green	dark
yellow brown	dark

RUBIFLAVIN
PC.
1. **Paper:**
    Whatman No. 1.
    Solvent:
    A. 2N ammonium hydroxide:tert.-amyl alcohol (1:1).
    B. Ethyl acetate:ethanol:water (3:1:3).
    Detection:
    R_f:

Solvent	R_f
A	0.66 (tailing)
B	0.90 (tailing)

Ref:
    A. Aszalos, M. Jelinek and B. Berk, Antimicrobial Agents and Chemotherapy, 1964 (1965) 68–74.

RUBRADIRIN
PC.
1. **Paper:**
    Schleicher and Schuell No. 589 blue ribbon.
    Solvent:
    Toluene:Skellysolve-C:methanol:0.1M phosphate buffer pH 7.0 (5:5:7:3).
    Equilibrated overnight; developed descending, 6 h.
    Detection:
    Bioautography vs. *Sarcina lutea.*
    R_f:
    0.6–0.8

Ref:

B.K. Bhuyan, S.P. Owen and A. Dietz, Antimicrobial Agents and Chemotherapy, 1964 (1965) 91–96.

CCD.

1. **Solvent:**

   Hexane:acetone:water (5:5:1), 200 transfers.

   Distribution:

   Pools made from tubes 84–95 and 96–113.

   Ref:

   C.E. Meyer, Antimicrobial Agents and Chemotherapy, 1964 (1965) 97–99.

SAFYNOL

TLC.

1. **Medium:**

   SilicAR (TLC-4GF, Mallinckrodt) 1 part, mixed with 40 parts Kieselgel (D5, A.H. Thomas).

   Solvent:

   A. Benzene:ethyl acetate:formic acid (75:24:1).

   B. Chloroform:acetone:formic acid (95:4:1).

   C. Ethyl ether:petroleum ether:formic acid (80:19:1).

   Detection:

   UV at 254 nm.

   R_f:

Solvent	R_f
A	0.21
B	0.17
C	0.50

   Ref:

   C.A. Thomas and E.H. Allen, Phytopath., 60 (1970) 261–263.

SARGANIN

PC.

1. **Paper:**

   Whatman No. 1.

   Solvent:

   A. 1-Butanol:water (84:16).

   B. As A + 0.25% p-toluenesulfonic acid.

   C. 1-Butanol:acetic acid:water (2:1:1).

   All systems developed 22 h.

   Detection:

   Bioautography vs. *Escherichia coli.*

   R_f:

Solvent	$R_f^{\star}$	
A	0.80	(major)
	0.90	(minor)
B	0.85	(major)
	0.92	(minor)
C	0.92	

*Estimated from drawing.

Ref:

N.G.M. Nadal, L.V. Rodriquez and C. Casillas, Antimicrobial Agents and Chemotherapy, 1964 (1965) 131–134.

SCLEROTHRICIN

PC.

1. **Paper:**

   Solvent:

   A. Butanol:methanol:ammonium hydroxide:water (10:4:3:3).

   B. n-Propanol:pyridine:acetic acid:water (15:10:3:10).

   Detection:

   Bioautography vs. *Bacillus subtilis* PCI-219.

   R_f:

Solvent	R_f (estimated from drawing)
A	0.35
B	0.45

   Ref:

   Y. Kono, S. Makino, S. Takeuchi and H. Yonehara, J. Antibiotics, 22 (1969) 583–589.

TLC.

1. **Medium:**

   Silica Gel G.

   Solvent:

   Chloroform:methanol:14% ammonium hydroxide (2:1:1).

   Detection:

   As PC (1).

   R_f:

   0.8 (estimated from drawing).

   Ref:

   As PC (1).

2. **Medium:**

   Alumina.

   Solvent:

   Ethanol:water (4:6).

   Detection:

   As PC (1).

R$_f$:

    0.35 (estimated from drawing).

Ref:

    As PC (1).

SCOPAFUNGIN

PC.

1. **Paper:**

    Solvent:

        A. 1-Butanol:water (84:16), 16 h.

        B. As A + 0.25% p-toluenesulfonic acid,
           16 h.

        C. 1-Butanol:acetic acid:water (2:1:1),
           16 h.

        D. As A + 2% piperidine, 16 h.

        E. 1-Butanol:water (4:96), 5 h.

        F. As E + 0.25% p-toluenesulfonic acid, 5 h.

    Detection:

        Bioautography vs. *Saccharomyces cerevisiae.*

    R$_f$:

Solvent	R$_f$*
A	0.18–0.50
B	0.65
C	0.85
D	0.18–0.50
E	0.10–0.35
F	0.10–0.35

    *Estimated from drawing.

    Ref:

        L.E. Johnson and A. Dietz, Appl. Microbiol.,
        22 (1971) 303–308.

TLC.

1. **Medium:**

    Silica Gel HF$_{254}$ (E. Merck) suspended in a
    soln. of buffer composed of 0.2 M disodium
    phosphate: 0.2 M potassium dihydrogen
    phosphate (1:1). Air dry, activate 2 h at
    130°C prior to use.

    Solvent:

        Methyl ethyl ketone:acetone:water
        (150:50:34).

    Detection:

        Spray with freshly prepared mixture of
        anisaldehyde:95% ethanol:conc. sulfuric
        acid:glacial acetic acid (0.5:9:0.5:0.1). Heat
        at 90–100°C for 5–10 min. Scopafungin
        appears as a dark blue spot.

    R$_f$:

    0.23

    Ref:

        M.E. Bergy and H. Hoeksema, J. Antibiotics,
        25 (1972) 39–43.

SENFOLOMYCINS

PC.

1. **Paper:**

    Whatman No. 1.

    Solvent:

        A. n-Heptane:diethylketone:tetrahydrofuran:
           water (8:3:3:8).

        B. Chloroform:carbon tetrachloride:
           methanol:water (4:4:1:8).

    Detection:

        Bioautography vs. *Bacillus subtilis* (pH 6.0).

    R$_f$:

Solvent	R$_f$ Senfolomycin A	B
A	0.75	0.54
B	0.47	0.15

    Ref:

        L.A. Mitscher, W. McCrae, S.E. DeVoe,
        A.J. Shay, W.K. Hausmann and N. Bohonos,
        Antimicrobial Agents and Chemotherapy,
        1965 (1966) 828–831.

SHARTRESIN

PC.

1. **Paper:**

    Leningradskaya M.

    Solvent:

        A. Methanol:ammonium hydroxide:water
           (20:1:4).

        B. Benzene:acetic acid:water (2:2:1).

        C. Benzene:methanol:water (1:1:2).

        D. n-Butanol:acetic acid:water (2:1:2).

    Detection:

    R$_f$:

Solvent	R$_f$
A	0.72
B	0.43
C	0.35
D	0.91

    Ref:

        D.Yu. Shenin, E.N. Sokolova and
        E.Yu. Konev, Antibiotiki, 15 (1970) 9–14.

SHINCOMYCINS

PC.

1. **Paper:**
   Solvent:
   A. Wet butanol.
   B. 3% Aq. ammonium chloride.
   C. 80% Phenol.
   D. 50% Acetone.
   E. Butanol:methanol:water (4:1:2).
   F. 1.5% Methyl orange.
   G. Benzene:methanol (4:1).
   H. Water.
   I. Butanol satd. water.
   J. Pyridine:propanol:acetic acid:water
   (10:15:3:12).
   Detection:
   R_f:

Solvent	R_f*
A	1.0
B	0.7
C	1.0
D	1.0
E	1.0
F	1.0
G	0.8
H	0.6
I	1.0
J	1.0

   *Estimated from drawing.
   Ref:
   N. Nishimura, K. Kumagai, N. Ishida, K. Saito,
   F. Kato and M. Azumi, J. Antibiotics, 18
   (1965) 251–258.

TLC.

1. **Medium:**
   Silica Gel containing 5% calcium sulfate.
   Solvent:
   A. Methanol:benzene (45:55).
   B. Chloroform:methanol (4:1).
   C. Acetone.
   D. Butanol:acetic acid:water (3:1:1).
   Detection:
   Spray with 10% sulfuric acid; heat at 120°C
   for 5 min. Shincomycins A and B give dark
   green and yellowish brown colors, respectively.
   R_f:

Solvent	R_f Shincomycin A	Shincomycin B
A	0.65	0.40
B	0.66	0.38
C	0.32	0.18
D	0.39	0.39

Ref:
N. Ishida, K. Kumagi and N. Nishimura,
U.S. Patent 3,534,138; October 13, 1970.

ELPHO.

1. **Medium:**
   Paper.
   Buffer:
   A. pH 5.0
   B pH 8.0
   Conditions:
   225 V/30 cm for 2 h.
   Mobility:
   A. Shincomycin A moves toward cathode.
   B. Shincomycin A moves slightly toward
   cathode.
   Ref:
   As PC (1).

SHOWDOMYCIN

PC.

1. **Paper:**
   Solvent:
   n-Butanol:water:acetic acid (4:5:1, upper
   phase), descending.
   Detection:
   UV absorption.
   R_f:
   0.41
   Ref:
   S. Roy-Burman, P. Roy-Burman and
   D.W. Visser, Cancer Res., 28 (1968)
   1605–1610.

2. **Paper:**
   Whatman No. 3 MM.
   Solvent:
   A. n-Butanol:ethanol:water (50:15:35).
   B. n-Butanol:formic acid:water (77:10:13).
   C. n-Butanol:methanol:water (20:7:8).
   All solvents developed ascending, 15–18 h.
   Detection:
   A. Bioautography vs. *Escherichia coli* K-12.
   B. UV.
   C. For analysis of showdomycin-^{14}C,
   papergrams are cut into 0.5–1.0 cm
   pieces and counted using a liquid
   scintillation spectrometer with a toluene
   phosphor soln.

R_f:

Solvent	R_f*
A	0.47
B	0.30
C	0.42

*Estimated from drawing.

Ref:

Y. Komatsu, J. Antibiotics, 24 (1971) 566–571.

SICCANIN

TLC.

1. **Medium:**

Eastman Chromagram Sheet 6061.

Solvent:

A. Benzene:acetone (10:1).

B. Benzene.

C. n-Hexane:ethanol (9:1).

All solvents developed to a height of 15 cm (10–30 min).

Detection:

Reagents:

a. 0.5 g benzidine dissolved in 1.4 ml conc. hydrochloric acid and 10 ml water, then made up to 100 ml.

b. 10% aq. sodium nitrite.

c. Mix (a):(b):acetone (2:2:1) immediately before use.

d. 0.5 N hydrochloric acid:acetone (1:1).

Procedure:

Dry sheet in warm air stream dipping into reagent (c) for 20 sec to develop red color of diazo compound. Remove excess reagent by blotting with filter paper immediately followed by dipping into reagent (d) for 40 sec. Blot excess hydrochloric acid and dry in warm air stream. Colors are as indicated under R_f. Quantitative determinations can be done by densitometric scan at 500–520 nm.

R_f:

	$R_{siccanin}$ in solvent systems			
	A	B	C	Color
Siccanin	1.00	1.00	1.00	dull red
Siccanochromene A	0.99	1.50	0.88	reddish brown
Siccanochromene B	0.85	0.50	0.67	reddish brown
Prechromene A	0.91	0.91	0.66	light brown

R_f values for siccanin in the solvent systems (A), (B) and (C) are approximately 0.64, 0.21 and 0.65, respectively.

Ref:

M. Arai, K. Hamano, K. Nose and K. Nakano, Annual Rept. Sankyo Res. Lab., 20 (1968) 93–98; M. Arai, K. Ishibashi and H. Okazaki, Antimicrobial Agents and Chemotherapy, 1969 (1970) 247–252.

SIOMYCINS

PC.

1. **Paper:**

Solvent:

Methanol:acetic acid:water (25:3:72).

Detection:

R_f:

Siomycin A	0.08–0.10
Siomycin B	0.30–0.31
Siomycin C	0.00

Ref:

M. Ebata, K. Miyazaki and H. Otsuka, J. Antibiotics, 22 (1969) 364–368.

TLC.

1. **Medium:**

Silica Gel G.

Solvent:

A. Chloroform:methanol (95:5).

B. Chloroform:methanol (90:10).

Detection:

R_f:

	R_f Siomycin		
Solvent	A	B	C
A	0.14	0.21	0.42
B	0.60	0.67	0.94

Ref:

As PC (1).

SISOMICIN
PC.
1. **Paper:**
   Whatman No. 1.
   Solvent:
   A. 80% methanol + 3% sodium chloride
      (w/v) (1:1), descending; paper buffered
      with 0.95 M sodium sulfate + 0.05 M
      sodium bisulfate dried before use.
   B. Propanol:pyridine:acetic acid:water
      (6:4:1:3), ascending.
   C. 80% phenol, ascending.
   D. Benzene:methanol (9:1), descending.
   E. n-Butanol:water:acetic acid (4:5:1),
      upper phase, ascending.
   F. Water satd. n-butanol + 2% p-toluene-
      sulfonic acid, descending 26 h.
   G. Chloroform:methanol:17% ammonium
      hydroxide (2:1:1), descending 16 h.
   Detection:
   A. Bioautography vs. *Staphylococcus aureus*
      ATCC 6538P.
   B. Ninhydrin spray (0.25% in pyridine:
      acetone, 1:1).
   R_f:

Solvent	R_f
A	0.49
B	0.29
C	0.45
D	0.00
E	0.00
F	0.51[*]
G	0.21[*]

   $$\frac{\text{*distance of zone from origin}}{\text{distance from origin to end of paper}}$$

   Ref:
   M.J. Weinstein, J.A. Marquez, R.T. Testa,
   G.H. Wagman, E.M. Oden and J.A. Waitz,
   J. Antibiotics, 23 (1970) 551–554;
   G.H. Wagman, R.T. Testa and J.A. Marquez,
   ibid, 555–558.

SPARSOGENIN
CCD.
1. **Solvent:**
   A. 1-Butanol:ethyl acetate:water
      (1.2:0.5:1.9), 300 transfers.
   B. 2-Butanol:water, 200 transfers.
   Distribution:
   A. K = 0.55
   B. K = 0.739

Ref:
   A.D. Argoudelis, C. DeBoer, T.E. Eble and
   R.R. Herr, U.S. Patent 3,629,406; December
   21, 1971.

SPARSOMYCIN
CCD.
1. **Solvent:**
   2-Butanol:water (1:1).
   Distribution:
   K = 0.74
   Ref:
   A.D. Argoudelis and R.R. Herr,
   Antimicrobial Agents and Chemotherapy,
   1962 (1963) 780–786.

SPHAEROPSIDIN
TLC.
1. **Medium:**
   Silica Gel GF$_{254}$ (E. Merck).
   Solvent:
   Ethyl acetate.
   Detection:
   A. UV absorbance.
   B. Spray with 10% phosphomolybdic acid
      and heat at 100°C.
   R_f:
   ca. 0.33
   Ref:
   J.M. Coats, M.E. Herr and R.R. Herr,
   U.S. Patent 3,585,111; June 15, 1971.

SPINAMYCIN
PC.
1. **Paper:**
   Toyo No. 51.
   Solvent:
   A. Acetone.
   B. Acetone:methanol (1:1).
   C. Methanol.
   D. Ethyl acetate.
   E. Ethyl acetate:chloroform (1:1).
   F. Butanol.
   G. Acetone:ethyl ether (1:1).
   Detection:
   R_f:

Solvent	R_f
A	1.00
B	0.72
C	0.62

D	1.00
E	0.95
F	1.00
G	1.00

Ref:

E.L. Wang, M. Hamada, Y. Okami and
H. Umezawa, J. Antibiotics, 19 (1966)
216–221.

TLC.

1. **Medium:**

Silica Gel.

Solvent:

A. Methanol.

B. Ethyl acetate:chloroform (1:1).

Detection:

R_f:

Solvent	R_f
A	0.66
B	0.27

Ref:

As PC (1).

SPORANGIOMYCIN

PC.

1. **Paper:**

Solvent:

A. Water satd. butanol.

B. As A + 2% p-toluenesulfonic acid.

C. As A + 2% conc. ammonia.

D. Butanol satd. water.

E. 20% Ammonium chloride.

F. Phenol:water (75:25).

G. n-Butanol:methanol:water (40:10:20),
   containing 0.75 g methyl orange.

H. n-Butanol:methanol:water (40:10:30).

I. Water:acetone (1:1).

J. Water satd. ethyl acetate.

Detection:

Bioautography vs. *Bacillus subtilis.*

R_f:

Solvent	R_f
A	0.88
B	0.83
C	0.82
D	0.10–0.50
E	0.00
F	0.98
G	0.94
H	0.91
I	0.10
J	0.88

Ref:

J.E. Thiemann, C. Coronelli, H. Pagani,
G. Beretta, G. Tamoni and V. Arioli,
J. Antibiotics, 21 (1968) 525–531.

SPOROCYTOPHAGE CAULIFORMIS
ANTIBIOTIC

PC.

1. **Paper:**

Solvent:

Water satd. butanol.

Detection:

A. Ninhydrin.

B. UV fluorescence.

R_f:

0.028 (ninhydrin +); 0.10 (fluorescent).

Ref:

German Patent No. 467,923; March 27, 1969.

SPOROVIRIDININ

PC.

1. **Paper:**

Solvent:

A. Butanol:pyridine:water:acetic acid
   (6:4:3:1).

B. Butanol:methanol:water (4:1:2).

Detection:

A. Bioautography.

B. UV light at 360 nm (yellowish-blue
   fluorescence; sporoviridin is not
   fluorescent).

R_f:

Solvent	R_f
A	0.51
B	0.37

Ref:

M. Suzuki, T. Takaishi and I. Takamori,
Derwent Farmdoc No. 41472
(JA.30481/69) published Sept. 12, 1969.

STAPHYLOMYCIN

PC.

1. **Paper:**

Solvent:

Propylene glycol:benzene, descending, 72 h.

Detection:

A. Bioautography vs. *Bacillus subtilis.*

B. Spray with 0.5% p-dimethylamino-
   benzaldehyde in 1 N hydrochloric acid
   and heat; red colored zones result.

R$_f$:

Factor S > factor M$_1$.

Ref:

H. Vanderhaeghe, P. Van Dijck, G. Parmentier
and P. De Somer, Antibiotics and
Chemotherapy, 7 (1957) 605–614.

STEFFISBURGENSIMYCIN
PC.

1. **Paper:**
Solvent:

A. 1-Butanol:water (84:16), 16 h.
B. As A + 0.25% p-toluenesulfonic acid,
16 h.
C. 1-Butanol:acetic acid:water (2:1:1), 16 h.
D. As A + 2% piperidine (v/v), 16 h.
E. 1-Butanol:water (4:96), 5 h.
F. As E + 0.25% p-toluenesulfonic acid, 5 h.

Detection:
R$_f$:

Solvent	R$_f$*
A	0.50–0.85
B	0.50–0.85
C	0.70–0.90
D	0.20–0.65
E	0.15–0.62
F	0.05–0.57

*Estimated from drawing.

Ref:

M.E. Bergy, J.H. Coats and F. Reusser, U.S.
Patent 3,309,273; March 14, 1967.

STREPTIMIDONE
CCD.

1. **Solvent:**

1-Butanol:cyclohexane:water (1:4:5),
25 transfers.

Distribution:

K = 1.10

Ref:

R.P. Frohardt, H.W. Dion, Z.L. Jakubowski,
A. Ryder, J.C. French and Q.R. Bartz,
J. Am. Chem. Soc., 81 (1959) 5500.

STREPTOLIN
PC.

1. **Paper:**

Eaton-Dikeman No. 613, buffered with
0.95 M sodium sulfate and 0.05 M sodium
acid sulfate and air dried before use.

Solvent:

75% Ethanol, 25°C, descending, 30–50 h.

Detection:

Bioautography vs. *Bacillus subtilis.*

R$_f$:

(Inches from origin; estimated from drawing)
Streptolin A   4.6
Streptolin B   6.5

Ref:

L.M. Larson, H. Sternberg and W.H. Peterson,
J. Am. Chem. Soc., 75 (1953) 2036.

STREPTOLYDIGIN
PC.

1. **Paper:**
Solvent:

A. n-Butanol:water (81:19).
B. n-Butanol:water:p-toluenesulfonic acid
(81:18.7:0.25).
C. n-Butanol:water:piperidine (81:17:2).
All solvents developed 16 h.
D. 1 M phosphate buffer, pH 7.0, descending,
4 h.

Detection:

Bioautography vs. *Mycobacterium avium*
ATCC 7992.

R$_f$:

Solvent	R$_f$*	
A	0.85	(tail)
B	0.90	(tail)
C	0.90	(tail)
D	0.15–0.30	

*Estimated from drawings.

Ref:

C. De Boer, A. Dietz, W.S. Silver and
G.M. Savage, Antibiotics Annual, (1955–
1956) 886–892.

STREPTOMYCES COLLINUS Lindenbein DIPEPTIDE ANTIBIOTIC
PC.

1. **Paper:**

Whatman No. 1.

Solvent:

A. Water-satd. 1-butanol + 2% p-toluenesulfonic acid.
B. Propanol:pyridine:acetic acid:water
(15:10:3:12).

Detection:

Bioautography vs. *Salmonella gallinarum.*

R_f:
Ref:

B.B. Molloy, D.H. Lively, R.M. Gale, M. Gorman, L.D. Boeck, C.E. Higgens, R.E. Kastner, L.L. Huckstep and N. Neuss, J. Antibiotics, 25 (1972) 137–140.

STREPTOMYCES RAMOCISSIMUS **ANTIBIOTIC**
TLC.

1. **Medium:**
    Silica Gel.
 Solvent:
    Acetone:ethyl acetate:water (12:8:1).
 Detection:
 R_f:
    Antibiotic separates into 3 components.
 Ref:
    Belgian Patent No. 771331; February 14, 1972.

STREPTOMYCES VIRIDOCHROMOGENES **ANTIBIOTIC**
PC.

1. **Paper:**
    Whatman No. 4 impregnated with acetone: water (7:3).
 Solvent:
    Benzene:chloroform:acetic acid:water (2:2:1:1).
 Detection:
 R_f:

Component A	0.35
Component B	0.25

 Ref:
    German Patent No. 1,954,047; published June 11, 1970.

STREPTOMYCIN
PC.

1. **Paper:**
    Whatman No. 1 or Eaton-Dikeman No. 613.
 Solvent:
    Water satd. n-butanol + 2% p-toluenesulfonic acid monohydrate; develop 24 h.
 Detection:
    Bioautography vs. *Bacillus subtilis*.
 R_f:
    Streptomycin > dihydroxystreptomycin > mannosidostreptomycin.

Ref:
D.H. Peterson and L.M. Reineke, J. Am. Chem. Soc., 72 (1950) 3598–3603.

2. **Paper:**
 Solvent:
    As PC (1).
 Detection:
    As PC (1).
 R_f:

	$R_{streptomycin}$
Streptomycin	1.00
Mannosidostreptomycin	0.37
Dihydroxystreptomycin	0.62
Hydroxystreptomycin	0.64

 Ref:
    J.N. Pereira, J. Biochem. and Microbiol. Tech. and Eng., 3 (1961) 79–85.

3. **Paper:**
    Whatman No. 20.
 Solvent:
    Equal vols of amyl alcohol containing 1% (v/v) di-2-ethyl hexyl phosphate and 0.5% sodium chloride in borate buffer (0.62 g boric acid, 0.21 g boraxe) are mixed. Adjust pH to 8.0 with sodium hydroxide while stirring for 30 min. Separate phases; dip paper in lower phase, blot, apply samples and dry several mins. While still wet develop with organic phase either ascending or descending.
 Detection:
    A. As PC (1).
    B. Spray or dip in alkaline α-naphthol-diacetyl color reagent [mix equal vols. of 40% (w/v) potassium hydroxide in 50% methanol, 2.5% (w/v) α-naphthol in methanol and 0.1% (w/v) diacetyl in methanol immediately before use in order given].
 R_f:

	$R_{streptomycin}$
Streptomycin	1.00 (R_f = 0.7)
Dihydrostreptomycin	0.83
Hydroxystreptomycin	0.73
Mannosidostreptomycin	0.43

 Ref:
    H. Heding, Acta Chem. Scand., 20 (1966) 1743–1746.

TLC.

1. **Medium:**

    Kieselgel G; heat at 110°C, 30 min. Spot compounds as phenyl hydrazones.

    Solvent:

    n-Butanol:water:methanol (40:20:10) + 1 g p-toluenesulfonic acid.

    Detection:

    Dry plate for 5 min at 110°C. Spray with a 1 + 4 dilution of the following mixture: sodium nitroprusside, 10 g; potassium permanganate, 0.15 g; 0.5 N sodium hydroxide, 2 ml; water, to 100 ml.

    R_f:

Streptomycin	0.60—0.62
Dihydroxystreptomycin	0.90—0.92

    Ref:

    P.A. Nussbaumer and M. Schorderet, Pharm. Acta Helv., 40 (1965) 205—209; ibid, 477—482.

2. **Medium:**

    Silica Gel G; heat at 110°C for 30 min and cool prior to use.

    Solvent:

    A. 3% Aq. sodium acetate.

    B. As A, but 4% aq. soln.

    Detection:

    1% Alcohol soln. of B.T.B. (yellowish spots on green background).

    R_f:

Compound	R_f Solvent A	B
Streptomycin	0.46	0.58
Dihydrodesoxystrepto-mycin	0.28	0.38
Dihydrostreptomycin	0.34	0.44

    Ref:

    T. Sato and H. Ikeda, Sci. Papers, Inst. Phys. Chem. Res., Tokyo, 59 (1965) 159—164.

3. **Medium:**

    Silica Gel G (Merck).

    Solvent:

    Water satd. n-butanol + 2% p-toluenesulfonic acid + 2% piperidine. Develop at 16°C, 3—5 h.

    Detection:

    Mix equal vols of 10% sodium hydroxide, 10% potassium ferricyanide and 10% sodium nitroprusside about 30 min prior to application to plate. Dry plate at 110°C, 15 min before spraying. Vermilion spots on a dark yellowish background.

    R_f:

	R_f		
Run	Streptomycin	Dihydro-streptomycin	Dihydrodesoxy-streptomycin
1	0.49	0.31	—
2	—	0.35	0.35
3	0.41	—	0.30

    Ref:

    T. Katayama and H. Ikeda, Sci. Papers, Inst. Phys. and Chem. Res., Tokyo, 60 (1966) 85—89.

STREPTONIGRIN

CCD.

1. **Solvent:**

    Ethyl acetate:3% phosphate buffer, pH 7.5; 100 transfers.

    Distribution:

    Peak at tube 34 (estimated from curve).

    Ref:

    K.V. Rao and W.P. Cullen, Antibiotics Annual (1959—1960) 950—953.

STREPTONIVICIN

PC.

1. **Paper:**

    Solvent:

    A. n-Butanol:water (81:19) + 0.25% p-toluenesulfonic acid.

    B. n-Butanol:water:acetic acid (50:25:25).

    C. n-Butanol:water:piperidine (78.4:18.6:2).

    D. Water:n-butanol (96:4).

    E. As D + 2% p-toluenesulfonic acid.

    Detection:

    R_f:

Solvent	R_f[*]
A	0.40—0.75
B	0.90
C	0.35—0.70
D	0.80
E	0.65

    [*]Estimated from drawing.

Ref:

H. Hoeksema, M.E. Bergy, W.G. Jackson, J.W. Shell, J.W. Hinman, A.E. Fonken, G.A. Boyack, E.L. Caron, J.H. Ford, W.H. Devries and G.F. Crum, Antibiotics and Chemotherapy, 6 (1956) 143–148.

STREPTOTHRICIN

streptothricin-like antibiotics

PC.

Circular paper chromatography.

1. **Paper:**

Filter paper circles. Samples spotted (ca. 4 μl) along an arc drawn 3.1 cm in diameter. Hydrochloride or sulfate derivatives used.

Solvent:

Propanol:pyridine:acetic acid:water (15:10:3:12), ca. 5.5 h, 23–24°C.

Detection:

A. Bioautography vs. *Bacillus subtilis*. (Sections cut out and tested.)

B. Ninhydrin spray.

R_f:

Antibiotic	Minimum No. of components	R_f HCL				$SO_4^=$			
Streptothricin	1	0.50				0.43			
Streptothricin VI	2	0.35,	0.50			0.32,	0.43		
Pleocidin complex	4	0.22,	0.35,	0.42,	0.50	0.20,	0.32,	0.37,	0.43
Viomycin	1	0.42				0.38			
Antibiotic 136	3	0.35,	0.40,	0.50		0.31,	0.43		
Streptolin A	2	0.24,	0.33			0.20,	0.33		
Streptolin B	3	0.30,	0.35,	0.50		0.27,	0.32,	0.43	
Antibiotic VIIa	3	0.30,	0.33,	0.44		0.27,	0.31,	0.41	
Antibiotic IXa	2	0.30,	0.44			0.27,	0.41		
Mycothricin complex	4	0.26,	0.35,	0.42,	0.50	0.23,	0.32,	0.37,	0.43
Geomycin	2	0.40,	0.33 (diffuse bands)			0.35,	0.26 (diffuse bands)		
Roseothricin A	2	0.30,	0.50			0.32,	0.43		
Roseothricin B	1	0.31				0.27			
Roseothricin C	1	0.28				0.24			

Ref:

M.I. Horowitz and C.P. Schaffner, Anal. Chem., 30 (1958) 1616–1620.

STREPTOVARICIN

PC.

1. **Paper:**

Schleicher and Schuell No. 589 (Blue Ribbon Special) impregnated with 0.2 M phosphate buffer at pH 4.1 and air dried.

Solvent:

Cyclohexane:chloroform:water (1:8:2). Equilibrate for 2 h in atmosphere of both phases and develop 5 h in organic phase.

Detection:

Bioautography vs. *Mycobacterium ranae*.

R_f:

Streptovaricin A	0.13
Streptovaricin B	0.37
Streptovaricin C	0.77
Streptovaricin D and E	0.88

Ref:

P. Siminoff, R.M. Smith, W.T. Sokolski and G.M. Savage, Amer. Rev. Tuberc., 75 (1957) 576–583.

2. **Paper:**

As PC (1). For quantitative determinations 0.25 in. wide strips used and standards applied as 0.025, 0.05, 0.10, 0.20, 0.30 and 0.50 μg streptovaricin A or 0.05, 0.10, 0.20, 0.40, 0.60 and 1.0 μg of B, C, or D. One set of standard used for every nine strips consisting of at least 3 replicates of each sample.

Solvent:

A. Methanol:benzene:water (1:1:2); equilibrate 16 h (chamber with both phases); develop 6 h.

B. Toluene:Skellysolve C:methanol:water
(5:5:7:3). Strips buffered with 0.2M
pH 4.1 phosphate buffer and dried prior
to use. Proceed as in A.

Detection:

Bioautography vs. *Mycobacterium ranae*
UC161, *Sarcina lutea* PCI1001 or *Bacillus
subtilis* UC564. Component potencies
estimated from satd. curves plotted as zone
width vs. logarithmic dose.

R_f:

Component	R_f* Solvent	
	A	B
A	0.35	0.02
B	0.65	0.07
C	0.72	0.15
D	0.82	0.60
E	0.88	0.75

*Estimated from drawings.

Ref:

W.T. Sokolski, N.J. Eilers and P. Siminoff,
Antibiotics Annual (1957–1958) 119–125.
See also H. Uamazaki, J. Antibiotics, 21
(1968) 204–208.

CCD.

1. **Solvent:**

Water:95% ethanol:cyclohexane:ethyl
acetate (1:1:1:1), 200 transfers.

Distribution:

3 components separate cleanly and a fourth
peak contains at least 2 components.

Ref:

G.B. Whitfield, E.C. Olson, R.R. Herr,
J.A. Fox, M.E. Bergy and G.A. Boyack,
Amer. Rev. Tuberc., 75 (1957) 584–587.

STREPTOVITACINS
PC.

1. **Paper:**

Schleicher and Schuell 589 (Blue Ribbon
special).

Solvent:

A. Water satd. ethyl acetate; paper pre-
impregnated with 0.1 M phosphate buffer
at pH 4.0; equilibrate 16 h; develop 6 h.
B. Upper phase of benzene:methanol:water
(1:1:2). Equilibrate and develop as A.
C. Butanol:water (84:16); develop 16 h
without equilibration.

Detection:

Bioautography vs. *Saccharomyces pastorianus*
ATCC 2366.

R_f:

Component	R_f* Solvent		
	A	B	C
A	0.35	0.0–0.1	0.52
B	0.45	0.0–0.1	0.55
C	0.55	0.0–0.1	0.60
D	0.72	0.0–0.1	0.68
E	0.87	0.0–0.1	0.75

*Estimated from drawing.

Ref:

W.T. Sokolski, N.J. Eilers and G.M. Savage,
Antibiotics Annual (1958–1959) 551–554.

2. **Paper:**

Whatman No. 1, 0.25 in. width.

Solvent:

As PC (1).

Detection:

Strips cut into 4 cm sections and exposed to
ethylene oxide vapors for 1 h. Each section
dropped into a tube containing 10 ml
Trichomonas vaginalis culture containing
10^4 cells/ml. After incubation at 37° for
48 h cells counted on a hemacytometer. Low
counts indicated antitrichomonal activity.

R_f:

Ref:

As PC (1).

3. Chromatography of streptovitacin A.
Paper:
Solvent:

Ethyl acetate:cyclohexane:pH 5.0 McIlvaines
buffer (7:1:8).

Detection:

R_f:

Ref:

T.E. Eble, M.E. Bergy, C.M. Large, R.R. Herr
and W.G. Jackson, Antibiotics Annual
(1958–1959) 555–559.

CCD.

1. Purification of streptovitacin A.
Solvent:

n-Amyl alcohol:isoamyl alcohol:water
(12:17:29).

Distribution:
Ref:
As PC (3).

STREPTOZOTOCIN
PC.
1. **Paper:**
Solvent:
A. n-Butanol:water (84:16).
B. As A + 0.25% (w/v) p-toluenesulfonic acid.
C. n-Butanol:acetic acid:water (2:1:1).
D. As A: piperidine (98:2).
E. Water:n-butanol (96:4).
F. As E + 0.25% p-toluenesulfonic acid.
Detection:
Bioautography.
R_f:

Solvent	R_f*
A	0.3
B	0.3
C	0.6
D	no zone
E	0.7
F	0.7

*Estimated from drawing.
Ref:
J.J. Vavra, C. De Boer, A. Dietz, L.J. Hanka and W.T. Sokolski, Antibiotics Annual (1959–1960) 230–235.

CCD.
1. **Solvent:**
Methyl ethyl ketone:water, 775 transfers.
Distribution:
Streptozotocin found in fractions 120–170.
Ref:
R.R. Herr, T.E. Eble, M.E. Bergy and H.K. Johnke, Antibiotics Annual (1959–1960) 236–240.

SUBSPORINS
TLC.
1. **Medium:**
Silica Gel G.
Solvent:
Chloroform:methanol:70% ethanol (7:3:5).
Detection:
R_f:
Subsporin C > B > A.

Ref:
M. Ebata, K. Miyazaki and Y. Takahashi, J. Antibiotics, 22 (1969).

SUBTILIN
CCD.
1. **Solvent:**
A. n-Butanol:water (1:1).
B. 20% Acetic acid:n-butanol (5:4).
C. 20% Acetic acid:iso-butanol (3:2).
D. 20% Acetic acid:n-butanol (1:1).
E. 4% Acetic acid:sec-butanol (6:5).
F. 20% Acetic acid:n-butanol (3:2).
Distribution:

Solvent	K
A	0.50
B	0.56, 0.55
C	0.33, 0.30, 0.28
D	0.45
E	0.33
F	0.40

Ref:
G. Alderton and N. Snell, J. Amer. Chem. Soc., 81 (1959) 701.

SUCCINIMYCIN
PC.
1. **Paper:**
Solvent:
A. n-Butanol:acetic acid:water (4:1:5).
B. Isopropanol:0.2M acetate buffer, pH 6.0 (70:30).
C. Ethanol:0.05M, pH 6.0 acetate buffer (80:20).
Detection:
Bioautography vs. *Bacillus subtilis*.
R_f:

Solvent	R_f
A	0.42
B	0.40
C	0.52

Ref:
T.H. Haskell, R.H. Bunge, J.C. French and Q.R. Bartz, J. Antibiotics, 16 (1963) 67–75.

ELPHO.
1. **Medium:**
Paper.
Buffer:
0.05M acetate, pH 4.0

Conditions:
360 V, 2.5 h.
Mobility:
7.9 cm.
Ref:
As PC (1).

CCD.

1. **Solvent:**
t-Butanol:aq. 0.1 M, pH 5.6 sodium acetate buffer, containing 142 g/l sodium sulfate (2·3).
Distribution:
Two peaks: major peak, K = 0.26; minor peak, K > 30.
Ref:
As PC (1).

SULFOCIDIN

PC.

1. **Paper:**
Solvent:
Aq. 3% ammonium chloride, descending.
Detection:
Bioautography vs. *Sarcina lutea*.
R_f:
0.0, 0.06, 0.13, 0.30
Ref:
M. Zief, R. Woodside, G.E. Horn, Antibiotics Annual (1957–1958) 886–892.

SULFOMYCINS

PC.

1. **Paper:**
Solvent:
A. Wet n-butanol.
B. 20% Aq. ammonium chloride.
C. 50% Aq. acetone.
D. n-Butanol:methanol:water:methyl orange [40:10:20 (v/v):1.5 w/v].
E. n-Butanol:methanol:water (40:10:20).
F. Benzene:methanol (4:1).
G. Water.
Detection:
Bioautography vs. *Bacillus subtilis*.
R_f:

Solvent	R_f (complex)
A	0.79
B	0.00
C	0.63

D	0.92
E	0.87
F	0.63
G	0.00

Ref:
Y. Egawa, K. Umino, Y. Tamura, M. Shimizu, K. Kaneko, M. Sakurazawa, S. Awataguchi and T.O. Kuda, J. Antibiotics, 22 (1969) 12–47.

2. **Paper:**
Toyo Roshi No. 51.
Solvent:
A. Ethyl acetate satd. with water.
B. n-Butanol satd. with water.
C. Chloroform:methanol (10:1).
All solvents developed ascending, 5 h.
Detection:
As PC (1).
R_f:

Solvent	R_f Sulfomycin		
	I	II	III
A	0.59	0.80	0.35
B	0.70	0.80	0.63
C	0.38	0.46	0.30

Ref:
As PC (1).

TLC.

1. **Medium:**
Kieselgel GF$_{254}$.
Solvent:
A. Ethyl acetate satd. with water.
B. Ethyl acetate:n-butanol (1:1) satd. with water.
C. Chloroform:methanol (10:1).
Detection:
As PC (1).
R_f:

Solvent	R_f Sulfomycin			
	I	II	III	Minor
A	0.13	0.26	0.05	—
B	0.87	0.93	0.84	—
C	0.38	0.46	0.30	0.42, 0.44, 0.49

Ref:
As PC (1).

TAIMYCINES
TLC.
1. **Medium:**
   A. MN Kieselgel G_{254}.
   B. Kieselgel G.
   C. Kieselgel $HF_{254-366}$.
   D. Alumina.
   Solvent:
   A. Butanol:acetone:water (4:5:1).
   B. Ethyl acetate:pyridine:isopropanol:water (7:2:3:2).
   C. Propanol:ethyl acetate:water (8:1:1).
   D. Butanol:pyridine:water (6:4:3).
   Detection:
   R_f:

		R_f Taimycine		
Medium	Solvent	A	B	C
A	A	0.40	0.30	0.70
B	A	0.60	0.30	0.75
C	A	0.35	0.25	0.50
A	B	0.50	0.50	0.80
B	C	0.45	0.25	0.50
D	D	0.50	0.30	0.70

   Ref:
   G. Cassinelli, E. Cotta and R. Mazzoleni, U.S. Patent 3,644,619; February 22, 1972.

TBILIMYCIN
CCD.
1. **Solvent:**
   A. Methanol:chloroform:borate buffer, pH 8.2 (2:2:1), 100 transfers.
   B. As A, but 220 transfers.
   Distribution:
   A. Kp = 1.93
   B. Tbilimycin peak, tube 145.
   Ref:
   D.Yu. Shenin, E.N. Sokolova and E.Yu. Konev, Antibiotiki, 15 (1970) 9–14.

TENNECETIN
PC.
1. **Paper:**
   Whatman No. 1.
   Solvent:
   Water satd. n-butanol, descending.
   Detection:
   Bioautography vs. *Saccharomyces carlsbergensis* K-20.

R_f:
   0.33
Ref:
   J. Burns and D.F. Holtman, Antibiotics and Chemotherapy, 9 (1959) 398–405.

TERTIOMYCINS
PC.
1. **Paper:**
   Solvent:
   A. Benzene:citrate buffer, pH 4.6.
   B. Butyl acetate:citrate buffer, pH 4.0.
   Detection:
   R_f:
   (Tertiomycin B)

Solvent	R_f
A	0.08–0.11
B	0.69–0.85

   Ref:
   T. Osato, K. Yagashita and H. Umezawa, J. Antibiotics, 8 (1955) 161–163.

2. **Paper:**
   Solvent:
   A. 1% Aq. ammonium hydroxide.
   B. 20% Dioxane.
   C. Butanol:acetic acid:water (70:5:25).
   D. Butanol:ammonium hydroxide:water (70:5:25).
   E. Ethyl acetate:acetic acid:water (88:6:6).
   F. Ethyl acetate:ammonium hydroxide:water (88:6:6).
   G. Water.
   H. Benzene:water (80:20).
   I. Butanol:methanol:water (4:1:2).
   J. 5% Acetone.
   K. 20% Ammonium chloride.
   L. Water satd. ether.
   M. 1% Acetic acid.
   N. Ethyl acetate.
   R_f:
   (Tertiomycin A)

Solvent	R_f
A	0.41
B	0.00
C	1.00
D	1.00
E	1.00
F	0.00
G	0.33

H	1.00
I	1.00
J	1.00
K	0.84
L	1.00
M	0.85
N	1.00

Ref:

A. Miyake, H. Iwasaki and T. Takewaka,
J. Antibiotics, 12 (1959) 59–64.

CCD.

1. **Solvent:**

Citrate buffer, pH 4.6:benzene; 30 transfers.

Distribution:

Peak found at tube 21.

Ref:

T. Osato, M. Ueda, S. Fukuyama,
K. Yagishita, Y. Okami and H. Umezawa,
J. Antibiotics, 8 (1955) 105–109.

TETRACYCLINES

This section includes data on chlortetracycline, 6-demethyltetracycline, oxytetracycline, tetracycline and various tetracycline derivatives and degradation products. Because the published data often includes a variety of these antibiotics in a given chromatographic system, the tetracyclines have been grouped by system rather than by compound. It may be necessary to examine each chromatographic category in order to locate a particular member of this family of antibiotics.

Many of the tetracyclines can be detected by exhibition of a bright yellow or orange fluorescence under UV light which is enhanced by gentle treatment with ammonia vapor. Bioautography against a number of susceptible organisms is useful in detecting trace quantities of these antibiotics.

PC.

1. **Paper:**

Whatman No. 4.

Solvent:

n-Butanol:acetic acid:water (4:1:5).

Detection:

A. UV fluorescence.

B. Bioautography vs. *Bacillus subtilis*.

R_f:

Oxytetracycline, 0.55

Ref:

P.P. Regna and I.A. Solomons, Ann. N.Y. Acad. Sci., 53, Art. 2 (1950) 229–237.

2. **Paper:**

Solvent:

A. Paper treated with McIlvaines buffer pH 3.5 as stationary phase; mobile phase, nitromethane:chloroform:pyridine: n-butanol (20:10:5:3).

B. Stationary phase as A, but pH 4.2; mobile phase, toluene:pyridine (20:3).

C. Stationary phase as B; mobile phase, ethyl acetate satd. with water.

Detection:

UV light.

R_f:

	R_f Solvent system	
Compound	A	B
12α-desoxytetracycline	0.70–0.75	–
10,12α-(0,0·diacetyl)-5-oxytetracycline	–	0.13–0.21

Ref:

German "Auslegeschrift" 1141638; published December 27, 1962.

3. **Paper:**

Eaton-Dikeman No. 613 soaked in 0.3 M pH 3 phosphate buffer and air-dried.

Solvent:

A. n-Butanol satd. with water.

B. n-Amyl acetate satd. with water, 48–72 h (solvent allowed to drip off paper).

Detection:

Bioautography vs. *Bacillus cereus* on pH 6.0 nutrient agar.

R_f:

	R_f Solvent system	
Compound	A	B
Tetracycline	0.40 ± 0.06	Oxytetracycline
Oxytetracycline	0.40 ± 0.06	> tetracycline;
Chlortetracycline	0.65 ± 0.05	chlorotetracycline moves off paper.

Ref:

N. Bohonos, A.C. Dornbush, L.I. Feldman, J.H. Martin, E. Pelcak and J.H. Williams, Antibiotics Annual (1953–1954) 49–55.

4. **Paper:**

Schleicher and Schuell No. 507.

Solvent:

Acetic acid:n-butanol:water (1:2:1).

Detection:

Bioautography.

R_f:

Chlortetracycline, 0.77

Ref:

R.J. Hickey and W.F. Phillips, Anal. Chem.,
26 (1954) 1640.

5. **Paper:**

Whatman No. 1.

Solvent:

Mix n-butyl acetate:methyl isobutyl ketone:
n-butanol:water (5 ml:15 ml:2 ml:22 ml).
Add 2 ml formic acid to the separated
organic phase. Develop ascending.

Detection:

Spray with 5% methanolic soln. of ferric
chloride.

R_f:

Chlortetracycline > tetracycline >
oxytetracycline.

Ref:

H. Fischbach and J. Levine, Antibiotics and
Chemotherapy, 5 (1955) 610–612.

6. **Paper:**

Whatman No. 1. Buffer paper with
McIlvaine's pH 3.5 buffer, blot firmly, spot
antibiotics and develop in solvent while still
damp.

Solvent:

Chloroform:nitromethane:pyridine (10:20:3),
ascending.

Detection:

UV fluorescence; greatly enhanced by
fuming with ammonia vapor.

R_f:

	R_f
Chlortetracycline	0.50
Tetracycline	0.28
Oxytetracycline	0.13
epi-Chlortetracycline	0.08
epi-Tetracycline	0.05

Ref:

G.B. Selzer and W.W. Wright, Antibiotics
and Chemotherapy, 7 (1957) 292–296.

7. **Paper:**

Solvent:

A. 0.3 M sodium phosphate (pH 3.0)/
n-butanol.

B. McIlvaines buffer (pH 4.7)/ethyl acetate.

C. 0.3 N phosphoric acid + 0.1% trichloro-
acetic acid/chloroform:n-butanol (9:1).

Detection:

R_f:

	R_f Solvent System		
	A	B	C
7-chloro-5a(11a)-dehydrotetra-cycline	0.49	0.87	0.39
5-epi-tetracycline	0.65	—	—

Ref:

J.R.D. McCormick, P.A. Miller, J.A. Growich,
N.O. Sjolander and A.P. Doerschuk, J. Amer.
Chem. Soc., 80 (1958) 5572.

8. **Paper:**

Whatman No. 1 impregnated by drawing
through 0.1 M disodium ethylenediaminetetraacetic acid and drying in air.

Solvent:

A. n-Butanol:acetic acid:water (4:1:5),
upper phase, descending, 16–20 h.

B. n-Butanol:ammonium hydroxide:water
(4:1:5), upper phase, descending,
16–20 h. Purge chamber with nitrogen
(to remove O_2) before use.

Detection:

Expose chromatogram to ammonia vapor
and view under UV light. Most compounds
give yellow to orange spot; iso compounds,
blue fluorescence; chlortetracycline, blue
fluorescence in solvent A.

R_f:

	R_f Solvent System	
	A	B
Tetracycline	0.65	0.39
4-Epitetracycline	0.65	0.15
Oxytetracycline	0.59	0.27
Chlortetracycline	0.76	0.47
Isochlortetracycline	0.67	0.47
Anhydrotetracycline	0.87	0.62
4-Epianhydrotetracycline	0.87	0.40
Demethylchlortetracycline	0.72	0.35
4-Epidemethylchlortetra-cycline	0.72	0.17
Isotetracycline	0.46	0.21
Anhydrodemethylchlor-tetracycline	0.89	0.70

4-Epianhydrodemethyl-
  chlortetracycline   0.92   0.44
Ref:
R.G. Kelly and D.A. Buyske, Antibiotics
and Chemotherapy, 10 (1960) 604–607.

9. **Paper:**
Whatman No. 1; paper is moistened with a
soln. composed as follows: 500 ml 0.1 N
citric acid, 208 ml 0.2 N disodium phosphate
containing 10 mg of sodium benzoate (as
preservative) and satd. with a solvent
mixture of nitromethane:chloroform:
pyridine (20:10:3).
Solvent:
Organic phase of above mixture, descending.
Detection:
R_f:

	R_f
Tetracycline	0.45
4-Epi-tetracycline	0.10
6-Demethyl-7-chlortetracycline	0.37
4-Epi-6-demethyl-7-chlortetracycline	0.12

Ref:
M.M. Noseworthy, U.S. Patent 3,009,956;
November 21, 1961.

10. **Paper:**
Whatman No. 4 satd. with aq. citrate-
phosphate buffer, pH 4.2.
Solvent:
Toluene:pyridine (20:3), satd. with water.
Detection:
R_f:

| 6-Demethyl-6-deoxytetracycline | 0.47 |
| C-4 epimer of above | 0.30 |

Ref:
As PC (9).

11. **Paper:**
Whatman No. 1; useful for radioactive
5-hydrotetracycline. Paper buffered with a
mixture of 0.3 M sodium dihydrogen
phosphate adjusted to pH 3.0 with
phosphoric acid, and air dried.
Solvent:
A. Ethyl acetate:phosphate-citrate buffer
   pH 4.5. Buffer composed of equal vols.
   of 0.4 M disodium phosphate and 4.5%
   citric acid. Develop descending 18 h.
B. Nitromethane:benzene:pyridine:pH 3.4
   buffer (20:10:3:3). Buffer composed of
   30 vols. of 0.2 M disodium phosphate and
   70 vols. of 2.24% citric acid. Develop
   descending 18 h.
Detection:
Scan with Geiger-Muller counter.
R_f:

| | Solvent | |
	A	B
5-hydroxytetracycline	0.58	0.24

Ref:
P.A. Miller and J.R.D. McCormick, U.S.
Patent 3,023,148; February 22, 1962.

12. **Paper:**
Whatman No. 1 satd. with disodium
phosphate-citric acid buffer at pH 3.5.
Solvent:
A. Nitromethane:chloroform:pyridine
   (20:10:3).
B. Nitromethane:toluene:butanol:pyridine
   (20:10:5:3).
Detection:
R_f:
0.35 in both solvents.
Ref:
R.K. Blackwood, U.S. Patent 3,026,354;
March 20, 1962.

13. **Paper:**
Whatman modified cellulose phosphate
cation-exchange paper.
Solvent:
0.1% (w/v) aq. ammonium chloride.
Detection:
R_f:

	R_f
Tetracycline	0.59
Epitetracycline	0.36
Chlortetracycline	0.61
Oxytetracycline	0.61
6-Demethylchlortetracycline	0.53
Epi-6-demethyl-chlortetracycline	0.32
6-Demethyl-6-desoxytetracycline	0.42
Epi-6-demethyl-6-desoxy-	
tetracycline	0.21
6-Methylene oxytetracycline	0.46
Anhydrotetracycline	0.14

Ref:
E. Addison and R.G. Clark, J. Pharm.
Pharmacol., 15 (1963) 268–272.

14. **Paper:**
    (Circular chromatography) Whatman No. 1, 28 cm diameter.

Solvent:
    McIlvaine's pH 4.5 buffer/chloroform: n-butanol (4:1), 90 min.

Detection:
    UV fluorescence.

R_f:

	R_f
Chlortetracycline	0.70—0.73
Demethylchlortetracycline	0.56—0.60
Tetracycline	0.47—0.50
Demethyltetracycline	0.38—0.41
Epimers	0.27—0.30

Ref:
    M. Urx, J. Vondrackova, L. Kovarik, O. Horsky and M. Herold, J. Chromatogr., 11 (1963) 62—65.

15. **Paper:**
    Treated with buffer, as below.

Solvent:
    A. pH 4.2 buffer/benzene:chloroform (1:1) satd. with water.
    B. pH 4.2 buffer/toluene:pyridine (20:3) satd. with pH 4.2 buffer.
    C. pH 3.5 buffer/nitromethane:chloroform: pyridine (20:10:3).
    D. pH 3.5 buffer/ethyl acetate satd. with water.

Detection:

R_f :

	R_f Solvent System			
	A	B	C	D
4a12a-anhydrotetracycline	0.86	0.88	0.90	1.00
12a(O-formyl) tetracycline	0.05	0.27	0.63	0.65
12a(O-formyl) chlortetracycline	—	0.52	—	—

Ref:
    C.R. Stephans, Jr. and R.K. Blackwood, U.S. Patent 3,081,346; March 12, 1963.

16. **Paper:**
    Leningrad "Quicky" soaked with McIlvaine's buffer pH 4.5 and dried.

Solvent:
    Ethyl acetate:water (1:1), 3—4 h.

Detection:
    UV fluorescence after exposing to ammonia vapors 5—10 sec.

R_f:
    From starting line; isotetracycline, epitetracycline, epichlortetracycline, isochlortetracycline, tetracycline, hydroxytetracycline, demethylchlortetracycline, chlortetracycline, anhydrotetracycline, anhydrochlortetracycline.

Ref:
    T.N. Lasnikova and N.G. Makarevich, Antibiotiki, 9 (1964) 579—583.

17. **Paper:**
    Leningrad "Quicky" treated with phosphate buffer pH 2.5 (0.3 M soln. phosphoric acid brought to pH 2.5 with strong soln. of potassium hydroxide). Paper is used while still damp.

Solvent:
    n-Butanol:acetic acid:water (4:1:5), 20 h.

Detection:
    UV fluorescence.

R_f:
    From starting line; isotetracycline, hydroxytetracycline, tetracycline, isochlortetracycline, demethylchlortetracycline, chlortetracycline, anhydrotetracycline.

Ref:
    As PC (16).

18. **Paper:**
    Paper satd. with 0.3 M phosphate buffer (pH 2.5) and air dried.

Solvent:
    A. n-Butanol satd. with water; equilibrate 4 h, develop overnight.
    B. Ethyl acetate satd. with water; equilibrate overnight.
    C. Chloroform:2-chloroethanol:water (2:1:1), organic phase; equilibrate overnight.

Detection:

R_f:

	R_f* Solvent System		
	A	B	C
5-Hydroxy-7-chlortetracycline	0.65	0.42	0.56
7-Chlortetracycline	0.65	0.03; 0.25	0.35; 0.65
Tetracycline	0.38	0.01; 0.05	0.16; 0.38
7-Chloro-6-demethyltetracycline	0.52	0.01; 0.15	0.23; 0.25
2-Acetyl-5-hydroxytetracycline	0.63	—	0.65
5-Hydroxytetracycline	0.38	0.08	0.17
Reduction product of oxychlortetracycline	0.37	0.08	0.17

*The double zones reflect the separation of the 4-epimers. In each case the natural product has the higher R_f value and its 4-epimer the lower.

Ref:

J.H. Martin, L.A. Mitscher, P.A. Miller,
P. Shu and N. Bohonos, Antimicrobial
Agents and Chemotherapy, 1966(1967)
563–567.

19. Paper:

Whatman No. 4 impregnated with 0.15 M
phosphate buffer pH 3.0 and dried.

Solvent:

n-Butanol:chloroform (9:1), 6 h, 22–25°C.

Detection:

R_f:

	R_f
Tetracycline	0.34–0.42
Chlortetracycline	0.57–0.68
Anhydrotetracycline	0.79–0.88

Ref:

J. Vondráčková and O. Štrauchová,
J. Chromatogr., 32 (1968) 780–781.

20. Paper:

Treated with buffer at pH 3.5 or 4.2 as
noted under solvent.

Solvent:

A. Pyridine:toluene (3:20) satd. with water,
pH 4.2 paper.

B. Toluene:1-butanol:nitromethane:pyridine
(10:5:20:3), pH 3.5 paper.

C. Ethyl acetate:nitromethane:chloroform
(40:25:7), pH 4.2 paper.

D. Ethyl acetate:chloroform:pyridine
(40:15:5), pH 4.2 paper.

E. Ethyl acetate satd. with water, pH 4.2
paper.

Detection:

R_f:

dl-6-demethyl-6-deoxytetracycline.

Solvent	R_f*
A	0.5
B	0.9
C	0.8
D	0.6
E	0.7

*Estimated from drawing.

Ref:

J.J. Korst, J.D. Johnston, K. Butler,
E.J. Bianco, L.H. Conover and
R.B. Woodward, J. Amer. Chem. Soc., 90
(1968) 439–457.

21. Paper:

Whatman No. 1 buffered at pH 4.5 with
0.05 M potassium citrate and hydrated by
dipping into an aq. soln. of 80% (v/v)
acetone and air drying to evaporate the
acetone.

Solvent:

Hexane:ethyl acetate (3:1), descending.

Detection:

A. UV light at 254 nm to detect absorbing
and fluorescent compounds. Spots are
outlined, the chromatogram exposed
momentarily to ammonia vapor and
re-examined under UV light.

B. Bioautography vs. Staphylococcus aureus
209P.

R_f:

Compound	R_f	Inhibitory activity	Fluorescence before ammonia	Fluorescence after ammonia
7-Chloro-6-demethyl-4-dedimethyl-aminotetracycline	0.80	+	dull orange	green
7-Chloro-6-demethyl-5a,6-anhydro-tetracycline	0.94	+	red-orange	orange
7-Chloro-6-demethyl-5a,6-anhydro-4-dedimethylaminotetracycline	0.98	+	red-orange	red-orange
9-Hydroxy-7-chloro-5-demethyl-4-dedimethylaminotetracycline	0.15	+	orange	orange
9-Hydroxy-7-chloro-6-demethyl-tetracycline	0.00	+	orange	orange

Ref:

S.L. Neidleman, R.W. Kinney,
F.L. Weisenborn, U.S. Patent 3,375,276;
March 26, 1968.

22. **Paper:**

Whatman No. 1 satd. with pH 3.0 phosphate
buffer and dried at room temperature.

Solvent:

n-Butanol satd. with water, 5–10°C,
ascending, 48 h.

Detection:

Air dry chromatograms and hang in
ammonia chamber for 15 sec to neutralize
acid. Expose to UV for 30 sec. Spray with
arsenomolybalate reagent and heat 10–15
min at 90°C. Greenish spots result.

R_f:

Chlortetracycline > tetracycline.

Ref:

Abou-Zeid A. Abou-Zeid, Indian J. Pharm.,
32 (1970) 59–61.

23. **Paper:**

Whatman No. 1 treated with 0.3 M
phosphate buffer pH 2.0 as stationary phase.

Solvent:

A. Butanol satd. with stationary phase.
B. Upper layer of n-butyl acetate:0.3 M
pH 2.0 phosphate buffer:5% trichloro-
acetic acid (5:4:1).

Detection:

R_f:

	Solvent	R_f
6-Demethyltetracycline-6-sulfuric acid ester	A	0.25
7-Chloro-6-demethyltetra-cycline-6-sulfuric acid ester	A	0.29
7-Chloro-6-demethyl-9-nitrotetracycline-6-sulfuric acid ester	A	0.29
5a,6-Anhydro-7-chloro-6-demethyltetracycline	B	0.68
5a,6-Anhydro-6-demethyl-tetracycline	A	0.72
	B	0.53
5a,6-Anhydro-7-chloro-6-demethyl-9-nitrotetra-cycline	A	0.70

Ref:

M. Tobkes and R.G. Wilkinson, U.S. Patent
3,549,681; December 22, 1970.

24. **Paper:**

Solvent:

A. 0.3 M sodium phosphate, pH 3.0/n-butyl
acetate.
B. 0.3 M sodium phosphate, pH 3.0/n-butanol.
C. McIlvaines buffer, pH 4.7/ethyl acetate.
D. 0.3 N phosphoric acid, 0.1% trichloro-
acetic acid/chloroform:n-butanol (9:1).

Detection:

R_f:

	6-demethyltetracycline
Solvent	R_f
A	0.30
B	0.30
C	0.27
D	0.22

Ref:
J.A. Growich, Jr., U.S. Patent 3,616,240; October 26, 1971.

TLC.

1. Circular Chromatography.

Medium:

A. Silica Gel G (according to Stahl). Plates activated at 110°C for 1 h and stored in a vacuum desiccator.

B. 9 g of EDTA dissolved in 60 ml water and 30 g Silica Gel G added. Plates coated to give a 250 μ thickness. Dry at room temperature before placing in oven and store as in (A).

Both A and B plates contain 1/8 in. dia. hole in center. Compounds spotted around center hole.

Solvent:

A. n-Butanol:oxalic acid:water (100 ml:5 g: 100 ml), organic phase.

B. n-Butanol:tartaric acid:water (100 ml: 6 g:100 ml), organic phase.

C. n-Butanol satd. with water.

Development carried out using 14 cm Petri dishes; Whatman No. 1 paper wick inserted in center hole and dipped into solvent, plate placed face down. Top of hole is covered with a vial. Development allowed to proceed until solvent front reaches 6.5 cm from center.

Detection:

A. UV light.

B. Spray with 5% methanolic soln. of ferric chloride. Dark grayish bands result.

R_f:

| | R_f (Medium-Solvent) | | |
	A-A	A-B	B-C
Tetracycline	0.38	0.26	0.23
Oxytetracycline	0.46	0.31	0.27
Chlortetracycline	0.49	0.35	0.30
Chlortetracycline HCl	0.49	0.35	0.30

Ref:
G.J. Kapadia and G.S. Rao, J. Pharm. Sci., 53 (1964) 223–224.

2. **Medium:**

Kieselguhr G impregnated with glycerol: phosphate-citrate buffer soln. (pH 3.7). Buffer is prepared by mixing 34 ml 0.2 M disodium hydrogen phosphate with 66 ml 0.1 M citric acid. For impregnation, 95 ml buffer is brought to 100 ml with glycerol. The plate is impregnated by placing the edge in the buffer solution in a chamber. After impregnation, air dry for 45 min at room temperature.

Solvent:

Chloroform:acetone (1:1) saturated with impregnating soln.

Detection:

UV light at 350 nm.

R_f:

Chlortetracycline > tetracycline > oxytetracycline.

Ref:
D. Sonamini and L. Anker, Pharm. Acta Helv., 39 (1964) 518–523.

3. **Medium:**

Coat plates with a mixture of Silica Gel G (after Stahl) and sodium ethylenediaminetetraacetate (sodium EDTA). Mix 30 g silica gel in a soln. of 9 g sodium EDTA in 50 ml water and coat to a thickness of 0.25 mm. Dry at 100°C for 30 min.

Solvent:

n-Butanol satd. with water.

Detection:

UV light after exposure to ammonia vapor.

R_f:

	R_f
Tetracycline	0.36
4-Epitetracycline	0.36
4-Epianhydrotetracycline	0.40
Anhydrotetracycline	0.50

Ref:
L. Rustici and M. Ferappi, Boll. Chim. Farm., 104 (1965) 305–308.

4. **Medium:**

Microcrystalline cellulose (50 g) is passed through a 100 mesh sieve and mixed in a mortar and pestle for 2 min with 180 ml of 0.05% ammonium chloride soln. A 0.25 ml layer is applied to glass plates, dried at room temperature for 10 min and heated at 90°C for 30 min. No special storage conditions are necessary.

Solvent:

0.1% Aq. ammonium chloride (pH 5.6), developed 20 min.

Detection:

(Anhydrotetracycline)

A. Qualitative: Visible yellow zones.

B. Quantitative: Individual zones scraped off and collected in 3 ml sintered glass funnels. Wash into 10 ml volumetric flasks with hot methanol and determine absorbance at 428 nm against a methanol blank. Average 5 determinations for each concentration and read against standard curve in range 10–60 mcg anhydrotetracycline per spot.

R_f:

0.35

Ref:

D.L. Simmons, C.K. Koorengevel, R. Kubelka and P. Seers, J. Pharm. Sci., 55 (1966) 219–220.

5. **Medium:**

Diatomaceous earth prepared as follows: Wash diatomaceous earth with hot 6 N hydrochloric acid until washings contain no calcium or iron. Wash with water to neutral pH and dry at 105°C. Triturate a slurry of 8 g of acid washed diatomaceous earth and 16 ml buffer [5 ml of 20% v/v PEG 400 in glycerin with 95 ml of 0.1 M ethylenediaminetetraacetic acid (EDTA) previously adjusted to pH 7.0 with ammonium hydroxide]. Pour plates, air dry for 35–50 min and use immediately.

Solvent:

Ethyl acetate:0.1 M EDTA previously adjusted to pH 7.0 (6:1); use organic layer. Equilibrate jar for 30 min prior to use.

Detection:

UV light.

R_f:

A. Anhydromethyl chlortetracycline > demethylchlortetracycline > demethyltetracycline > epidemethylchlortetracycline.

B. Chlortetracycline > demethylchlortetracycline > tetracycline.

C. Anhydrotetracycline > chlortetracycline > tetracycline > epitetracycline.

D. Anhydrochlortetracycline > chlortetracycline > tetracycline > epichlortetracycline.

Ref:

P.P. Ascione, J.B. Zagar and G.P. Chrekian, J. Pharm. Sci., 56 (1967) 1393–1395.

6. **Medium:**

Kieselguhr; prepared as follows: 500 g kieselguhr stirred with 3 l hydrochloric acid (1:2) for 2 h, decanted, filtered by suction, and repeated 3 times. For decanting wash with water until chlorides are eliminated, dry at 100°C, and sift through sieve No. 200 ASTM. A slurry of 40 g of kieselguhr is made with 80 ml of aq. 5% EDTA neutralized to pH 7.5 or 9.0 with 20% sodium hydroxide. A 0.3 mm coating is made, dried at room temperature for 1 h and then at 100°C for 1 h.

Solvent:

A. Acetone:water (10:1).

B. Acetone:ethyl acetate:water (20:10:3).

Detection:

UV light at 366 nm.

R_f:

	R_f (pH-solvent)	
	7.5-B	9.0-A
Anhydrotetracycline	0.88	0.84
Tetracycline	0.71	0.69
Epi-anhydrotetracycline	0.46	0.55
Epitetracycline	0.38	0.22

Ref:

A.A. Fernandez, V.T. Noceda and E.S. Carrera, J. Pharm. Sci., 58 (1969) 443–446.

7. **Medium:**

Silica Gel G buffered with phosphate buffer, pH 3.0.

Solvent:

n-Butanol satd. with water.

Detection:

A. UV light.

B. Bioautography vs. *Bacillus subtilis* NRRL B-543.

R_f:

Chlortetracycline > tetracycline.

Ref:

As PC (22).

8. Medium:

Microgranular cellulose (Whatman), 30 g/
75 ml distilled water. Apply 0.5 mm layer,
air dry for 10 min at room temperature,
then heat at 90°C for 30 min.

Solvent:

Spray plate uniformly with 10 ml of buffer
(0.1 M disodium EDTA—0.1% ammonium
chloride) and immediately develop with
buffer satd. chloroform for 16 cm (about
45 min). Air dry.

Detection:

Expose to ammonia for 2 min and view
under short wave UV.

R_f:

	R_f
Tetracycline hydrochloride	0.0–0.25
Anhydrotetracycline hydrochloride	0.93
4-Epi-anhydrotetracycline hydrochloride	0.48

Ref:

P.B. Lloyd and C. Cornford, J. Chromatogr.,
53 (1970) 403—405.

9. Medium:

Kieselguhr G (Merck) prepared as follows:
50 g kieselguhr slurried in a mixture of 0.1 M
aq. EDTA: 20% v/v PEG 400 in glycerin
(95:5). Coat plates with 0.25 ml layer, dry
at room temperature 4 h overnight.

Solvent:

A. Methyl ethyl ketone satd. with
   McIlvaine's pH 4.7 buffer.
B. Dichloromethane:ethyl formate:ethanol
   (9:9:2) satd. with McIlvaine's pH 4.7
   buffer.

Detection:

A. UV light.
B. Spray reagents:
   1. Fast Blue B (Diazo-Reagent). Spray
      soln. A: 0.5% aq. freshly prepared soln.
      of fast blue B. Spray soln. B: 0.1 N aq.
      sodium hydroxide.
   2. Diazotized p-nitroaniline. Spray soln.
      A: just before spraying 5% aq. sodium
      nitrite soln. (1.5 ml) is added to 0.3%
      p-nitroaniline in 8% hydrochloric acid
      (25 ml). Spray soln. B: 20% aq. sodium
      carbonate soln. After spraying with
      soln. A, spray with soln. B taking
      care not to make the plate transparent
      with excess of the sprays.
   3. Modified Sakaguchi Reagent. Boric
      acid (5 g) is dissolved in water (150 ml)
      and conc. sulfuric acid (350 ml). The
      reagent is stored in a glass-stoppered
      bottle in a refrigerator and is used cold.
   4. Diphenylpicrylhydrazyl (DPPH)
      reagent. Soln. A: methanolic soln. of
      DPPH (~1 mg/2 ml). Soln. B: 25%
      aq. sodium hydroxide.

R_f:

	R_f* Solvent System		Color** (and limit of detection, mcg)			
	A	B	Reagent 1	Reagent 2	Reagent*** 3	Reagent 4
Tetracycline	0.53	0.36	Pk	Y	Y	Pk
Chlortetracycline	0.76	0.60	Pk	Y	Y	Y-Pk
Demethylchlortetracycline	0.73	0.44	Pk	Y	Y	Pk-Y
Oxytetracycline	0.60	0.20	Y	Pk-Y	Y	Br-Y
Methacycline	0.44	0.29	Pk-Br	Y	Y	Y
Doxycycline	0.53	0.57	Pk-Br	Y	Y	Pk
4-Epi-tetracycline	0.20	0.12	Y	Y	Y	Pk-Y
Anhydrotetracycline	0.93	0.83	Pk	Y	Y	Y-Pk
Epi-anhydrotetracycline	0.47	0.50	Y-Pk	Y	Y	Y-Pk
4-Epi-chlortetracycline	0.33	0.21	Y-Pk	Y	Y	Pk-Y
Anhydrotetracycline	0.83	0.57	Pk	Y	Y	Y

*R_f values vary considerably with tank temperature, especially in case of stored plates. If very low R_f values
are obtained, the chromatograms, after brief drying may be rechromatographed in the same solvent system.
**Pk = pink, Y = yellow, Br = brown.
***Colors change with excess of spray reagent and with time.

Ref:

N.D. Gyanchandani, I.J. McGilveray and
D.W. Hughes, J. Pharm. Sci., 59 (1970)
224–228.

10. **Medium:**

Kieselguhr (E. Merck) prepared as follows:
Slurry 40 g Kieselguhr with 80 ml of 5% aq.
EDTA neutralized to pH 7.5 with either
20% sodium hydroxide or conc. ammonium
hydroxide. Coating, 0.3 mm; dry overnight.

Solvent:

Acetone:ethyl acetate:water (80:40:12),
develop to height of 15 cm.

Detection:

A. Isolate band, measure absorbance of
extracted material at 430 nm.

B. Spray with 0.5% aq. Fast Blue Salt B and
heat for 3 min at 110°C. Purple-pink
spots result. For quantitation, these can
be analyzed by densitometry and
compared with known concentrations.

R_f:

Ref:

C. Radecka and W.L. Wilson, J. Chromatogr.,
57 (1971) 297–302.

11. **Medium:**

Diatomaceous earth.

Solvent:

Ethyl acetate satd. with 0.1 M EDTA.

Detection:

R_f:

6-methylenetetracycline > tetracycline >
6-deoxy-5-oxytetracycline > 5-oxytetra-
cycline > 6-methylene-5-oxytetracycline.

Ref:

W. Sobiczewski and M. Domradzki, Chemia
Analityczna, 16 (1971) 131–134.

12. **Medium:**

Talc suspended in citrate-phosphate buffer
(pH 3.5–4.5) plates sprayed with 0.1 M
EDTA, pH 7.0 before use.

Solvent:

As TLC (1).

Detection:

R_f:

6-methylenetetracycline > 5-oxytetracycline
> tetracycline > 6-deoxy-5-oxytetracycline >
6-methylene-5-oxytetracycline.

Ref:

Ibid, TLC (11) 433–437.

CCD.

1. **Solvent:**

0.01 N hydrochloric acid:n-butanol,
230 transfers.

Distribution:

Tetracycline peak at tube 66 (K = 0.40);
2-acetyl-2-decarboxy tetracycline peak at
tube 109 (K = 0.9).

Ref:

G.C. Lancini and P. Sensi, Experientia, 20
(1964) 83–84.

2. **Solvent:**

0.01 N hydrochloric acid:n-butanol (1:1),
100 transfers.

Distribution:

Chlortetracycline peak, tube 52; K = 1.11.
Oxytetracycline peak, tube 30; K = 0.435.
Phases analyzed by assaying against *Bacillus
megatherium*.

Ref:

R.J. Hickey and W.F. Phillips, Anal. Chem.,
26 (1954) 1640–1642.

TETRAMYCIN

PC.

1. **Paper:**

Schleicher and Schull No. 2043 bmgl.

Solvent:

A. Water satd. n-butanol.

B. 20% Ammonium chloride.

C. 3% Ammonium chloride.

D. 75% Aq. phenol.

E. 50% Aq. acetone.

F. n-Butanol:methanol:water:methyl orange
(40:10:20:1.5 g).

G. n-Butanol:methanol:water (40:10:20).

H. Benzene:methanol (80:20).

I. Distilled water.

J. n-Butanol:acetic acid:water (40:10:50).

K. n-Butanol:pyridine:water (60:40:30).

L. Dimethyl formamide:water (10:90).

M. Dimethyl formamide:water (50:50).

N. 70% Aq. propanol.

Detection:

Bioautography vs. *Candida albicans*.

R_f:

Solvent	R_f
A	0.30
B	0.04
C	0.59
D	0.82
E	0.93
F	0.62
G	0.54
H	0.00
I	0.59
J	0.65
K	0.55
L	0.62
M	0.90
N	0.70

Ref:

K. Dornberg, R. Fugner, G. Bradler and
H. Thrum, J. Antibiotics, 24 (1971)
172–177.

TETRANACTIN
TLC.
1. **Medium:**
   Silica Gel.
   Solvent:
   A. Benzene:acetone (4:1).
   B. Chloroform:ethyl acetate (1:2).
   C. n-Hexane:diethyl ether (1:2).
   Detection:
   R_f:

Solvent	R_f
A	0.12
B	0.31
C	0.21

Ref:

K. Ando, H. Oishi, S. Hirano, T. Okutomi,
K. Suzuki, H. Okazaki, M. Sawada and
T. Sagawa, J. Antibiotics, 24 (1971)
347–352.

TETRANGOMYCIN
PC.
1. **Paper:**
   Solvent:
   A. n-Amyl acetate:dibutyl ether:water
      (20:6:11).
   B. n-Heptane:diethyl ketone:tetrahydrofuran:
      0.2 M acetic acid (50:3:3:50).
   Detection:
   R_f:

Solvent	R_f
A	0.90
B	0.80

Ref:

M. Dann, D.V. Lefemine, F. Barbatschi,
P. Shu, M.P. Kunstmann, L.A. Mitscher
and N. Bohonos, Antimicrobial Agents and
Chemotherapy, 1965 (1966) 832–835.

TLC.
1. **Medium:**
   Eastman Chromagram Type K301R.
   Solvent:
   Ethyl acetate.
   Detection:
   R_f:
      0.47
   Ref:
   As PC (1).

TETRIN
PC.
1. **Paper:**
   Solvent:
   A. Water satd. n-butanol.
   B. 3% Ammonium chloride.
   C. 50% Acetone.
   D. 70% Propanol.
   Detection:
   UV fluorescence.
   R_f:

Solvent	R_f
A	0.15–0.22
B	0.50–0.69
C	0.82–0.90
D	0.65–0.69

Ref:

D. Gottlieb and H.L. Pote, Phytopath., 50
(1960) 817–822.

THAIMYCINS
TLC.
1. **Medium:**
   A. Silica Gel G.
   B. Silica Gel HF.
   C. Aluminum oxide G.
   Solvent:
   A. Butanol:acetone:water (4:5:1).
   B. Propanol:ethyl acetate:water (8:1:1).

C. Ethyl acetate:pyridine:isopropanol:water
   (7:2:3:2).
D. Butanol:pyridine:water (6:4:3).

Detection:

R_f:

Medium	Solvent	R_f Thaimycins A	B	C
A	A	0.60	0.30	0.75
A	B	0.45	0.25	0.50
B	C	0.50	0.50	0.80
C	D	0.50	0.30	0.70

Ref:

G. Cassinelli, E. Cotta, G. D'Amico,
C.D. Bruna, A. Grein, R. Mazzoleni,
M.L. Ricciardi and R. Tintinelli, Arch.
Microbiol., 70 (1970) 197–210.

THIOLUTIN

PC.

1. **Paper:**

   As aureothricin, PC (1).

   Solvent:

   As aureothricin, PC (1).

   Detection:

   As aureothricin, PC (1).

   R_f:

   0.45

   Ref:

   As aureothricin, PC (1).

THIOPEPTINS

PC.

1. **Paper:**

   Solvent:

   A. Ethyl acetate:n-hexane:2N ammonium
      hydroxide (4:1:1).
   B. Methanol:acetic acid:water (25:3:72).

   Detection:

   R_f:

Thiopeptin	R_f Solvent A	B
A_1	0.95	0.18
A_2	0.85	0.25
A_3	0.57	0.52
A_4	0.57	0.38
B	0.00	0.23

Ref:

N. Miyairi, T. Miyoshi, H. Aoki, M. Kohsaka,

H. Ikushima, K. Kunugita, H. Sakai and
H. Imanaka, 176th Meeting Japan Antibiotics Res. Assn., November 20, 1970.

TLC.

1. **Medium:**

   A. Silica Gel G.
   B. Spotfilm (Silica Gel, Tokyo-kasei Co.).

   Solvent:

   A. Chloroform:methanol (9:1).
   B. Chloroform:methanol (19:1).
   C. Chloroform:n-butanol (6:1).

   Detection:

   R_f:

Thiopeptin	R_f Solvent Medium A A	B	Medium B C
A_1	0.83	0.48	0.73
A_2	0.70	0.42	0.62
A_3	0.60	0.37	0.48
A_4	0.50	0.30	0.38
B	0.10	0.00	0.00

Ref:

N. Miyairi, T. Miyoshi, H. Aoki, M. Kohsaka,
H. Ikushima, K. Kunugita, H. Sakai and
H. Imanaka, Antimicrobial Agents and
Chemotherapy, 1 (1972) 192–196.

THIOSTREPTON

PC.

1. **Paper:**

   Whatman No. 1.

   Solvent:

   A. Acetone:water (70:30), ascending, 5 h.
   B. Acetone:propanol:water (40:40:20),
      ascending, 7 h.
   C. 0.2N acetic acid, ascending, 6 h.

   Detection:

   Bioautography vs. *M. pyogenes var. aureus.*

   R_f:

Solvent	R_f
A	0.50
B	0.80
C	0.08

Ref:

J.F. Pagano, M.J. Weinstein, H.A. Stout and
R. Donovick, Antibiotics Annual (1955–
1956) 554–559.

TILOMYCIN
CCD.
1. **Solvent:**
    Upper phase, t-butanol; lower phase,
    4% sodium chloride; 200 transfers.
    Distribution:
    Single, symmetrical peak with maximum at
    tube 148.
    Ref:
    M. Misiek, O.B. Fardig, A. Gourevitch,
    D.C. Johnson, I.R. Hooper and J. Lein,
    Antibiotics Annual (1957–1958) 852–855.

TOBRAMYCIN
see nebramycin factor 6.

TOLYPOMYCIN R
PC.
1. **Paper:**
    Solvent:
    n-Hexane:benzene:acetone:water
    (30:10:18:32).
    Detection:
    R_f:
    0.65
    Ref:
    T. Kishi, H. Yamana, M. Muroi and K. Mizuno,
    163rd Meeting Japan Antibiotics Res. Assn.,
    September 27, 1968.

TLC.
1. **Medium:**
    Silica Gel, containing 2% oxalic acid.
    Solvent:
    Ethyl acetate containing 1% oxalic acid.
    Detection:
    R_f:
    0.2
    Ref:
    As PC (1).

TOLYPOMYCIN Y
PC.
1. **Paper:**
    Whatman No. 1.
    Solvent:
    A. n-Hexane:benzene:ethanol:water
       (1:3:1:3).
    B. n-Hexane:benzene:acetone:water
       (30:10:18:22).

C. n-Hexane:ether:acetone:water
   (15:5:8:12).
All solvents developed ascending.
Detection:
A. As visible colored spots.
B. Bioautography vs. *Staphylococcus aureus.*
R_f:

Solvent	R_f
A	0.78
B	0.68
C	0.27

Ref:
T. Kishi, H. Yamana, M. Muroi, S. Harada,
M. Asai, T. Hasegawa and K. Mizuno,
J. Antibiotics, 25 (1972) 11–15.

TLC.
1. **Medium:**
    As Tolypolycin R, TLC(1).
    Solvent:
    A. Ethyl acetate:acetone (1:1), containing
       1% oxalic acid.
    B. Ethyl acetate containing 1% oxalic acid.
    C. Acetone containing 1% oxalic acid.
    Detection:
    As PC (1).
    R_f:

Solvent	R_f
A	0.05
B	0.00
C	0.20

Ref:
As PC (1).

TOMAYMYCIN
TLC.
1. **Medium:**
    Kieselgel (E. Merck).
    Solvent:
    A. Ethyl acetate.
    B. Ethyl acetate:chloroform (1:1).
    C. Chloroform:methanol (50:1).
    D. Ethyl acetate:benzene (1:1).
    Detection:
    R_f:

Solvent	R_f
A	0.50
B	0.21
C	0.24
D	0.02

Ref:

K. Arima, M. Kosaka, G. Tamura, H. Imanaka and H. Sakai, 174th Meeting Japan Antibiotics Res. Assn., July 7, 1970.

TREHALOSAMINE
PC.
1. **Paper:**
   Toyo Roshi No. 50.
   Solvent:
   Butanol:acetic acid:water (4:1:5), ascending.
   Detection:
   Ninhydrin.
   R_f:
   0.14
   Ref:
   S. Umezawa, K. Tatsuta and R. Muto, J. Antibiotics, 20 (1967) 388–389.

TRICHOMYCIN
PC.
1. **Paper:**
   Whatman No. 1.
   Solvent:
   As aureofungin, PC (1) A–F.
   Detection:
   R_f:

Solvent	R_f
A	0.60
B	0.58
C	0.17, 0.14
D	0.72
E	0.94
F	0.32

   Ref:
   As aureofungin, PC (1).

2. **Paper:**
   Whatman No. 1.
   Solvent:
   A. Water satd. n-butanol, descending, 16 h.
   B. n-Butanol:pyridine:water (1:0.6:1), ascending, 16 h.
   C. 50% Aq. acetone, ascending, 10 h.
   D. Methanol:water:ammonium hydroxide (20:4:1), descending, 5.5 h.
   E. 60% Aq. isopropanol, ascending, 16 h.
   Detection:
   Bioautography vs. *Saccharomyces cerevisiae.*
   R_f:

Solvent	R_f
A	0.26
B	0.75
C	0.78
D	0.67, 0.42
E	0.99

Ref:
P.V. Divekar, V.C. Vora and A.W. Khan, J. Antibiotics, 19 (1966) 63.

TRIENINE
PC.
1. **Paper:**
   Solvent:
   A. Butanol:acetic acid:water (4:1:5).
   B. 5% Dimethylformamide in methanol.
   Detection:
   R_f:

Solvent	R_f
A	0.55
B	0.70

   Ref:
   A. Aszalos, R.S. Robison, P. Lemanski and B. Berk, J. Antibiotics, 21 (1968) 611–615.

TLC.
1. **Medium:**
   Eastman chromagram ITLC.
   Solvent:
   Methanol.
   Detection:
   R_f:
   0.0
   Ref:
   A. Aszalos, R.S. Robison, F. Pansy and B. Berk, U.S. Patent 3,632,749; January 4, 1972.

TRIOSTIN
PC.
1. **Paper:**
   Solvent:
   A. Petroleum ether:benzene:methanol:water (66.7:33:3:80:20).
   B. 25% Ethanol.
   C. Amyl acetate satd. with water.
   Detection:
   R_f:

Solvent	R_f
A	0.40
B	0.26
C	0.76

Ref:

T.S. Maksimova, I.N. Kovsharova and
U.V. Proshlyakova, Antibiotiki, 10 (1965)
298–304.

2. Paper:
Solvent:

Dibutyl ether:s-tetrachloroethane:10%
sodium o-cresotinate (2:1:3).

Detection:

A. Bioautography vs. *Bacillus subtilis.*
B. Radioactive triostin detected by scanning.

R_f:

Triostin C > A (estimated 0.5, 0.3
respectively, from drawing).

Ref:

T. Yoshida and K. Katagiri, Biochem., 8
(1969) 2645–2651.

TLC.
1. Circular TLC.
Medium:

As quinomycins, TLC (1).

Solvent:

As quinomycins, TLC (1).

Detection:

R_f:

Triostin C > B > A.

Ref:

As quinomycins, TLC (1).

2. Medium:
A. Aluminum oxide GF_{254}, circular
chromatography.
B. Silica Gel GF_{254}, ascending.

Solvent:

A. Lower phase of ethyl acetate:s-
tetrachloroethane:water (3:1:3).

Detection:

UV light.

R_f:

Both systems separate triostins A from C.

Ref:

As PC (2).

TRYPANOMYCIN A₂
PC.
1. Paper:
Schleicher and Schuell No. 2043b.

Solvent:

A. Water satd. butanol.
B. Methanol.
C. 50% Acetone.
D. Acetone:benzene:water (12:3:2).
E. Butanol:methanol:water (4:1:2).
Solvents A–D, ascending; E, circular.

Detection:

Bioautography vs. *Escherichia coli* C600.

R_f:

Solvent	R_f
A	0.65
B	0.90
C	0.48
D	0.87
E	0.70

Ref:

W. Fleck, D. Straus, C. Schönfeld,
W. Jungstand, C. Seiber and H. Prauser,
Antimicrobial Agents and Chemotherapy,
1 (1972) 385–391.

TLC.
1. Medium:
Silica Gel D (Merck).

Solvent:

Chloroform:acetone:methanol:water
(200:20:50:50).

Detection:

Color of zone.

R_f:

0.46

Ref:

As PC (1).

TSUSHIMYCIN
TLC.
1. Medium:
Silica Gel G.

Solvent:

A. n-Butanol:acetic acid:water (3:1:1).
B. Ethanol:14% aq. ammonia (4:1).

Detection:

A. Bioautography.
B. Sulfuric acid.

R_f:

Solvent	R_f
A	0.37–0.40
B	0.16–0.19

Ref:

J. Shoji, S. Kozuki, S. Okamoto,
R. Sakazaki and H. Otsuka, J. Antibiotics,
21 (1968) 439–443.

TUBERACTINOMYCINS
TLC.
1. **Medium:**
   Silica Gel G.
   Solvent:
   10% Aq. ammonium acetate:acetone:10% ammonium hydroxide (9:10:0.5).
   Detection:
   R_f:
   0.44
   Ref:
   A. Nagata, T. Ando, R. Izumi, H. Sakakibara, T. Take, K. Hayano and J. Abe, J. Antibiotics, 21 (1968) 681–687.

2. **Medium:**
   As TLC (1).
   Solvent:
   A. As TLC (1), but (9:10:1).
   B. Phenol:water:conc. ammonium hydroxide (30:10:0.6).
   Detection:
   R_f:

	R_f Solvent	
	A	B
Tuberactinomycin	0.53	0.13
Tuberactinomycin-N	0.53	0.28

   Ref:
   T. Ando, R. Izumi, K. Matsura, A. Nagata and J. Abe, 175th Meeting Japan Antibiotics Res. Assn., September 25, 1970.

3. **Medium:**
   Kieselgel G (Merck).
   Solvent:
   A. 10% Ammonium acetate:acetone:10% ammonium hydroxide (9:10:1).
   B. As TLC (2), B.
   Detection:
   R_f:

Tuberactinomycin	R_f* Solvent	
	A	B
A	0.50	0.13
B**	0.25	0.13
N	0.50	0.30
O	0.25	0.30

   * Estimated from drawing.
   **Identical to viomycin.

Ref:
R. Izumi, T. Noda, T. Ando, T. Take and A. Nagata, J. Antibiotics, 25 (1972) 201–207.

TUMIMYCIN
TLC.
1. **Medium:**
   Eastman Si-Gel Chromagram.
   Solvent:
   Methanol:chloroform (1:9).
   Detection:
   R_f:
   0.65 (major); 0.55 (minor).
   Ref:
   A. Aszalos, R.S. Robison, N.V. Kraemer, J. Henshaw and M.S. Giannini, German "Offenlegungsschrift" 2139261, 1972.

TYLOSIN
PC.
1. **Paper:**
   As relomycin, PC (1).
   Solvent:
   As relomycin, PC (1).
   Detection:
   As relomycin, PC (1).
   R_f:
   0.48
   Ref:
   As relomycin, PC (1).

2. **Paper:**
   Solvent:
   A. Methyl ethyl ketone on pH 4 buffered paper.
   B. Methyl ethyl ketone.
   C. n-Butanol satd. with water on pH 4 buffered paper.
   D. n-Butanol satd. with water.
   E. Water containing 7% sodium chloride and 2.5% methyl ethyl ketone.
   F. Ethyl acetate satd. with water on pH 4 buffered paper.
   Detection:
   R_f:

Solvent	R_f
A	0.46
B	0.81
C	0.90
D	0.84
E	0.57
F	0.89

Ref:

R.L. Hamill and W.M. Stark, J. Antibiotics, 17 (1964) 133—139.

TLC.

1. Two dimensional and one dimension chromatography.

Medium:

Silica Gel GF$_{254}$ (Merck), 0.25 mm thick.

Solvent:

A. First dimension; chloroform:acetone (60:40).

B. Second direction; ethyl acetate:methanol (85:15).

Detection:

A. UV absorbance at 254 nm.

B. Consecutive spraying with the following:

1. Iodoplatinate. 1 g of Pt Cl$_4$.2HCl.6H$_2$O and 20 g potassium iodide are dissolved in 8 ml conc. hydrochloric acid and diluted to 400 ml with distilled water. Chromatograms are sprayed until uniformly pink with faint brown color for tylosin.

2. Draggendorf's reagent modified by Meunier and Macheboeuf. Soln. (a): 0.85 g basic bismuth nitrate, 10 ml acetic acid (96%) and 40 ml distilled water. Soln. (b): 20 g potassium iodide dissolved in 50 ml water. Both solutions mixed and kept in a brown bottle. 10 ml acetic acid and 35 ml water added to 5 ml of mixture just before spraying. This reagent makes tylosin spots more pronounced.

3. Satd. soln. of silver sulfate in 10% sulfuric acid. After this spray, tylosin spots become orange brown against a dark background.

R$_f$:

Solvent	R$_f$
A	0.12
B	0.60

Ref:

M. Debackere and K. Baeten, J. Chromatogr., 61 (1971) 125—132.

TYROTHRICIN

TLC.

1. **Medium:**

Kieselgel G.

Solvent:

n-Butanol:acetic acid:water (100:10:30), 3 h.

Detection:

Dry plates 2—3 min in air followed by 10 min at 45°C. Suspend in a jar containing solution of 100 ml potassium permanganate, 1.5% to which has been added 100 ml of 10% hydrochloric acid heated about 50°C. The plate is exposed to the chlorine vapor for approximately 20 min and excess chlorine removed by exposing the plate to a stream of air. Spray plate with a mixture prepared by adding 160 mg of o-tolidine in 30 ml conc. acetic acid and diluting to 500 ml.

R$_f$:

0.34

Ref:

P.A. Nussbaumer, Pharm. Acta Helv., 89 (1964) 647—652.

UMBRINOMYCIN

PC.

1. **Paper:**

Whatman No. 4.

Solvent:

n-Butanol:water:acetic acid (4:5:1).

Detection:

Bioautography vs. *Staphylococcus aureus* 209P.

R$_f$:

0.9

Ref:

Belgian patent 708601; published June 27, 1968.

VALIDAMYCINS

TLC.

1. **Medium:**

Silica Gel G.

Solvent:

A. n-Propanol:acetic acid:water (4:1:1).

B. Benzene:ethyl acetate (1:1).

Detection:

Aq. potassium permanganate, 1%.

R$_f$:

	R_f* Solvent	
	A	B
Validamycin A	0.30	0.7
Validamycin B	0.43	

*Estimated from drawing.

Ref:

T. Iwasa, Y. Kameda, M. Asai, S. Horii and
K. Mizuno, J. Antibiotics, 24 (1971)
119–123.

GLC.

1. **Apparatus**:

   Hitachi Model 063 with FID.

   Column:

   Glass, 2 m × 3 mm I.D. packed with 1%
   silicone OV-1 on Chromosorb W AW DMCS.

   Temperature:

   Column, 250°C; injection, 300°C.

   Carrier gas:

   He at 60 ml/min.

   Silylation procedure:

   Approximately 1 mg sample dissolved in
   100 μl pyridine. Bis(trimethylsilyl)acetamide,
   100 μl and trimethyl chlorosilane, 50 μl
   added. Heat at 70–80°C for 30 min.

   Chromatography:

   Peaks, in min, estimated from graph are:

Validamycin A	4
Validamycin B	5
Validamycin C	27
Validamycin D	4.5
Validamycin E	23
Validamycin F	24

   Ref:

   S. Horh, Y. Kameda and K. Kawahara,
   J. Antibiotics, 25 (1972) 48–53.

VANCOMYCIN

PC.

1. **Paper**:

   Whatman No. 1.

   Solvent:

   A. 5% Aq. ammonium chloride, descending.
   B. 90% Phenol:m-cresol:pyridine:acetic
   acid:water (25:25:1:1:25), descending.

   Detection:

   Bioautography vs. *Bacillus subtilis* or
   Corynebacterium xerosis.

   R_f:

Solvent	R_f
A	0.85
B	0.35, 0.59

Ref:

M.P. Kunstmann, L.A. Mitscher, J.N. Porter,
A.J. Shay and M.A. Darken, Antimicrobial
Agents and Chemotherapy, 1968 (1969)
242–245.

2. **Paper**:

   Whatman 3 MM washed extensively with M
   ammonium acetate, then water, and dried
   before use.

   Solvent:

   A. Ethanol:ammonium acetate (5:2), 18 h.
   B. Isobutyric acid:aq. 0.5 M ammonia (5:3),
   18 h.

   Detection:

   R_f:

	R $_{vancomycin}$ Solvent	
	A	B
Iodinated vancomycin	1.02	1.01

   Ref:

   H.R. Perkins and M. Nieto, Biochem. J.,
   116 (1970) 83–92.

TLC.

Qualitative and quantitative.

1. **Medium**:

   A. Qualitative; Silica Gel G activated 105°C
   for 10 min before use.
   B. Quantitative; Kieselguhr G (Merck), no
   preactivation. Range, 2–10 mcg.

   Solvent:

   A. Benzene:n-butanol:water (20:20:100),
   aq. phase.
   B. Methanol:water (1:99).

   Detection:

   A. Qualitative: Spray with 20% sodium
   carbonate solution followed by Folin-
   Ciocalteau reagent. Gray-blue zones result.
   Detection limit < 0.1 mcg.
   B. Quantitative: Developed with solvent A.
   Plates dried in warm air stream and
   immediately sprayed with 20% aq.
   sodium carbonate, dried thoroughly and
   sprayed with fresh Folin-Ciocalteau
   reagent diluted 1:3 and dried 15 min in
   warm air stream. Scan with integrating

densitometer (Photovolt model 520 M with TLC stage used; slit 0.1 mm × 6 mm; 420 nm filter; search unit, 1 mm; response setting, 10). Read each spot against standard curve.

R_f:

Solvent	R_f^*
A	0.98
B	0.54

*Silica Cel G.

Ref:

J.R. Fooks, I.J. McGilveray and R.D. Strickland, J. Pharm. Sci., 57 (1968) 314–317.

VARIOTIN

CCD.

1. Solvent:

70% Methanol:carbon tetrachloride (1:1), 60 transfers.

Distribution:

Variotin found in tubes 29–38.

Ref:

N. Tanaka, K. Sashikata and H. Umezawa, J. Gen. Appl. Microbiol., 8 (1962) 192–200.

VENTURICIDINS

TLC.

1. Medium:

Silica Gel.

Solvent:

Ethyl acetate.

Detection:

R_f:

Compound	R_f
Venturicidin A	0.49
Venturicidin B	0.41
Venturicidin X	0.80

Ref:

H. Zachner and W. Keller, U.S. Patent 3,636,198; January 18, 1972.

VERMICULINE

TLC.

1. Medium:

Silica Gel (Silufol).

Solvent:

A. Chloroform:methanol (98:2).
B. Chloroform:acetone (8:2).
C. Benzene:acetone (7:3).
D. Benzene:acetone (8:2).
E. Benzene:methanol (9:1).
F. Benzene:acetic acid (1:1).
G. Ethyl acetate:acetic acid (10:1).

Detection:

A. Bioautography vs. *Bacillus subtilis* SDPC 1:220.
B. Concentrated sulfuric acid.
C. Potassium permanganate.

R_f:

Solvent	R_f
A	0.71
B	0.47
C	0.52
D	0.23
E	0.44
F	0.48
G	0.59

Ref:

J. Fuska, P. Nemec and I. Kuhr, J. Antibiotics, 25 (1972) 208–211.

VERRUCARINES

TLC.

1. Medium:

A. Aluminum oxide.
B. Kieselgel G.

Solvent:

A. Chloroform:methanol (98:2).
B. Chloroform:methanol (97:3).

Detection:

A. Iodine vapor.
B. UV light.

R_f:

	R_f (Medium-solvent)			Color	
	(A-A)	(B-A)	(B-B)	Iodine	UV
Verrucarine A	0.70	0.28	0.59	yellow brown	pale
Verrucarine B	0.83	0.47	0.69	yellow brown	pale
Verrucarine C	0.74	0.28	0.52	yellow brown	brightly fluorescent
Verrucarine D	0.70	0.28	0.55	yellow brown	dark
Verrucarine E	0.00	0.00	0.09	violet	dark
Verrucarine F	—	0.54	—	light yellow brown	dark
Verrucarine G	—	0.49	—	brown	not visible

Ref:

E. Härri, W. Loeffler, H.P. Sigg, H. Stähelin, Ch. Stoll, Ch. Tamm and D. Weisinger, Helv. Chim. Acta, 45 (1962) 840—853.

2. **Medium:**

Kieselgel G.

Solvent:

A. Chloroform:methanol (98:2).

B. Benzene:tetrahydrofuran (85:15).

C. Ether (twice).

Detection:

Iodine vapor.

R_f:

	R_f Solvent		
	A	B	C
Verrucarine B	0.58	0.63	0.37
Verrucarine H	0.59	0.72	0.51
Verrucarine J	0.59	0.64	0.42

Ref:

B. Böhner, E. Fetz, E. Härri, H.P. Sigg, Ch. Stoll and Ch. Tamm, Helv. Chim. Acta, 48 (1965) 1079—1087.

VERSICOLIN

PC.

1. **Paper:**

Whatman No. 1.

Solvent:

A. n-Butanol:acetic acid:water (6:1:2).

B. Benzene:acetic acid:water (6:7:3).

C. Petroleum ether, 40—60°C:methanol (1:1).

D. Ether satd. with water.

E. Toluene:petroleum ether, 40—60°C: methanol (5:4:1).

All solvents developed ascending.

Detection:

Bioautography.

R_f:

Solvent	R_f
A	1.00
B	0.88
C	0.97
D	0.85
E	0.50

Ref:

A.K. Dhar and S.K. Bose, Appl. Microbiol., 16 (1968) 749—752.

TLC.

1. **Medium:**

Silica Gel G (E. Merck).

Solvent:

A. Petroleum ether, 40—60°C:benzene.

B. Chloroform:benzene (3:1).

C. Benzene:methanol (4:1).

D. Benzene:methanol:acetic acid (80:20:1).

E. Benzene:methanol:ammonia (80:20:1).

Detection:

Permanganate-BPB reagent.

R_f:

Solvent	R_f
A	0.00
B	0.80
C	0.50
D	0.40
E	0.20

Ref:

As PC (1).

VIOMYCIN

TLC.

1. **Medium:**

Kieselgel G (Merck).

Solvent:

10% Aq. ammonium acetate:acetone:10% ammonium hydroxide (9:10:0.5).

Detection:

R_f:

0.24

Ref:

A. Nagata, T. Ando, R. Izumi, H. Sakakibara, T. Take, K. Hayano and J. Abe, J. Antibiotics, 21 (1968) 681—687.

ELPHO.

1. **Medium:**

Whatman No. 1 paper.

Buffer:

Sodium veronal, 6.23 g + sodium acetate, 4.11 g in 1 liter water adjusted to pH 8.0 with N hydrochloric acid.

Conditions:

300 V (11.5 V/cm), 3 h.

Detection:

Ninhydrin.

Mobility:

Separates from co-crystalline polypeptide.

Ref:
> Z. Kotula, P. Bukowski, Z. Kowszyk-
> Gindifer, Med. Dosw. Mikrobiol., 22 (1970)
> 95–100.

XANTHOCIDIN
PC.
1. **Paper:**
   Solvent:
   > A. Wet butanol.
   > B. 3% Ammonium chloride.
   > C. 75% Phenol.
   > D. 50% Acetone.
   > E. Butanol:methanol:water:methyl orange
   >   (40 ml:10 ml:20 ml:1.5 g).
   > F. Butanol:methanol:water (40:10:20).
   > G. Benzene:methanol (80:20).
   > H. Water.
   > All solvents developed ascending.

   Detection:
   > Bioautography vs. *Xanthomonas oryzae.*

   R_f:

Solvent	R_f*
A	0.75
B	0.82
C	0.75
D	0.80
E	0.70
F	0.75
G	0.50
H	0.75

   *Estimated from drawing.

   Ref:
   > K. Asahi, J. Nagatsu and S. Suzuki,
   > J. Antibiotics, 19 (1966) 195–199.

XANTHOMYCIN A
PC.
1. **Paper:**
   > Eaton-Dikeman 613 (0.5 in. wide strips).

   Solvent:
   > 1-Butanol containing 1% (v/v) 1 N
   > hydrochloric acid.

   Detection:
   > Bioautography vs. *Bacillus subtilis.*

   R_f:
   > 0.0, 1.0.

   Ref:
   > K.V. Rao and W.H. Peterson, J. Amer. Chem.
   > Soc., 76 (1954) 1335; D. Dougall and
   > E.P. Abraham, Nature, 176 (1955) 256.

YAZUMYCIN
PC.
1. **Paper:**
   Solvent:
   > A. n-Propanol:pyridine:acetic acid:water
   >   (10:15:3:10).
   > B. 80% Methanol:piperidine (10:1) adjusted
   >   to pH 9.3 with acetic acid.
   > C. Water satd. n-butanol containing 2%
   >   p-toluenesulfonic acid.
   > D. n-Butanol:acetic acid:water (2:1:1).

   Detection:

   R_f:

Solvent	R_f
A	0.42
B	0.53
C	0.09
D	0.16

   Ref:
   > K. Akasaki, H. Abe, A. Seino and S. Shirato,
   > J. Antibiotics, 21 (1968) 98–105.

TLC.
1. **Medium:**
   > Silica Gel.

   Solvent:
   > A. Chloroform:methanol:17% ammonium
   >   hydroxide (2:1:1), upper layer.
   > B. n-Propanol:pyridine:acetic acid:water
   >   (15:10:3:10).

   Detection:

   R_f:

Solvent	R_f
A	0.3–0.3
B	0.6

   Ref:
   > As PC (1).

YEMINIMYCIN
PC.
1. **Paper:**
   Solvent:
   > A. Petroleum ether, b.p. 40–60°C.
   > B. Petroleum ether, b.p. 100–120°C.
   > C. Distilled water.
   > D. n-Butanol:water (1:1).
   > E. Methanol.
   > F. n-Butanol:acetic acid:water (4:1:5).
   > G. Ethyl acetate:water (1:1).
   > H. Chloroform satd. with water.
   > I. Ethyl acetate:petroleum ether.

J. Ethanol.

K. Chloroform.

L. Ethyl acetate.

M. Acetone.

Detection:

A. Bioautography vs. *Bacillus subtilis* NRRL-B-543 or *Penicillium chrysogenum* Q176.

B. Spray with dilute potassium permanganate and heat.

R_f:

Solvent	R_f^*
A	0.00
B	0.00
C	0.25
D	0.30
E	0.50
F	0.65
G	0.70
H	0.70
I	0.70
J	0.80
K	0.95
L	0.95
M	0.95

*Estimated from drawing.

Ref:

I.B. Shimi, A. Dewedar and N. Abdallah, J. Antibiotics, 24 (1971) 283–289.

ZORBAMYCIN; ZORBONOMYCINS

TLC.

1. **Medium:**

   MN-Polygram CEL 300 (Brinkman).

   Solvent:

   A. Sodium citrate, 0.05 M, pH 6.9 buffer.

   B. 0.1 M Aq. ammonium chloride adjusted to pH 7.5 with aq. ammonium hydroxide.

   C. 0.2 M Aq. ammonium chloride adjusted to pH 7.5 with aq. ammonium hydroxide.

Detection:

Bioautography vs. *Bacillus subtilis*, *Klebsiella pneumoniae* or *Staphylococcus aureus*.

R_f:

	R_f^*		
	Solvent A	Solvent B	Solvent C
Zorbamycin	0.40	0.40–0.55	—
Zorbonomycin B	—	0.25	0.50–0.55
Zorbonomycin C	—	0.10	0.40–0.50

*Estimated from drawing.

Ref:

A.D. Argoudelis, M.E. Bergy and T.R. Pyke, J. Antibiotics, 24 (1971) 543–557.

ZYGOMYCINS

PC.

1. **Paper:**

   Toyo Roshi No. 131.

   Solvent:

   A. 50% Aq. phenol, descending, 44 h.

   B. n-Butanol:acetic acid:water (2:1:2).

   C. As B, but (4:1:5).

Detection:

A. Bioautography vs. *Bacillus subtilis*.

B. Ninhydrin.

C. Sakaguchi reaction.

R_f:

Compound	R_f Solvent		
	A	B	C
Zygomycin A	4 cm from origin*	0.33	0.01
Zygomycin B	14 cm from origin**	—	—

* Sachaguchi (–).

** Sachaguchi (+).

Ref:

K. Nakazawa, M. Shibata, E. Higashide, T. Kanzaki, H. Yamamoto, A. Miyake, H. Hitomi, S. Horii, T. Yamaguchi, T. Araki, K. Tsuchiya, Y. Oka, A. Imai, U.S. Patent 3,089,827; May 14, 1963.

ZYGOSPORINS

TLC.

1. **Medium:**

   Silica Gel.

Solvent:
   A. Chloroform:methanol (9:1).
   B. Toluene:methanol (10:1).
Detection:
R_f:

	R_f Solvent	
	A	B
Zygosporin A	0.50	—
Zygosporin D	0.40	—
Zygosporin E	0.55	—
Zygosporin F	0.57	0.28
Zygosporin G	0.57	0.35

Ref:

M. Minato, M. Matsumoto and T. Katayama, 167th Meeting Japan Antibiotics Res. Assn., May 28, 1969.

NUMBERED ANTIBIOTICS

15
PC.

1. **Paper:**

   Whatman No. 1.

   Solvent:

   Propanol:pyridine:acetic acid:water (15:10:3:12), descending, 48 h, 25°C; front runs off end of paper.

   Detection:

   Bioautography vs. *Klebsiella pneumoniae.*

   R_f:

Component	R_f*
15A	0.53
15B	0.41
15C	0.30
15D	0.24
15E	0.17
15F	0.13

   *Distance of spot from origin/distance of origin to end of paper.

   Ref:

   M.J. Weinstein, G.H. Wagman and G. Luedemann, U.S. Patent No. 3,458,626; July 26, 1969.

19A
PC.

1. **Paper:**

   Whatman No. 1; buffer as stationary phase.

Solvent:
   A. Ethyl acetate:0.1 M phosphate buffer, pH 3—9.
   B. Isopropanol:water (70:30).
   C. Sodium chloride:water:methanol (2.0%:25:75).
   D. Butanol:0.1 M phosphate (pH 7.0).
   E. Methyl isobutyl ketone:0.1 M phosphate (pH 5.0).
All solvents developed descending.
Detection:
   Bioautography.
R_f:

Solvent System	R_f
A (pH 3)	1.00
A (pH 5)	1.00
A (pH 6)	0.69
A (pH 7)	0.70
A (pH 8)	0.08
A (pH 9)	0.00
B	0.54
C	0.79
D	0.08
E	0.60

Ref:

I. Putter and F.J. Wolf, Antimicrobial Agents and Chemotherapy, 1961 (1962) 454—461.

67-694
TLC.

1. **Medium:**

   Silica Gel (Analtech "Uniplate").

   Solvent:

   A. Chloroform:methanol:17% ammonia (2:1:1).
   B. Butanol:acetic acid:water (3:1:1).
   C. Chloroform:methanol (4:1).
   D. Chloroform:methanol (3:2).

   Detection:

   Bioautography vs. *Sarcina lutea.*

   R_f:

Solvent	R_f
A	0.98
B	0.37
C	0.45
D	0.48

   Ref:

   M.J. Weinstein, G.H. Wagman and J.A. Marquez, German "Offenlegungsschrift" 2,102,718; July 29, 1971.

106-7
PC.
1. **Paper:**
   Solvent:
   A. Ethanol:water (4:1).
   B. Butanol:water:acetic acid (4:2:1).
   Detection:
   Ninhydrin (0.2% in 93% ethanol). Gives characteristic yellow-blue color.
   R_f:

Solvent	R_f
A	0.33
B	0.37

   Ref:
   U.K. Patent No. 757,089; September 12, 1956.

136
PC.
1. **Paper:**
   Whatman No. 1.
   Solvent:
   1-Butanol satd. with water containing 2% p-toluenesulfonic acid.
   Detection:
   Bioautography vs. *Bacillus subtilis.*
   R_f:
   Component 136A > B > C > D > E.
   Ref:
   W.F. Phillips and H.S. Ragheb, J. Chromatogr., 19 (1965) 147–159.

289F, 289FO, Acetyl 289F.
PC.
1. **Paper:**
   A. Toyo No. 50, developed ascending.
   B. Circular aluminum oxide paper.
   Solvent:
   A. Acetonitrile.
   B. Butyl acetate:dibutyl ether (3:1).
   C. Ethyl acetate satd. with water.
   Detection:
   A. Yellow colored zones.
   B. Coloration with nickel acetate.
   R_f:

	Paper	Solvent	R_f
289F	A	A	0.14
	A	B	0.71
289FO	A	A	0.40–0.45
	A	B	0.80–0.85
	B	C	0.28–0.39
Acetyl 289F	B	C	1.00

   Ref:
   South Africa Appl. No. 695196; July 16, 1969.

TLC.
1. **Medium:**
   Silica Gel (Kieselgel G, Merck).
   Solvent:
   A. Ethanol:14% ammonia (4:1).
   B. Ethanol:pyridine (4:1).
   Detection:
   As PC (1); A, B.
   R_f:

Compound	Solvent	R_f
289F	A	0.81
	B	0.06
Acetyl 289F	B	0.55

   Ref:
   As PC (1).

460
PC.
1. **Paper:**
   Whatman No. 1.
   Solvent:
   A. Propanol:pyridine:acetic acid:water (15:10:3:12).
   B. Propanol:acetic acid:water (50:40:5).
   Detection:
   Bioautography.
   R_f:

	R_f Solvent	
	A	B
1	0.20	0.13
2	0.25	0.20
3	0.95	0.93

   Ref:
   M.J. Weinstein, G.H. Wagman, J.A. Marquez and G. Luedemann, U.S. Patent No. 3,454,696; July 8, 1969.

1985/11
PC.
1. **Paper:**
   Solvent:
   As 3035/48, PC (1).
   Detection:
   R_f:
   0.20, 0.26, 0.41, 0.54

Ref:

As 3035/48, PC (1).

2814P
PC.

1. **Paper:**
   Solvent:

   As eurocidin, PC (1).
   Detection:
   R_f:

   0.58
   Ref:

   As eurocidin, PC (1).

3035/48
PC.

1. **Paper:**
   Solvent:

   n-Butanol:acetic acid:water:pyridine
   (15:3:12:10).
   Detection:
   R_f:

   0.20, 0.24, 0.32, 0.43
   Ref:

   R.A. Zhukova, R.V. Kirsanova, L.A. Kovaleva,
   T.V. Kotenko, W.I. Kuznetsova,
   A.A. Medvedova, B.V. Sokolov, M.D. Paikin,
   M.A. Frolova and Y.D. Shenin, Mikro-
   biologiya, 35 (1966) 312—318.

3950
PC.

1. **Paper:**
   Solvent:

   As echinomycin, PC (2), A, B, C.
   Detection:
   R_f:

Solvent	R_f
A	0.26, 0.76
B	0.32, 0.54
C	0.60, 0.80

   Ref:

   As echinomycin, PC (2).

4205
PC.

1. **Paper:**
   Whatman No. 1.
   Solvent:

   1-Butanol:acetic acid:water (4:1:5), organic
   phase, ascending, 17.5 h.

Detection:

A. 0.25% Ninhydrin in acetone.
B. Bioautography vs. *Staphylococcus albus*
   or *Escherichia coli.*
R_f:

4205A, 0.69; 4205B, 0.67.
Ref:

M. Shaw, R. Brown and A.G. Martin, Appl.
Microbiol., 14 (1966) 79—85.

TLC.

1. **Medium:**
   Silica Gel G (E. Merck).
   Solvent:

   n-Butanol:acetic acid:water (2:1:1); develop
   to 15 cm from origin.
   Detection:

   A. Heat plates at 120—150°C for 10—15
      min; while hot, spray with 0.2% ninhydrin
      in 95% n-butanol + 5% acetic acid.
   B. After ninhydrin spray, re-heat again for
      a short time at 120—150°C and spray
      with a satd. soln. of potassium dichronate
      in conc. sulfuric acid.
   R_f:

   4205A, 0.67; 4205B, 0.63; 4205C, 0.66.
   Ref:

   As PC (1); also E. Ehrhardt and F. Cramer,
   J. Chromatogr., 7 (1962) 405—407.

6270
PC.

1. **Paper:**
   Solvent:

   As echinomycin, PC (2), A, B, C.
   Detection:
   R_f:

Solvent	R_f
A	0.76
B	0.31
C	0.80

   Ref:

   As echinomycin, PC (2).

16,511 R.P.
TLC.

1. **Medium:**
   Kieselgel $H_{254, 336}$; buffered at pH 5 with
   M/15 phosphate.
   Solvent:

   Ethyl acetate.

Detection:

A. UV light.

B. Bioautography vs. *Neisseria catarrhalis* or *Sarcina lutea.*

R_f:

Component	R_f
16,511A	0.1
16,511B*	0.2
16,511C	0.35
16,511D	0.60

*Major zone = 18,051 R.P.

Ref:

South Africa Patent No. 671147; July 19, 1967.

17,967 R.P.

TLC.

1. **Medium:**

A. Silica Gel F_{254} (Merck).

B. Silica Gel H (Merck), buffered with M/3 phosphate, pH 8.0.

Solvent:

A. Chloroform:methanol:acetone (78:20:2).

B. Chloroform:methanol (87:13).

C. Acetone:dioxane (50:50).

Detection:

A. UV light.

B. Bioautography vs. *Bacillus subtilis.*

R_f:

Medium	Solvent	R_f
A	A	0.6
A	B	0.4
B	C	0.6

Ref:

Netherlands Patent No. 69,06827; November 11, 1969.

18,051 R.P.

see 16,511 R.P.

18631 R.P.

PC.

1. **Paper:**

A. Arches 302.

B. As A, but buffered with M/3 phosphate, pH 7.

Solvent:

A. Water satd. butanol.

B. Benzene:methanol (4:1).

C. Ammonium chloride (30 g/l).

D. Butanol:acetic acid:water (4:1:5), upper phase.

E. Ethyl acetate:cyclohexane (1:1) satd. with water.

F. Chloroform.

Detection:

Bioautography vs. *Staphylococcus albus.*

R_f:

Paper	Solvent	R_f
A	A	0.95
	B	0.95
	C	0.05
	D	1.00
	E	0.50
B	F	0.50

Ref:

Netherlands Patent No. 69,02381; August 18, 1969.

TLC.

1. **Medium:**

A. Aluminum oxide.

B. Silica Gel G.

Solvent:

A. Methanol:water (95:5).

B. As PC (1), D.

C. Carbon tetrachloride:ethanol:acetic acid (90:6:6).

Detection:

As PC (1).

R_f:

Medium	Solvent	R_f
A	A	0.27
B	B	1.00
B	C	0.50

Ref:

As PC (1).

19,402 R.P.

PC.

1. **Paper:**

Arches 302.

Solvent:

A. n-Butanol:acetic acid (60:40).

B. n-Butanol:acetic acid:water (60:40:1).

C. Ethyl acetate:pyridine:water (50:40:30).

Detection:

Bioautography vs. *Staphylococcus aureus* 209P.

R_f:

Solvent	R_f
A	0.62
B	0.40
C	0.30

Ref:

Netherlands Patent No. 68, 02093; August 23, 1968.

TLC.

1. **Medium:**

   A. Kieselgel G.

   B. Kieselgel G + alumina G (70:30).

   C. Kieselgel H.

   Solvent:

   A. Isopropanol:2 N ammonium hydroxide (70:30).

   B. Isopropanol:n-butanol:water (50:40:30).

   C. Dioxane:water (60:20).

   Detection:

   As PC (1).

   R_f:

Medium	Solvent	R_f
A	A	0.36
B	B	0.39
C	C	0.20

   Ref:

   As PC (1).

24010

TLC.

1. **Medium:**

   Silica Gel.

   Solvent:

   A. n-Butanol:acetic acid:water (4:1:5, 4:1:2, 2:1:1).

   B. n-Butanol:ethanol:water (10:3:7).

   Detection:

   A. Anisaldehyde:sulfuric acid; heat.

   B. Potassium permanganate:sodium carbonate reagent.

   C. UV light.

   D. Bioautography vs. *Bacillus subtilis*.

   R_f:

   One spot under all conditions.

   Ref:

   M. Mizuno, Y. Shimojima, T. Sugawara and I. Takeda, J. Antibiotics, 24 (1971) 896–899.

A204

PC.

1. **Paper:**

   Whatman No. 1.

   Solvent:

   A. Water:methanol:acetone:benzene (72:24.5:4:0.5).

   B. 10% Aq. n-propanol.

   C. Water:methanol:acetic acid (12:3:1); adjust to pH 10.5 with ammonium hydroxide then to pH 7.3 with phosphoric acid.

   Detection:

   Bioautography vs. *Bacillus subtilis*.

   R_f:

Solvent	R_f
A	0.14
B	0.87
C	0.33

   Ref:

   Belgium Patent No. 728,382; August 13, 1969.

TLC.

1. **Medium:**

   Silica Gel.

   Solvent:

   Ethyl acetate.

   Detection:

   Sulfuric acid with vanillan.

   R_f:

   0.8

   Ref:

   As PC (1).

A-396-I

TLC.

1. **Medium:**

   Silica Gel GF (Merck).

   Solvent:

   Chloroform:methanol:4% ammonia (2:1:1), upper layer.

   Detection:

   R_f:

   0.5 (estimated from drawing).

   Ref:

   S. Shoji, S. Kozuki, M. Mayama, Y. Kawamura and K. Matsumoto, J. Antibiotics, 23 (1970) 291.

A/672
PC.
1. **Paper:**
   Solvent:
   A. Water:satd. n-butanol.
   B. Water-satd. n-butanol containing 2% p-toluenesulfonic acid.
   C. Water-satd. butanol containing 2% conc. ammonia.
   D. n-Butanol-satd. water.
   E. 20% Aq. ammonium chloride.
   F. Phenol:water (75:25).
   G. n-Butanol:methanol:water (40:10:20), containing 0.75 g methyl orange.
   H. n-Butanol:methanol:water (40:20:20).
   I. Water:acetone (1:1).
   J. Water-satd. ethyl acetate.
   Detection:
   Bioautography vs. *Bacillus subtilis.*
   R_f:

Solvent	R_f
A	0.0
B	0.0
C	0.05
D	0.85
E	0.20
F	0.90
G	0.20
H	0.20
I	0.0
J	0.0

Ref:
   J.E. Thiemann, G. Beretta, C. Coronelli and H. Pagani, J. Antibiotics, 22 (1969) 119–125.

A4993A; A4993B
PC.
1. **Paper:**
   Whatman No. 1.
   Solvent:
   A. Propanol:pyridine:acetic acid:water (15:10:3:12).
   B. n-Butanol satd. with 2% p-toluenesulfonic acid.
   C. As B + 2% piperidine.
   Detection:
   R_f:

	R_f Solvent		
	A	B	C
A4993A	0.75	0.45	0.53
A4993B	0.60	0.31	0.32

Ref:
   R.L. Hamill and M.M. Hoehn, U.S. Patent No. 3,629,405; December 21, 1971.

A16884
PC.
1. **Paper:**
   Whatman No. 1.
   Solvent:
   A. Propanol:acetonitrile:water (1:1:1).
   B. Ethanol:water (80:20) containing 1.5% sodium chloride. Paper impregnated with 1 N sodium sulfate.
   C. Methanol:propanol:water (6:2:1); paper buffered with 0.75 M potassium phosphate, pH 4.0.
   D. Propanol:pyridine:acetic acid:acetonitrile: water (45:30:9:40:36).
   E. t.-Amyl alcohol:acetone:water (2:1:2).
   F. Ethyl acetate:acetic acid:water (3:1:1).
   G. Methyl ethyl ketone:water (92:8); paper buffered with 0.1 N sodium acetate, pH 4.6.
   H. Propanol:water (70:30).
   I. Butanol satd. with water.
   J. As I + 2% p-toluenesulfonic acid.
   Detection:
   Bioautography vs. *Salmonella gallinarum.*
   R_f:

Solvent	R_f
A	0.79
B	0.58
C	0.21
D	0.40
E	0.40
F	0.36
G	0.00
H	0.30
I	0.00
J	0.60

Ref:
   Belgium Patent No. 754,424; August 5, 1970.

TLC.
1. **Medium:**
   A. Silica Gel.
   B. Cellulose.
   Solvent:
   Acetonitrile:water (70:30).
   Detection:
   Ninhydrin spray.

R$_f$:

Medium	R$_f$
A	0.47
B	0.45

Ref:

As PC (1).

A16886B
PC.
1. **Paper:**
Whatman No. 1.
Solvent:
Propanol:pyridine:acetic acid:acetonitrile:
water (45:30:9:40:36), 16 h, 25°C.
Detection:
A. Bioautography vs. *Pseudomonas
solanacearum* Lilly culture X185.
B. Radioactive A16886B detected by
scanning.
R$_f$:
Resolves factor A from B.
Ref:
J.G. Whitney, D.R. Brannon, J.A. Mabe and
K.J. Wicker, Antimicrobial Agents and
Chemotherapy, 1 (1972) 247–251.

A16886-I; A16886-II
PC.
1. **Paper:**
Solvent:
A. As A16884, PC (1), B.
B. As A16884, PC (1), I.
C. As A16884, PC (1), J.
D. Water satd. methyl isobutyl ketone.
E. As D + 2% p-toluenesulfonic acid.
F. As D + 2% piperidine.
G. Acetonitrile.
H. Propanol:acetonitrile:methanol:water
(4:3:2:1).
I. Propanol:pyridine:acetic acid:water
(15:10:3:12).
J. As A16884, PC (1), D.
K. Butanol:acetic acid:water (3:1:1).
L. As A16884, PC (1), F.
M. As A16884, PC (1), H.
N. As A16884, TLC (1).
Detection:
A. Ninhydrin.
B. Bioautography vs. *Salmonella gallinarum.*
R$_f$:

Solvent	R$_f$ A16886-I	A16886-II
A	0.38	0.33
B	0.00	0.00
C	0.39	0.32
D	0.00	0.00
E	0.00	0.00
F	0.00	0.00
G	0.00	0.00
H	0.00	0.00
I	0.32	0.27
J	0.21	0.15
K	0.20	0.17
L	0.29	0.22
M	0.17	0.17
N	0.72	0.65

Ref:
Netherlands Patent No. 7,011,805; February
16, 1971.

TLC.
1. **Medium:**
A. Silica Gel.
B. Cellulose.
Solvent:
A. Acetonitrile:water (70:30).
B. Acetonitrile:isopropanol:water (1:1:1).
Detection:
As PC (1).
R$_f$:

Component	R$_f$ (Medium-Solvent) A-A	B-B
16886-I	0.51	0.36
16886-II	0.42	0.29

Ref:
As PC (1).

A-21101
TLC.
1. **Medium:**
Silica Gel.
Solvent:
Toluene:ethyl acetate (2:1).
Detection:
Spray with phosphomolybdic acid; heat
5 min at 100°C.
R$_f$:
0.24, 0.31, 0.36, 0.31

Ref:

Belgian Patent No. 719522; February 14, 1969.

A22765
PC.
1. **Paper:**

Solvent:

A. n-Butanol:acetic acid:water (4:1:5).

B. As A, but (4:1:2).

C. As A, but (1:1:2).

D. n-Propanol:pyridine:water (60:4:40).

E. n-Propanol:acetic acid:2.5% aq. sodium chloride (10:1:8).

F. n-Propanol:acetic acid:water (25:2:25).

G. n-Butanol:ethanol:acetic acid:water (25:25:3:47).

H. Acetone:acetic acid:water (60:3:37).

I. Methanol:0.1 N hydrochloric acid (3:1).

Detection:

Bioautography vs. *Staphylococcus aureus* or *Bacillus subtilis*.

R_f:

Solvent	R_f
A	0.25
B	0.35
C	0.85
D	0.50
E	0.65
F	0.69
G	0.70
H	0.72
I	0.75

Ref:

E. Gaumann, E. Vischer and H. Bickel, German Patent No. 1129259; May 10, 1962.

AB-664α
PC.
1. **Paper:**

Whatman No. 1.

Solvent:

m-Cresol:pyridine:acetic acid:water (200:1:1:100), lower phase, descending.

Detection:

Wash papergrams with ethyl ether to remove cresol; bioautography vs. *Bacillus subtilis* at pH 6.0.

R_f:

0.4–0.5

Ref:

W.K. Hausmann and S.O. Thomas, U.S. Patent No. 3,495,003; February 10, 1970.

ABBOTT 29119
PC.
1. **Paper:**

Solvent:

A. 0.1 M Aq. ammonium hydroxide satd. with methyl isobutyl ketone.

B. 0.5 M Aq. ammonium chloride satd. with p-dioxane.

Detection:

Bioautography vs. *Bacillus subtilis*.

R_f:

Solvent	R_f
A	0.35
B	0.60

Ref:

P.P. Hung, C.L. Marks and P.L. Tarchew, Appl. Microbiol., 13 (1965) 216–217.

AC 98
PC.
1. **Paper:**

Whatman No. 1.

Solvent:

5% Aq. ammonium chloride.

Detection:

Bioautography vs. *Bacillus subtilis* or *Corynebacterium xerosis*.

R_f:

AC 98 mixture:	0.01–0.15, 0.15–0.45, 0.45–0.70.
AC 98 complex A:	0.04, 0.23, 0.57.
AC 98 complex B:	0.03, 0.18, 0.63.

Ref:

S.E. DeVoe and M.P. Kunstmann, U.S. Patent No. 3,495,004; February 10, 1970.

AC541A; AC541B
PC.
1. **Paper:**

Solvent:

90% phenol:m-cresol:acetic acid:pyridine: water (100:25:4:4:75).

Detection:

R_f:

AC541A	0.40
AC541B	0.58

Ref:
W.K. Hausmann, V. Zbinovsky and A.J. Shay, U.S. Patent No. 3,522,349; July 28, 1970.

AF 283α
PC.
1. **Paper:**
   Solvent:
   A. 5% Ammonium chloride.
   B. 90% Phenol:water plus 2% dichloroacetic acid (added to bottom phase).
   C. m-Cresol:90% phenol:0.2 M morpholine: 0.2 M acetic acid (5:5:7:3).
   D. m-Cresol satd. with water plus 2% hepta-fluorobutyric acid (added to lower phase).
   E. sec-Butanol:acetic acid:water (1000:375: 500).
   Detection:
   Bioautography vs. *Corynebacterium xerosis.*
   R_f:

Solvent	R_f
A	0.32
B	0.65
C	0.25
D	0.24
E	0.24

   Ref:
   Australian Patent Appl. 23,886/67; June 29, 1967.

AF 283β
PC.
1. **Paper:**
   Solvent:
   A. 3% Aq. ammonium chloride.
   B. m-Cresol satd. with water with 2% perfluorobutyric acid added.
   C. Chloroform:pyridine:acetic acid:water (10:4:4:5).
   D. sec-Butanol:pyridine:s-collidine:water (3:6:6:3).
   E. 90% Phenol:2% dichloroacetic acid (1:1).
   Detection:
   Bioautography vs. *Corynebacterium xerosis.*
   R_f:

Solvent	R_f
A	0.20
B	0.58
C	0.01
D	0.01
E	0.80

Ref:
As AF 283α.

AO-341
PC.
1. **Paper:**
   Solvent:
   Isoamyl alcohol:methyl isobutyl ketone: acetic acid:water (100:150:50:200).
   Detection:
   R_f:
   0.20
   Ref:
   H.A. Whaley, E.L. Patterson, W.K. Hausmann and J.N. Porter, U.S. Patent No. 3,777,244; April 9, 1968.

B4-81
PC.
1. **Paper:**
   Solvent:
   As BD-12, PC (1), A–L.
   Detection:
   As BD-12, PC (1).
   R_f:

Solvent	R_f
A	0.00
B	1.00
C	0.72
D	0.10
E	0.58
F	0.08
G	0.00
H	0.12
I	0.24
J	0.17
K	0.45
L	0.07

   Ref:
   As BD-12, PC (1).

B-2847-Y; B-2847-R; B-2847-RB
PC.
1. **Paper:**
   Whatman No. 1.
   Solvent:
   A. n-Hexane:benzene:ethanol:water (1:3:1:3).
   B. n-Hexane:benzene:acetone:water (30:10:18:22).

C. n-Hexane:diethyl ether:acetone:water (15:5:8:12).

All solvents developed ascending.

Detection:

Bioautography vs. *Staphylococcus aureus*.

R_f:

Solvent	R_f	
	B-2847-Y	B-2847-R
A	0.78	—
B	0.60	0.65
C	0.27	—

Ref:

Netherlands Patent No. 68,02679; August 26, 1968.

TLC.

1. **Medium:**
   Solvent:
   A. 1% Oxalic acid containing ethyl acetate: acetone (1:1).
   B. 1% Oxalic acid containing ethyl acetate.
   C. 1% Oxalic acid containing acetone.
   Detection:
   R_f:

Solvent	R_f	
	B-2847-Y	B-2847-R
A	0.05	0.70
B	0.00	0.20
C	0.20	—

   Ref:
   As PC (1).

2. **Medium:**
   Kieselgel.
   Solvent:
   Ethyl acetate:acetone (1:1).
   Detection:
   R_f:
   0.65
   Ref:
   German Patent No. 2015076; October 8, 1971.

B-15645
PC.

1. **Paper:**
   Solvent:
   A. n-Butanol:water:pyridine (4:7:3), ascending.
   B. n-Butanol:water (1:1), ascending.

Detection:

R_f:

Solvent	R_f
A	0.72
B	0.35

Ref:

Japanese Patent No. 20559/1970; July 13, 1970.

TLC.

1. **Medium:**
   Silica Gel HF$_{254}$ (Merck).
   Solvent:
   Ethyl acetate:ethanol (4:1).
   Detection:
   R_f:
   0.35
   Ref:
   As PC (1).

BA-6903
CCD.

1. **Solvent:**
   Chloroform:methanol:water:ligroin (3:4:1:1), 100 transfers.
   Distribution:
   Main component found in tubes 20—40 based on O.D. at 275 nm and activity vs. *Bacillus subtilis*.
   Ref:
   K.V. Rao and S.C. Brooks, Antimicrobial Agents and Chemotherapy, 1961 (1962) 491—494.

BD-12
PC.

1. **Paper:**
   Solvent:
   A. Wet butanol.
   B. 1.5% Aq. ammonium chloride.
   C. Phenol:water (3:1).
   D. 50% Aq. acetone.
   E. n-Butanol:methanol:water:methyl orange (40:10:20 ml:1.5 g).
   F. n-Butanol:methanol:water (40:10:20).
   G. Benzene:methanol (4:1).
   H. Water.
   I. n-Propanol:pyridine:acetic acid:water (60:40:10:30) + 1.2 g sodium p-hydroxy-benzene sulfonate/140 ml.

J. Wet butanol + 2% p-toluenesulfonic acid.

K. n-Butanol:pyridine:acetic acid:water
(15:10:3:12).

L. Butanol:acetic acid:water (4:1:5).

Detection:

Bioautography vs. *Bacillus subtilis.*

R_f:

Solvent	R_f
A	0.00
B	0.93
C	0.87
D	0.08
E	0.60
F	0.09
G	0.00
H	0.05
I	0.36
J	0.29
K	0.54
L	0.21

Ref:

Y. Ito, Y. Ohashi, Y. Sakurai, M. Sakurazawa,
H. Yoshida, S. Awataguchi and T. Okuda,
J. Antibiotics, 21 (1968) 307–312.

CP 21,635

PC.

1. Paper:

Solvent:

A. 5% Aq. ammonium chloride.

B. Methanol:1.5% aq. sodium chloride
(4:1); paper buffered with 0.95 M
sodium sulfate + 0.05 M sodium bisulfate.

C. Water satd. methyl isobutyl ketone:
piperidine (100:1).

D. Water satd. methyl isobutyl ketone:
glacial acetic acid (100:1).

E. Benzene satd. with 25% aq. methanol.

Detection:

A. Bioautography vs. *Staphylococcus aureus.*

B. UV light.

R_f:

Solvent	R_f
A	0.29
B	0.81
C	0.88
D	0.86
E	0.36

Ref:

F.C. Sciavolino, J.B. Routien, E.J. Tynan

and W.D. Celmer, U.S. Patent No.
3,655,876; April 11, 1972.

TLC.

1. Medium:

Silica Gel.

Solvent:

A. Ethyl acetate.

B. Chloroform:acetone (1:1).

C. Ethyl acetate:methanol (1:1).

D. Chloroform:methanol (9:1).

E. Butanol.

Detection:

A. As PC (1), A.

B. As PC (1), B.

C. Sulfuric acid.

D. Van Urk's reagent (0.125 g p-dimethylaminobenzaldehyde and 0.1 ml of 5%
ferric chloride in 100 ml of 65% sulfuric
acid).

R_f:

Solvent	R_f
A	0.15
B	0.32
C	0.37
D	0.62
E	0.70

Ref:

As PC (1).

E-749-C

PC.

1. Paper:

Solvent:

A. n-Butanol:acetic acid:water (4:1:2).

B. n-Propanol:pyridine:acetic acid:water
(15:10:3:12).

Detection:

R_f:

Solvent	R_f
A	ca. 0.11
B	0.45–0.55

Ref:

J. Shoji, S. Kozuki, M. Ebata and H. Otsuka,
J. Antibiotics, 21 (1968) 509–511.

G-253

PC.

1. Paper:

Solvent:

Water satd. chloroform.

Detection:

R_f:

Component	R_f
G-253A	0.40—0.50
G-253B$_1$	0.27—0.38
G-253B$_2$	0.13—0.17
G-253B	0.06—0.10
G-253C	0.01—0.06
G-253C$_1$	0.00

Ref:

S. Nomura, H. Yamamoto, I. Umesawa,
A. Matsumae and T. Hata. J. Antibiotics, 20
(1967) 55—61.

TLC.

1. **Medium:**

Kieselgel G.

Solvent:

A. Methanol:ethyl acetate (4:25).

B. Methanol:ethyl acetate:benzene (1:5:5).

Detection:

R_f:

	R_f	
Component	Solvent A	Solvent B
G-253B$_1$	0.67	0.25
G-253B$_2$	0.65	0.23
G-253C$_1$	0.63	0.21

Ref:

As PC (1).

K-288

PC.

1. **Paper:**

Solvent:

A. Wet butanol.

B. 20% Ammonium chloride.

C. 72% Phenol.

D. 50% Acetone.

E. Butanol:methanol:water:methyl orange
(40 ml:10 ml:20 ml:1.5 g).

F. Butanol:methanol:water (40:10:20).

G. Benzene:methanol (80:20).

H. Water.

Detection:

R_f:

Solvent	R_f*
A	0.05
B	0.95
C	0.90
D	0.95
E	0.45
F	0.35
G	0.05
H	0.05

*Estimated from drawing.

Ref:

K. Matsumoto, J. Antibiotics, 14 (1961)
141—146.

ELPHO.

1. **Medium:**

Paper.

Buffer:

A. pH 5.0 buffer.

B. pH 8.0 buffer.

Conditions:

Mobility:

A. Slight movement towards cathode*.

B. Slight movement towards anode*.

*Estimated from drawing.

Ref:

As PC (1).

L. A. 5352

PC.

1. **Paper:**

Solvent:

A. 3% Aq. ammonium chloride.

B. Methanol:0.1 N hydrochloric acid (3:1).

C. Butanol:ethanol:acetic acid:water
(25:25:3:47).

D. Butanol:acetic acid:water (1:1:2).

E. Water satd. butanol.

F. As D, but (4:1:2).

G. As D, but (2:1:1).

Detection:

Bioautography vs. *Micrococcus aureus*.

R_f:

Solvent	R_f
A	0.80
B	0.75
C	0.87
D	0.88
E	0.17
F	0.54, 0.72
G	0.35, 0.45

Ref:

P. Sensi and M.T. Timbal, Antibiotics and
Chemotherapy, 9 (1959) 160—166.

L. A. 5937
PC.
1. **Paper:**
    Solvent:
        As L. A. 5352 (A–G).
    Detection:
        As L. A. 5352.
    R_f:

Solvent	R_f
A	0.80
B	0.75
C	0.83
D	0.90
E	0.20
F	0.14, 0.37, 0.46
G	0.07, 0.17, 0.31

    Ref:
        As L. A. 5352, PC (1).

LA-7017
PC.
1. Circular paper chromatography.
    Paper:
    Solvent:
        A. Benzene:acetic acid:water (20:25:5).
        B. Benzene:butanol:water (18:2:20).
        C. Chloroform:carbon tetrachloride, satd.
           with water:methanol (5:4:1).
        D. Water satd. diisoamyl ester:butanol
           (20:10).
    Detection:
        Bioautography vs. *Staphylococcus aureus*
        209P.
    R_f:
        Useful for comparing LA-7017 with
        aburamycin and NSCA-649.
    Ref:
        E.V. Kruglyak, V.N. Borisova and
        M.G. Brazhnikova, Antibiotiki, 8 (1963)
        1064–1067.

LL-21220
TLC.
1. **Medium:**
    Silica Gel F_{254} (E. Merck).
    Solvent:
        A. Methanol.
        B. Acetone.
        C. Ethyl acetate.

Detection:
    A. UV quenching.
    B. 1% Aq. potassium permanganate spray.
R_f:

Solvent	R_f
A	0.52
B	0.47
C	0.06

Ref:
    D.B. Borders, F. Barbatschi, A.J. Shay and
    P. Shu, Antimicrobial Agents and
    Chemotherapy, 1969 (1970) 233–235.

LL-AB664
PC.
1. **Paper:**
    Whatman No. 1.
    Solvent:
        m-Cresol:acetic acid:pyridine:water
        (200:1:1:100), lower phase, descending.
    Detection:
        Wash air-dried strips with diethyl ether to
        remove cresol; bioautography vs. *Klebsiella
        pneumoniae* at pH 7.9 or *Bacillus subtilis*
        at pH 6.0.
    R_f:
        0.45–0.50
    Ref:
        K.J. Sax, P. Monnikendam, D.B. Borders,
        P. Shu, L.A. Mitscher, W.K. Hausmann and
        E.L. Patterson, Antimicrobial Agents and
        Chemotherapy, 1967 (1968) 442–448.

LL-AC541
PC.
1. **Paper:**
    Whatman No. 1.
    Solvent:
        90% Phenol:m-cresol:acetic acid:pyridine:
        water (100:25:4:4:75).
    Detection:
    R_f:
        0.58
    Ref:
        V. Zbinovsky, W.K. Hausmann, E.R. Wetzel,
        D.B. Borders and E.L. Patterson, Appl.
        Microbiol., 16 (1968) 614–616.

LL-AO341A; LL-AO341B
PC.
1. **Paper:**
    Whatman No. 1.
   Solvent:
    Isoamyl alcohol:methyl isobutyl ketone:
    acetic acid:water (2:3:1:4), upper layer,
    descending.
   Detection:
    Bioautography vs. *Bacillus subtilis*.
   R_f:
    LL-AO341A   0.35
    LL-AO341B   0.22
   Ref:
    H.A. Whaley, E.L. Patterson, M. Dann,
    P. Shu, M.E. Swift, J.N. Porter and G. Redin,
    Antimicrobial Agents and Chemotherapy,
    1966 (1967) 587–590.

LL-AV290
PC.
1. **Paper:**
    Whatman No. 1.
   Solvent:
    A. 5% Aq. ammonium chloride.
    B. Pyridine:s-collidine:sec.-butanol:water
       (2:2:1:1).
    C. Methanol:1.5% aq. sodium chloride
       (4:1); paper buffered with 0.95 M sodium
       sulfate + 0.05 M sodium bisulfate.
    D. 90% Phenol:m-cresol:pyridine:acetic
       acid:water (25:25:1:1:25).
    All solvents developed descending.
   Detection:
    Bioautography vs. *Bacillus subtilis* or
    Corynebacterium xerosis.
   R_f:

Solvent	R_f
A	0.75
B	0.58
C	0.54
D	0.20

   Ref:
    M.P. Kunstmann, L.A. Mitscher, J.N. Porter,
    A.J. Shay and M.A. Darken, Antimicrobial
    Agents and Chemotherapy, 1968 (1969)
    242–245.

LL-BL136
   (cf: SF-701)

PC.
1. **Paper:**
   Solvent:
    A. Water satd. 1-butanol containing 2%
       p-toluenesulfonic acid.
    B. Pyridine:s-collidine:tetramethyl-
       ammonium hydroxide:water (50:25:1:125).
    C. Phenol:m-cresol:acetic acid:pyridine:
       water (100:25:4:4:75).
    D. 1-Butanol:methanol:water:p-toluene-
       sulfonic acid (40:10:20:1).
   Detection:
   R_f:

Solvent	R_f
A	0.21
B	0.70
C	0.55, 0.68
D	0.63

   Ref:
    D.B. Borders, J.P. Kirby, E.R. Wetzel,
    M.C. Davies and W.K. Hausmann, Anti-
    microbial Agents and Chemotherapy, 1
    (1972) 403–407.

MSD-235
PC.
1. **Paper:**
    Whatman No. 3 MM.
   Solvent:
    n-Butanol satd. with 0.1 N ammonium
    hydroxide, 17 h, 25°C.
   Detection:
    Bioautography vs. *Escherichia coli*.
   R_f:

Component	Cm from origin
MSD-235S$_1$	3–5
MSD-235S$_2$	10
MSD-235S$_3$	16

   Ref:
    L. Chaiet, T.W. Miller, F. Tausig and
    F.J. Wolf, Antimicrobial Agents and
    Chemotherapy, 1963 (1964) 28:32.

NSCA-649
PC.
1. Circular paper chromatography.
   Paper:
   Solvent:
    As LA-7017, PC (1), A–D.

Detection:

As LA-7017, PC (1).

R$_f$:

Useful for comparing NSCA-649 with
LA-7017 and aburamycin.

Ref:

As LA-7017, PC (1).

O-2867

PC.

1. **Paper:**

Toyo Roshi No. 51.

Solvent:

n-Butanol:acetic acid:water (4:1:2).

Detection:

Bioautography vs. *Pellicularia oryzae.*

R$_f$:

O-2867-α 0.66
O-2867-β 0.53

Ref:

T. Sato, K. Yamaguchi, M. Katagiri,
J. Awaya, Y. Iwai, S. Omura and T. Hata,
J. Antibiotics, 24 (1971) 774–778.

ELPHO.

1. **Medium:**

Paper.

Buffer:

A. McIlvaine's buffer, pH 2.0.
B. Pyridine:acetic acid:water (1:10:289),
   pH 3.7.
C. M/15 phosphate, pH 8.0.

Conditions:

200 V, 2.5 h.

Mobility:

Buffer	Mobility	
	O-2867-α	O-2867-β
A	Toward cathode	Toward cathode
B	Origin	Origin
C	Toward anode	Toward anode

Ref:

As PC (1).

PA-108; PA-133A; PA-133B; PA-148

PC.

1. **Paper:**

Treated with formamide as stationary phase.

Solvent:

A. Benzene:cyclohexane (1:1).
B. Benzene.
C. Benzene:chloroform (3:1).
D. Benzene:chloroform (4:1).
All solvents developed at 24°C.

Detection:

R$_f$:

	R_f Solvent			
	A	B	C	D
PA-108	0.05	0.58	0.89	0.90
PA-133A	0.75	0.75	0.95	0.95
PA-133B	0.20	0.24	0.76	0.90
PA-148	0.03	0.18	0.58	0.90

Ref:

K. Murai, B.A. Sobin, W.D. Celmer and
F.W. Tanner, Antibiotics and Chemotherapy,
9 (1959) 485–490.

CCD.

1. **Solvent:**

Benzene:cyclohexane:95% ethanol:water
(5:5:8:2).

Distribution:

	Distribution coefficient
PA-108	0.43
PA-133A	1.50
PA-133B	0.50
PA-148	0.57

Ref:

As PC (1).

R-468

PC.

1. **Paper:**

Solvent:

A. Water satd. n-butanol.
B. 3% Ammonium chloride.
C. 50% Aq. phenol.
D. 50% Aq. acetone.
E. Butanol:methanol:water:methyl orange
   (40 ml:10 ml:20 ml:1.5 g).
F. Butanol:methanol:water (4:1:2).
G. Benzene:methanol (4:1).
H. Water.
I. Butanol satd. water.
J. n-Propanol:pyridine:acetic acid:water
   (15:10:3:12).

Detection:
R_f:

Solvent	R_f*
A	0.05
B	1.00
C	0.35
D	0.75
E	0.50
F	0.45
G	0.00
H	1.00
I	1.00
J	0.60

*Estimated from drawing.

Ref:

T. Nishikawa and N. Ishida, J. Antibiotics, 18 (1965) 132–133.

ELPHO.

1. Medium:

Buffer:

A. M/15 phosphate, pH 5.0.

B. M/15 phosphate, pH 8.0.

Conditions:

225 V/20 cm, 3 h.

Mobility:

A. Toward cathode.

B. Slightly toward cathode.

Ref:

As PC (1).

Ro 5-2667; Ro 7-7730; Ro 7-7731

TLC.

1. Medium:

A. MN-polygram cel 300 (Brinkmann).

B. As A, but buffered by dipping plate into 0.2 M ammonium sulfate and allowing excess liquid to drip off plate.

Solvent:

A. 2-Propanol:water (7:3).

B. 1-Butanol:acetic acid:water (4:1:5).

Detection:

R_f:

	R_f (Medium-Solvent)	
	A-B	B-A
Ro 5-2667	0.07	0.06
Ro 7-7730	0.19	0.13
Ro 7-7731	0.02	0.04

Ref:

H. Maehr and J. Berger, Biotech. and Bioeng., 11 (1969) 1111–1123.

S-520

TLC.

1. Medium:

Silica Gel GF.

Solvent:

A. n-Butanol:acetic acid:water (3:1:1).

B. Chloroform:methanol (4:1).

Detection:

R_f:

	R_f Solvent	
	A	B
S-520	0.58 ± 0.05	–
DNP-S-520	–	(I) 0.80
		(II) 0.20
Acetyl-S-520	–	(I) 0.70
		(II) 0.10

Ref:

J. Shoji, S. Kozuki, M. Mayama and N. Shimaoka, J. Antibiotics, 23 (1970) 429–431; J. Shoji and R. Sakazaki, ibid, 432–436.

S-583-A-II; S-583-A-III; S-583-B.

TLC.

1. Medium:

Metal-free Silica Gel plate.

Solvent:

A. Chloroform:methanol (85:15).

B. Benzene:ethyl formate:formic acid (3:2:2).

Detection:

R_f:

Solvent A: S-583-B HCl (streak) > S-583-A-III HCl > S-583-A-II HCl.

Solvent B: S-583-A-II HCl > S-583-B HCl > S-583-A-III HCl.

Ref:

J. Shoji, S. Kozuki, H. Nishimura, M. Mayama, K. Motokawa, Y. Tanaka and H. Otsuka, J. Antibiotics, 21 (1968) 643–648.

S-666

PC.

1. Paper:

Solvent:

n-Butanol:acetic acid:water (4:1:5).

Detection:

R$_f$:

Single spot.

Ref:

Derwent Farmdoc 55495; July 22, 1970.

SF-689
ELPHO.

1. **Medium:**

Buffer:

pH 1.9

Conditions:

3000 V, 20 min.

Mobility:

Migrates 4.5 cm toward cathode.

Ref:

Japanese Patent No. 6076/1970; February 28, 1970.

SF-701
PC.

1. Circular.

Paper:

Solvent:

n-Butanol:pyridine:acetic acid:water (15:10:3:12).

Detection:

R$_f$:

0.39

Ref:

T. Tsuruoka, T. Shoumura, N. Ezaki, T. Niwa and T. Niida, J. Antibiotics, 21 (1968) 237—238.

TLC.

1. **Medium:**

A. Silica Gel.

B. Cellulose.

Solvent:

A. Chloroform:methanol:17% ammonium hydroxide (2:1:1), upper layer.

B. n-Butanol:acetic acid:water (2:1:1).

C. n-Propanol:pyridine:acetic acid:water (15:10:3:12).

D. Wet butanol containing 2% p-toluene-sulfonic acid.

E. Phenol:water (6:4).

Detection:

R$_f$:

Medium	Solvent	R$_f$
A	A	0.72
	B	0.15
B	C	0.66
	B	0.40
	D	0.23
	E	0.42

Ref:

As PC (1).

SF-733
PC.

1. **Paper:**

Solvent:

A. n-Butanol satd. with water containing 2% p-toluenesulfonic acid.

B. n-Butanol:pyridine:acetic acid:water (6:4:1:3).

Detection:

A. Ninhydrin.

B. Bioautography vs. *Bacillus subtilis.*

R$_f$:

Solvent	Distance of zone from origin, cm
A	14.8
B	8.0

Ref:

Netherlands Patent No. 68,18105; June 20, 1969; T. Shomura, N. Ezaki, T. Tsuruoka, T. Niwa, E. Akita and T. Niida, J. Antibiotics, 23 (1970) 155—161.

TLC.

1. **Medium:**

Silica Gel.

Solvent:

A. t-Butanol:acetic acid:water (2:1:1).

B. n-Butanol:acetic acid:water (3:1:1).

C. n-Butanol:pyridine:water (6:4:3).

Detection:

As PC (1).

R$_f$:

Solvent	R$_f$
A	0.40
B	0.16
C	0.50

Ref:

As PC (1), 1.

ELPHO.
1. **Medium:**
   Paper.
   Buffer:
   pH 1.8 buffer.
   Conditions:
   3300 V, 15 min.
   Mobility:
   Migrates 15 cm toward cathode.
   Ref:
   As PC (1), 1.

SF-767-A; SF-767-L.
PC.
1. **Paper:**
   Solvent:
   A. As SF-733, A.
   B. As SF-733, B.
   C. n-Propanol:pyridine:acetic acid:water
   (15:10:3:12).
   Detection:
   As SF-733, A, B.
   R_f:

| Solvent | Distance of zone from origin | |
	SF-767-A	SF-767-L
A	3.9	2.5
B	6.1	5.7
C	11.4	9.7

   Ref:
   German Patent No. 1926458; February 12,
   1970.

TLC.
1. **Medium:**
   Silica Gel G (Merck).
   Solvent:
   A. As SF-733, A.
   B. As SF-733, C.
   Detection:
   R_f:

| Derivative | Solvent | |
	A	B
n-Acetyl SF-767-A	0.89	1.00
n-Acetyl SF-767-L	0.78	1.00

   Ref:
   As PC (1).

ELPHO.
1. **Medium:**
   Paper.

Buffer:
   pH 1.8
Conditions:
   3000 V, 20 min.
Detection:
Mobility:
   Both compounds migrate 11.5 cm to the
   cathode.
Ref:
   As PC (1).

SF-837
TLC.
1. **Medium:**
   A. Silica Gel.
   B. Alumina.
   Solvent:
   A. Benzene:acetone (2:1).
   B. n-Butanol:acetic acid:water (3:1:1).
   C. Methanol.
   D. Ethyl acetate:benzene (2:1).
   E. Ethyl acetate.
   Detection:
   R_f:

| | R_f (Medium-Solvent) | | | | |
	A-A	A-B	A-C	B-D	B-E
SF-837	0.45	0.67	0.82	0.34	0.78
SF-837-A_2	0.51	0.68	0.83	0.40	0.84
SF-837-A_3	0.50	0.68	0.83	0.45	0.87
SF-837-A_4	0.55	0.69	0.84	0.52	0.91

   Ref:
   T. Tsuruoka, T. Shomura, N. Ezaki, E. Akita,
   S. Inoue, S. Fukatsu, S. Amano, H. Watanabe
   and T. Niida, Belgian Patent No. 745-430;
   July 16, 1970; T. Niida, T. Tsuruoka,
   N. Ezaki, T. Shomura, E. Akita and S. Inouye,
   J. Antibiotics, 24 (1971) 319–320.

T-2636 Antibiotics
TLC.
1. **Medium:**
   Kieselgel F_{254} (Merck).
   Solvent:
   A. Chloroform:methanol (93:7).
   B. Ethyl acetate:acetone (95:5).
   C. Methyl ethyl ketone:ethyl ether (1:3).
   D. Benzene:acetone (1:1).
   Detection:
   A. Conc. sulfuric acid.

B. Iodine vapor.

C. Bioautography vs. *Sarcina lutea* PCI 1001.

R_f:

Component	R_f Solvent			
	A	B	C	D
A	0.87	0.77	0.85	0.82
B	0.85	0.67	0.78	0.81
C	0.51	0.51	0.57	0.69
D	0.41	0.47	0.53	0.56
E	0.33	0.35	0.35	0.49
F	0.22	0.27	0.25	0.40
M	0.00	0.00	0.00	0.00

Ref:

S. Harada, T. Kishi and K. Mizuno,
J. Antibiotics, 24 (1971) 13–22; T. Fugono,
S. Harada, E. Higashide and T. Kishi, ibid,
23–28.

TA 2407

PC.

1. **Paper:**

Toyo No. 131.

Solvent:

A. Water satd. n-butanol.

B. 20% Aq. ammonium chloride.

C. 75% Phenol.

D. 50% Acetone.

E. Butanol:methanol:water (4:1:2).

F. As E:methyl orange (70 ml:1.5 g).

G. Water.

H. Ethyl acetate:conc. ammonium hydroxide: water (3:1:1).

All solvents developed ascending.

Detection:

R_f:

Solvent	R_f
A	1.00
B	0.33
C	1.00
D	1.00
E	1.00
F	1.00
G	0.66
H	0.90

Ref:

Japanese Patent No. 956/1970; January 15, 1970.

TLC.

1. **Medium:**

Silica Gel GF$_{254}$.

Solvent:

A. Benzene.

B. Chloroform.

C. Ethyl acetate.

D. Hexane:ethyl acetate (7:3).

E. Benzene:ethyl acetate (4:1).

F. Benzene:ethyl acetate (1:1).

G. Ether:isopropyl ether (1:1).

H. Isopropyl ether.

Detection:

R_f:

Solvent	R_f
A	0.00
B	0.04
C	0.90
D	0.28
E	0.28
F	0.63
G	0.57
H	0.33

Ref:

As PC (1).

U-12,898

PC.

1. **Paper:**

Solvent:

A. 1-Butanol:water (84:16), 16 h.

B. As A + 0.25% p-toluenesulfonic acid, 16 h.

C. 1-Butanol:acetic acid:water (2:1:1), 16 h.

D. As A + 2% piperidine, 16 h.

E. 1-Butanol:water (4:96), 5 h.

F. As E + 0.25% p-toluenesulfonic acid, 5 h.

G. As A + 2% p-toluenesulfonic acid, 64 h.

H. Methanol:15% sodium chloride (4:1), paper impregnated with 0.1 M sodium sulfate, 5 h.

Detection:

Bioautography vs. *Bacillus subtilis.*

R_f:

Solvent	$R_f^\star$
A	0.05
B	0.05
C	0.15
D	0.00

E   0.90
F   0.90
G   0.15
H   0.50

*Estimated from drawing.

Ref:

D.J. Mason, A. Dietz and L.J. Hanka,
Antimicrobial Agents and Chemotherapy,
1962 (1963) 607—613.

CCD.

1. **Solvent:**

    1-Butanol:water.

   Distribution:

    Distribution coefficient of p-toluenesulfonic
    acid salt was 0.38.

   Ref:

    M.E. Bergy, T.E. Eble, R.R. Herr, C.M. Large
    and B. Bannister, ibid, 614—618.

U-13,714

PC.

1. **Paper:**

    Whatman No. 1.

   Solvent:

    As U-12,898, A, B, C, E, F.

   Detection:

    Bioautography vs. vaccinia-chick-embryo
    kidney monolayer.

   R_f:

Solvent	R_f*
A	0.00
B	0.00
C	0.30
E	0.68
F	0.65

   *Estimated from drawing.

   Ref:

    J.J. Vavra and A. Dietz, Antimicrobial
    Agents and Chemotherapy, 1964 (1965)
    75—79.

CCD.

1. **Solvent:**

    2-Butanol:water (1:1), 1000 transfers.

   Distribution:

    Peak found in tube 365; K = 0.57.

   Ref:

    M.E. Bergy and R.R. Herr, Antimicrobial
    Agents and Chemotherapy, 1964 (1965)
    80—82.

U-13,933

PC.

1. **Paper:**

   Solvent:

    As U-12,898, A—F.

   Detection:

    Bioautography vs. KB cells.

   R_f:

Solvent	R_f*
A	0.80
B	0.85
C	0.90
D	0.90
E	0.87
F	0.90

   *Estimated from drawing.

   Ref:

    A.D. Argoudelis, J.H. Coats and R.R. Herr,
    Antimicrobial Agents and Chemotherapy,
    1965 (1966) 801—803.

U-20,661

PC.

1. **Paper:**

   Solvent:

    A—F as U-12,898, PC (1), A—F.
    G. 0.1 M potassium phosphate buffer,
      pH 7.0; 5 h.
    H. 0.075 N ammonium hydroxide satd. with
      methyl isobutyl ketone; 5 h.
    I. Benzene:methanol:water (1:1:2). Paper
      equilibrated with vapor phase at 25°C;
      developed 5 h with upper phase.

   Detection:

    Bioautography vs. *Sarcina lutea*.

   R_f:

Solvent	R_f*
A	0.50—0.85
B	0.50—0.85
C	0.70—0.90
D	0.20—0.70
E	0.15—0.65
F	0.10—0.60
G	0.00—0.20
H	0.30—0.50
I	0.05—0.25

   *Estimated from drawing.

   Ref:

    M.E. Bergy and F. Reusser, Experientia, 23
    (1967) 254—255.

U-21,963
PC.
1. Paper:
Solvent:

As U-12,898, PC (1), A–F.

Detection:

Bioautography.

R_f:

Solvent	R_f*
A	0.37–0.50
B	0.50–0.80
C	0.75–0.93
D	no zone
E	0.75–0.90
F	0.75–0.90

*Estimated from drawing.

Ref:

T.R. Pyke and A. Dietz, Appl. Microbiol., 14 (1966) 506–510. J.H. Coats, C.E. Meyer and T.R. Pyke, U.S. Patent No. 3,627,882; December 14, 1971.

U-22,324
TLC.
1. Medium:
Silica Gel G.

Solvent:

1-Butanol:acetic acid:water (2:1:1).

Detection:

Bioautography vs. *Sarcina lutea.*

R_f:

Ref:

F. Reusser, J. Biol. Chem., 242 (1967) 243–247.

U-22,956
PC.
1. Paper:
Whatman No. 1.

Solvent:

As U-12,898, PC (1), A–F.

Detection:

Bioautography vs. *Salmonella gallinarum.*

R_f:

Solvent	R_f*
A	0.20–0.43
B	0.45–0.60
C	0.83
D	no zone
E	0.85
F	0.85

*Estimated from drawing.

Ref:

D.J. Mason, W.L. Lummis and A. Dietz, Antimicrobial Agents and Chemotherapy, 1964 (1965) 110–113.

VD 844
TLC.
1. Medium:
Solvent:

Ethyl acetate:water (pH 2).

Detection:

Bioautography vs. *Neisseria gonorrheae.*

R_f:

0.15–0.20

Ref:

W. von Daehne, W.O. Godtfredsen and L. Tybring, J. Antibiotics, 22 (1969) 233–236.

YA 56-X; YA 56-Y
PC.
1. Paper:
Toyo No. 51A.

Solvent:

A. Water satd. butanol.
B. Acetone:water (1:1).
C. Phenol:water (3:1).
D. n-Butanol:methanol:water (4:1:2).
E. n-Butanol:methanol:water:methyl orange (40 ml:10 ml:20 ml:1.5 g).
F. n-Butanol:pyridine:acetic acid:water (15:10:3:12).
G. n-Butanol:acetic acid:water (4:1:5).

All solvents developed ascending.

Detection:

Bioautography vs. *Bacillus subtilis.*

R_f:

	R_f	
Solvent	YA 56-X	YA 56-Y
A	0.00	0.00
B	0.05	0.05
C	0.93	0.93
D	0.10	0.10
E	0.47	0.47
F	0.30	0.45
G	0.23	0.31

Ref:

Y. Ito, Y. Ohashi, Y. Egawa, T. Yamaguchi, T. Furumai, K. Enomoto and T. Okuda, J. Antibiotics, 24 (1971) 727–731.

YC 73
PC.
1. **Paper:**
   Toyo Roshi No. 51A.
   Solvent:
   A. Wet n-butanol.
   B. 20% Aq. ammonium chloride.
   C. 50% Aq. acetone.
   D. n-Butanol:methanol:water (4:1:2).
   E. Benzene:methanol (4:1).
   F. Water.
   All solvents developed ascending.
   Detection:
   Bioautography vs. *Staphylococcus aureus*.
   R_f:

Solvent	R_f
A	0.73
B	0.65
C	0.85
D	0.69
E	0.82
F	0.73

   Ref:
   Y. Egawa, K. Umino, S. Awataguchi,
   Y. Kawano and T. Okuda, J. Antibiotics, 23
   (1970) 267–270.

TLC.
1. **Medium:**
   Kieselgel GF$_{254}$.
   Solvent:
   A. Chloroform.
   B. Ethyl acetate.
   Detection:
   A. Visible color.
   B. Bioautography.
   R_f:

Solvent	R_f
A	0.19
B	0.57

   Ref:
   As PC (1).

ELPHO.
1. **Medium:**
   Paper.
   Buffer:
   M/15 phosphate, pH 5.0 and pH 8.0.
   Conditions:
   10 V/cm, 2.5 h.

Mobility:
   YC 73 moves slightly to the cathode with
   both buffers.
Ref:
   As PC (1).

YL 704 Series
TLC.
1. **Medium:**
   A. Kieselgel GF$_{254}$.
   B. Aluminum oxide:Kieselgel GF$_{254}$ (4:1).
   Solvent:
   A. Ethyl acetate:n-hexane:conc. ammonium
      hydroxide (8:2:1).
   B. Benzène:acetone (3:2).
   Detection:
   R_f:

	R_f (Medium-Solvent)		
	A-A	A-B	B-B
YL 704A$_1$	0.68	0.60	0.59
YL 704A$_2$	0.68	0.53	0.42
YL 704B$_1$	0.53	0.47	0.50
YL 704B$_2$	0.53	0.41	0.33

   Ref:
   Belgian Patent No. 750,572; May 19, 1970.

INDEX BY COMPOUND

Aabomycin A_1, 19

Alblastmycin, 19

Aburamycin, 133

2-Acetamidophenoxazine-3-one, 147

N-acetyl hybrimycin A_1, 125

N-acetyl hybrimycin A_2, 125

N-acetyl hybrimycin B_1, 125

N-acetyl hybrimycin B_2, 125

2-acetyl-5-hydroxytetracycline, 185

N-acetyl neamine, 125

N-acetyl neomycin B, 124, 125

N-acetyl neomycin C, 124, 125

Acrylamidine, 20

Actinobolin, 20

Actinoleukin, 20

Actinomycins, 20–25

Actinomycin monolactone, 22, 25

Actinomycin A, 20, 21, 22

Actinomycin B, 20, 21, 22, 23

Actinomycin B_{VIc}, 22

Actinomycin C, 20, 21, 22, 23, 25

Actinomycin C_0, 21, 24

Actinomycin C_1, 21, 24, 25

Actinomycin C_{1a}, 21

Actinomycin C_2, 21, 22, 24, 25

Actinomycin C_2a, 21

Actinomycin C_3, 21, 22, 24, 25

Actinomycin C_3a, 21

Actinomycin C_4, 21

Actinomycin C_0a, 24

Actinomycin D, 20, 21, 22, 23, 24

Actinomycin D–H^3, 23

Actinomycin F Group, 25

Actinomycin F_1, 25

Actinomycin F_2, 25

Actinomycin I_0, 24

Actinomycin I_0a, 24

Actinomycin I_1, 24

Actinomycin I_2, 24

Actinomycin I_3, 24

Actinomycin L, 23

Actinomycin S_1, 23

Actinomycin S_2, 23

Actinomycin S_3, 23

Actinomycin U_1, 23

Actinomycin U_2, 23

Actinomycin U_3, 23

Actinomycin U_4, 23

Actinomycin X, 22

Actinomycin X_0, 24

Actinomycin X_0a, 24

Actinomycin X_1, 24

Actinomycin X_1a, 24

Actinomycin X_2, 24

Actinomycin X_3, 24

Actinomycin X_4, 24

Actinomycin Z_0, 24

Actinomycin Z_1, 24

Actinomycin Z_2, 24

Actinomycin Z_3, 24

Actinomycin Z_4, 24

Actinomycin Z_5, 24

Actinomycin I, 22

Actinomycin II, 22

Actinomycin III, 22

Actinomycin IV, 22

Actinomycin V, 22

Actinomycin VIa, 22

Actinomycin VIb, 22

Actinomycin VIc, 22

Actinomycin VId, 22

Actinomycin VIe, 22

Actinomycinic acid, 22, 25

Actinospectacin, 25–26

Actinoxanthin, 26

Adriamycin, 26

Albocycline, 26–27

Albomycin, 27–28

Albomycin δ_1, 27

Albomycin δ_2, 27

Aldgamycin E, 28

Alveomycin, 28

Amaromycin, 28

Ambutyrosine (cf. butyrosin), 28

Tetra-N-acetyl-ambutyrosine A, 28

Tetra-N-acetyl-ambutyrosine B, 28

Amicetin, 28–29

Amidinomycin, 29

Amidomycin, 29

7-aminocephalosporanic acid (7ACA), 47, 49, 51

3-amino-3-deoxy-D-glucose, 29

6-Amino-penicillanic acid, 51; 137, 138, 139, 140, 146
2-Aminophenoxazin-3-one, 146, 147
Aminopyrrolnitrin, 161
Amphotericin A, 29—30
Amphotericin B, 29—30
Ampicillin, 139, 140, 142
Angolamycin, 30
5a,6-Anhydro-7-chloro-6-demethyl-9-nitrotetracycline, 186
5a,6-Anhydro-7-chloro-6-demethyltetracycline, 186
Anhydrochlortetracycline, 184, 188
Anhydrodemethylchlorotetracycline, 182
5a,6-Anhydro-6-demethyl-tetracycline, 186
Anhydroerythromycin, 71, 72
Anhydroerythromycin A, 72
Anhydroerythromycin C, 72
Anhydroerythronolide, 72
Anhydromethylchlortetracycline, 188
Anhydrotetracycline, 182, 184, 185, 187, 188, 189
Anthelvencins, 30—31
Anthramycin, 31
Anticapsin, 31
Antimycin A, 31
Antimycin A$_0$, 31
Antimycin A$_1$, 31
Antimycin A$_2$, 31
Antimycin A$_3$, 31
Antimycin A$_4$, 31
Antimycin A$_5$, 31
Antimycin A$_6$, 31
Antimycin B, 31
Antimycoin, 32
Antimycoin A, 32
Antiviral substance from *Penicillium cyaneo-fulvum* Biourge, 32
Aquayamycin, 32
Aranoflavin A, 32
Aranoflavin B, 32
Aristeromycin, 32—33
Armentomycin, 33
Ascocholin α, 33
Ascocholin β, 33
Asperlin, 33
Atroventin, 33—34
Aureofungin, 34
Aureothricin, 34
Avilamycin, 34

Axenomycin A, 34
Axenomycin B, 34
Axenomycin D, 34—35
Ayamycin A$_1$, 35
Ayamycin A$_2$, 35
Ayamycin A$_3$, 35
5-Azacytidine, 35
Azalomycin B, 35
Azalomycin F, 35—36
Azalomycin F$_3$, 35—36
Azalomycin F$_4$, 35—36
Azalomycin F$_5$, 35—36
α-Azidobenzylpenicillin, 139, 141
Azirinomycin, 36
Azomultin, 36
Azotobacter chroococcum antibiotic, 36—37
Azotomycin, 37

Bacimethrin, 37
Bacitracin, 37—38, 125, 126
Bacitracin A, 37
Bacitracin B, 37
Bamicetin, 38
Bandamycin A, 38
Bandamycin B, 38
Benzylpenicillic acid, 143
Benzylpenicillin (cf. penicillin G), 137, 138, 139, 142, 143, 145
Benzylpenicillin acetonyl ester, 141
Benzylpenicillin acetoxymethyl, 141
Benzylpenicillin amide, 141
Benzylpenicillin cyanomethyl ester, 141
Benzylpenicillin diethylaminoethyl ester, 141
Benzylpenicillin methyl ester, 141
Benzylpenicillin phenacyl ester, 141
Benzylpenicillin thiomethyl ester, 141
Benzylpenicilloic acid, 141, 143
Blasticidin, 38—39
Blasticidin S, 39
Bleomycin A, 39
Bleomycin B, 39
Bleomycin-Copper Chelates, 39—40
Bleomycin Cu-At-1, 39—40
Bleomycin Cu-Bt-1, 39—40
Bleomycin Cu-At-2, 39—40
Bleomycin Cu-At-3, 39—40
Bleomycin Cu-At-4, 39—40
Bleomycin Cu-At-5, 39—40

Bleomycin Cu-At-6, 39—40
Bleomycin Cu-Bt-2, 39—40
Bleomycin Cu-Bt-3, 39—40
Bleomycin Cu-Bt-4, 39—40
Bleomycin Cu-Bt-5, 39—40
Bluensomycin, 40
Boseimycin, 40
Bottromycin A, 41
Bottromycin B, 41
Bramycin, 41
Bresein, 41—42
6-Bromopenicillanic acid, 145
Bulgerin, 42
Butyryl holothin, 90

Candicidin, 42
Capreomycin, 42—43
Capreomycin I, 42
Capreomycin IA, 42
Capreomycin IB, 42
Capreomycin II, 42
Capreomycin IIA, 42
Capreomycin IIB, 42
O-Carbamyl-d-serine, 43
Carbomycin (cf. magnamycin), 43—44
Carbomycin B, 43—44
4-carboxy-n-butyl-penicillin, 137
Cefazolin, 44—45
Celesticetin, 45—46
Celesticetin B, 45
Celesticetin C, 45
Celesticetin D, 45
Cenococcum antibiotic, 46
Cephaloglycin, 46
Cephaloglycin metabolites, 46
Cephalosporins (See also specific
    derivatives), 46—52
Cephalosporin C, 46, 47, 48, 49, 50, 51
Cephalosporin C-dibenzhydrylester, 49
Cephalosporin C nucleus (7-ACA) (See:
    7-amino cephalosporanic acid), 47, 51,
    137
Cephalosporin C_A, 47, 50, 51
Cephalosporin C_C, 47, 51
Cephalosporin C_C nucleus, 51
Cephalosporin N, 46, 48, 137
Cephalosporin P, 48
Cephalosporin P_1, 48
Cephalosporin P_2, 48
Cephalosporin P_3, 48

Cephalosporin P_4, 48
Cephalosporin P_5, 48
Cephalosporin derivatives:
    7-Aminocephalosporanic acid-
        benzhydrylester, 49
    Iso-7-aminocephalosporanic acid-
        benzylester, 49
    Iso-7-aminocephalosporanic acid-
        benzhydrylester, 49
    N-t-butyloxycarbonyl-cephalosporin
        C-dibenzylester, 49
    N-phenylacetyl, 47, 51
    N-phthalyl-cephalosporin-C-9-
        benzhydrylester, 49
    N-phthalyl-cephalosporin-C-9-
        benzhydrylester-1′-methylester, 49
    N-phthalyl-D-α-aminoadipic acid-
        benzhydrylester-e-methylester, 50
    N-phthalyl-DL-α-aminoadipic acid-
        dimethylester, 50
    N-phthalyl-D-α-aminoadipic acid-e-
        methylester, 50
    N-phthalyl-cephalosporin C-
        dibenzhydrylester, 49
    Piperidine-(6)-carbonic-acid-(2)-
        benzylester, 49
Cephalosporum graminius antibiotic, 52
Cephalothin, 48
    Deacetyl cephalothin, 48
Chalcidin, 52
Chalcidin Fraction II, 52
Chalcidin Fraction III, 52
Champamycin A, 52
Champamycin B, 52
Champavitin, 52—53
Chelocardin, 53
Chloramphenicol, 53—55
Chloramphenicol palimitate, 54, 55
Chloramphenicol stearate, 54
Chloramphenicol succinate, 54, 55
7-chloro-5a-(11a)-dehydrotetracycline,
    182
7-chloro-6-demethyl-5a,6-anhydrotetra-
    cycline, 186
7-chloro-6-demethyl-5a,6-anhydro-4-
    dedimethyl-aminotetracycline, 186
7-chloro-6-demethyltetracycline, 185
7-chloro-6-demethyl-4-dedimethylamino-
    tetracycline, 186

7-chloro-6-demethyl-9-nitrotetracycline-6-sulfuric acid ester, 186
7-chloro-6-demethyltetracycline-6-sulfuric acid ester, 186
6-chloropenicillanic acid, 145
2-Chloropyrrolnitrin, 161
Chlortetracycline (See also specific derivatives), 55, 181, 182, 183, 184, 185, 186, 187, 188, 189, 190
Chromin, 55
Chromomycins, 55—56
Chromomycin A group, 56
Chromomycin A_1, 55—56
Chromomycin A_2, 55—56
Chromomycin A_3, 55—56
Chromomycin A_3-Ac, 56
Chromomycin A_3-formate, 56
Chromomycin A_3-Me, 56
Chromomycin A_3-Me-Ac, 56
Chromomycin A_3 hemi-succinate, 56
Chromomycin A_4, 56
Chromomycin A_5, 56
Chromomycin B group, 56
Chromomycin C group, 56
Chromomycin F, 56
Chromomycin O_1, 56
Chromomycin O_2, 56
Chrothiomycin, 57
Cineromycin B, 57
Cirramycins, 57—59
Cirramycin A, 57, 58, 59
Cirramycin A_1, 58, 59
Cirramycin A_1 derivatives, 58
Cirramycin A_2, 58, 59
Cirramycin A_3, 58, 59
Cirramycin A_4, 58, 59
Cirramycin A_5, 58, 59
Cirramycin B, 57, 59
Citromycin, 59
Clindamycin, 108
Cloxacillin, 140, 142, 143, 145
Coformycin, 59—60
Colisan, 60
Colisan, acetylated, 60
Colisan, deaminated, 60
Colistin, 60
Comirin, 60—61
Copiamycin, 61
Coumermycins, 61—65
Coumermycin complex, 61

Coumermycin A_1, 62
Coumermycin D-1, 61
Coumermycin D-1a, 62
Coumermycin D-1b(c), 62
Coumermycin D-1d, 62
Coumermycin D-2, 61, 62
Coumermycin D-3, 61, 62
Coumermycin D-4, 62
Cranomycin, 62
Cremeomycin, 62
Curamycin, 63
Cyanein, 63
Cyathin A_3, 63
Cyathin A_4, 63
Cyathin B, 63
Cyathin B_3, 63
Cyathin C_5, 63
Cyathin No. 1, 63
Cyclamidomycin, 64
Cycloserine, 64
Danubomycin, 64—65
Daunomycin, 65
Deacetyl cephalosporin C, 47, 51
(-) Dehydrogriseofulvin, 86
Dehydro-1-thiogriseofulvin, 86
Demethylchlortetracycline, 182, 183, 184, 188, 189
N-demethylclindamycin, 108
1'-Demethylclindamycin, 108
Demethyldecarbamylnovobiocin, 130
dl-6-demethyl-6-deoxytetracycline, 185
6-demethyl-6-desoxytetracycline, 183
4-demethylgriseofulvin, 85
6-demethylgriseofulvin, 85, 86
N-demethyl-N-hydroxymethylclindamycin (compound A), 108
Demethylnovobiocin, 130
Demethyltetracycline, 184, 186, 188
6-Demethyltetracycline-6-sulfuric acid ester, 186
Deoxyherqueinone, 65
6-Deoxy-5-oxytetracycline, 190
Desacetyl cephaloglycin, 46
Desacetyl cephaloglycin lactone, 46
12α-desoxytetracycline, 181
Desalicetin, 45—46
Descarbamyl novobiocin, 130
Desertomycin, 65
Desmethylherqueichrysin, 89
Desmycosin, 66

Detoxin, 66–67
Dextochrysin, 67
Diacetyloleandomycin, 132
1,2-Diacetyloleandomycin, 132
1,3-Diacetyloleandomycin, 132
2,3-Diacetyloleandomycin, 132
10,12α-diacetyl-5-oxytetracycline, 181
Dianemycin, 67
Diazomycin A, 67
Diazomycin B, 67
Diazomycin C, 67
Dicloxacillin, 142, 145
Dienomycin, 67
Dihydrodesoxystreptomycin, 175
Dihydrostreptomycin, 68, 174, 175
Dihydroxystreptomycin, 174, 175
Distamycin A, 30, 68
Diumycin A, 68
Diumycin B, 68
Doricin, 68
Doxycycline, 189

Echanomycin, 68
Echinomycin, 68
Edeine A, 69
Edeine A₁, 69
Edeine A₂, 69
Edeine B, 69
Endomycin A, 69
Endomycin B, 69
Enduracidin, 69–70
Enhygrofungin, 70
Enomycin, 70
4-Epianhydroemethylchlortetracycline,
    183
4-Epianhydrotetracycline, 182, 187, 188,
    189
4-Epi-chlortetracycline, 182, 184, 189
4-Epidemethylchlortetracycline, 182, 183,
    188
Epi-6-demethyl-6-desoxytetracycline, 183
Epi-Tetracycline, 182, 183, 184, 188, 189
5-Epitetracycline, 182
Ericamycin, 70
Erizomycin, 70
Erythrolosamine, 72
Erythromycin, 71–72
Erythromycin A, 71, 72
Erythromycin B, 71, 72
Erythromycin C, 71, 72

Erythromycin acetate, 71
Erythromycin estolate, 72
Erythromycin ethyl carbonate, 72
Erythromycin ethyl succinate, 72
Erythromycin gluceptate, 72
Erythromycin lactobionate, 72
Erythromycin stearate, 72
Esein, 72–73
Ethoxy-carbonyl-acetamido-cephalospor-
    anic acid, sodium salt, 50
Eurocidin, 73
Everninomicins, 73–74
Everninomicin A, 73, 74
Everninomicin B, 73, 74
Everninomicin C, 73, 74
Everninomicin D, 73, 74
Everninomicin E1, 74
Everninomicin E2, 74
Everninomicin E3, 74
Everninomicin E4, 74
Everninomicin F, 73
Exfoliatin, 74

Ferramido chloromycin (FACM), 74–75
Ferrimycin A, 75
Ferrimycin A₁, 75
Ferrimycin A₂, 75
Ferrimycin B, 75
Fervenulin, 75
Filipin complex, 75–76
Filipin I, 76
Filipin II, 76
Filipin III, 76
Filipin IV, 76
Flavofungin, 76
Flavomycoin, 76
3′-Fluoro-3′-dechloropyrrolnitrin, 161
4′-Fluoropyrrolnitrin, 161
Fluorpyrrolnitrin, 160
Folimycin, 76–77
Formycins, 77
Formycin A, 77
Formycin B, 77
12a(O-formyl) chlortetracycline, 184
12a(O-formyl) tetracycline, 184
Foromacidin A, 77
Foromacidin B, 77
Foromacidin C, 77
Foromacidin D, 77
Fumigachlorin, 77

Fungichromin, 77–78
Furanomycin, 78
Fusarium antibiotic, 78

Gatavalin, 78
Gelbecidin, 78–79
Geldanamycin, 79
Genimycin, 79
Gentamicins, 79–82
Gentamicin A, 81, 82
Gentamicin A_1, 81, 82
Gentamicin B, 81, 82
Gentamicin B_1, 81, 82
Gentamicin C_1, 80, 81, 82
Gentamicin C_1a, 80, 81, 82
Gentamicin C_2, 80, 81, 82
Gentamicin X, 81, 82
Geomycin, 82–83, 176
Glebomycin, 83
Gliotoxin, 83
Gluconimycin, 83
2-Glycine-oxytocin, 134
3-Glycine-oxytocin, 134
4-Glycine-oxytocin, 134
Gougeroxymycin, 83–84
Gramicidins, 84–85
Gramicidin J, 84, 85
Gramicidin S, 85
Grisein, 85
Griseofulvin, 85, 86, 87
Griseofulvins, 85–87
(+) Griseofulvin, 86
Griseofulvin acid, 85
Griseolutein A, 87–88
Griseolutein B, 87–88

Halomicin, 88
Halomicin A, 88
Halomicin B, 88
Halomicin C, 88
Halomicin D, 88
Hamycin, 88–89
Herqueichrysin, 89
Hetacillin, 142
Hikizimycin, 89
Histidomycin A, 89
Histidomycin B, 89
Hodydamycin, 89–90
Holomycin, 90
HON(δ-hydroxy-γ-oxo-L-norvaline), 90

Hondamycin, 90–91
Hordecin, 91
Hortadine A, 91
Hortadine B, 91
Hybrimycins (See N-acetyl hybrimycins)
9-Hydroxy-7-chloro-5-demethyl-4-
    dedimethylaminotetracycline, 186
9-Hydroxy-7-chloro-6-demethyltetra-
    cycline, 186
5-Hydroxy-7-chlortetracycline, 185
Hydroxymycin, 91–92
Hydroxystreptomycin, 92, 174
Hydroxytetracycline (See oxytetra-
    cycline), 184
5-Hydroxytetracycline, 183, 185
(+)-5′-Hydroxy-1-thiogriseofulvin, 86
Hygromycin, 92
Hygrostatin, 92

Ikutamycin, 92–93
Ilicicolin A, 93
Ilicicolin B, 93
Ilicicolin C, 93
Ilicicolin D, 93
Ilicicolin E, 93
Ilicicolin F, 93
Ilicicolin G, 93
Ilicicolin H, 93
Iodinin (See 1,6-phenazinediol-5,10
    dioxide)
Isochlortetracycline, 182, 184
Isogriseofulvin, 87
Isonovobiocin, 130
Isopyrrolnitrin, 161
Isotetracycline, 182, 184
Iturine, 93

Janiemycin, 93–94
Josamycin, 94
Julymicins, 94–95
Julymycin B-0, 95
Julymycin B-I, 95
Julymycin B-II, 95
Julymycin B-III, 95
Julymycin B-IV, 95
Julymycin S.V., 95
Juvenimicins, 95
Juvenimicin A, 95
Juvenimicin A_1, 95
Juvenimicin A_2, 95

Juvenimicin A$_3$, 95
Juvenimicin A$_4$, 95
Juvenimicin B$_1$, 95
Juvenimicin B$_2$, 95
Juvenimicin B$_3$, 95
Juvenimicin B$_4$, 95

Kalafungin, 96
Kanamycins, 96—98
Kanamycin A, 96, 97, 98
Kanamycin B, 96, 97
Kanamycin C, 96, 97
Kanamycin derivatives:
   Tetra-N-benzylkanamycin, 97, 98
   Tetra-N-cinnamylkanamycin, 97, 98
   Tetra-N-phenylethylkanamycin, 97, 98
   Tetra-N-phenylpropylkanamycin, 97, 98
   Tetra-N-2-chlorobenzylkanamycin, 97,
     98
   Tetra-N-2-hydroxybenzylkanamycin
     Na$_2$, 97, 98
   Tetra-N-2-methoxybenzylkanamycin,
     97, 98
   Tetra-N-2,4-dichlorobenzylkanamycin,
     97, 98
   Tetra-N-2,4-dimethoxybenzylkana-
     mycin, 97, 98
   Tetra-N-2-hydroxy-3-methoxybenzyl-
     kanamycin Na$_2$, 97, 98
   Tetra-N-3-hydroxybenzylkanamycin,
     97, 98
   Tetra-N-3-nitrobenzylkanamycin, 97,
     98
   Tetra-N-4-isopropylbenzylkanamycin,
     97, 98
   Tetra-N-4-methoxybenzylkanamycin,
     97, 98
   Tetra-N-4-methylbenzylkanamycin,
     97, 98
   Tetra-N-4-chlorobenzylkanamycin,
     97, 98
Kanchanomycin, 98
Kasugamycin, 99
Ketomycin, 99
Kidamycin, 99—100
Kikumycin A, 100
Kikumycin B, 100
Kinamycin A, 100—101
Kinamycin B, 100—101
Kinamycin C, 100—101

Kinamycin D, 100—101
Kirromycin, 101
Kobenomycin, 101—102
Komamycin A, 102
Komamycin B, 102
Kujimycin A, 102
Kujimycin B, 102
Kundrymycin, 102

Lactenocin, 102
Lagosin, 102—103
Largomycin, 103
Laspartomycin, 103—104
Lateriomycin F, 104
Lemacidine B$_1$, 104
Lemacidine B$_2$, 104
Lemacidine B$_3$, 104
Lemonomycin, 104—105
Leucinamycin, 105
Leucomycin, 105—106
Leucomycin A$_1$, 106
Leucomycin A$_2$, 106
Leucopeptin, 106
Leucylnegamycin, 106
Leupeptin, 106
Levomycin, 106—107
Levorin A, 107
Libanomycin (See lybanomycine)
Licheniformin A, 107
Licheniformin B, 107
Licheniformin C, 107
Lincomycin, 107—109
Lincomycin B, 108, 109
Lincomycin, S-ethyl homolog, 108
Lipoxamycin, 109
Lividomycin, 110
Lividomycin A, 110
Lividomycin B, 110
Lomofungin, 111
Lybanomycine A, 111
Lybanomycine B, 111
Lybanomycine C, 111
Lydimycin, 111

Marcarbomycin, 112
Macrocin, 112
Macromomycin, 112
Magnamycin (cf. carbomycin), 112—113
Mannosidostreptomycin, 113, 174

Maridomycins, 113
Maridomycin I, 113
Maridomycin II, 113
Maridomycin III, 113
Maridomycin IV, 113
Maridomycin V, 113
Maridomycin VI, 113
Megalomicins, 113–114
Megalomicin A, 114
Megalomicin B, 114
Megalomicin C_1, 114
Megalomicin C_2, 114
Melinacidins, 114–115
Melinacidin II, 115
Melinacidin III, 115
Melinacidin IV, 115
Methacycline, 189
Methicillin, 140, 142, 145
Methoxy carbonyl-acetylamino-cephalo-
    sporanic acid, 50
3'-Methyl-3'-dechloropyrrolnitrin, 161
6-Methylene oxytetracycline, 183, 190
6-Methylenetetracycline, 190
Methylpenicillin, 139
Methymycin, 115
Miamycin, 115
Micromonospora chalcea antibiotic, 115
Micromonosporin, 115–116
Micropolysporin A, 116
Micropolysporin B, 116
Miniatomicin M_2, 116–117
Miniatomicin M_3, 116–117
Minimycin, 117
Mitochromin A, 117
Mitochromin B, 117
Mitochromin C, 117
Mitochromin D, 117
Moenomycins, 118–119
Moenomycin A, 118, 119
Moenomycin B, 119
Moenomycin B_1, 118
Moenomycin B_2, 118
Moenomycin C, 118, 119
Moenomycin D, 118
Moenomycin E, 118
Moenomycin F, 118
Moenomycin G, 118
Moenomycin H, 118
Monamycins, 119–120
Monamycin A, 119, 120

Monamycin B, 119, 120
Monamycin B_1, 119
Monamycin B_2, 119
Monamycin B_3, 119
Monamycin C, 119
Monamycin D_1, 119
Monamycin D_2, 119
Monamycin E, 119
Monamycin F, 119
Monamycin G_1, 119
Monamycin G_2, 119
Monamycin G_3, 119
Monamycin H_1, 119
Monamycin H_2, 119
Monamycin I, 119
Monazomycin, 120
Monensin A, 120
Monensin B, 120
Monensin C, 120
Monensin D, 120
Monoacetyloleandomycin, 132
1-monoacetyloleandomycin, 132
2-monoacetyloleandomycin, 132
3-monoacetyloleandomycin, 132
Mycobacillin, 120–121
Mycobactocidin Fraction B, 121
Mycobactocidin Fraction D, 121
Mycophenolic acid, 121
Mycorhodin A, 121
Mycorhodin B, 121
Mycothricin complex, 176
Mycotrienin, 121

Naematolin, 121
Nafcillin, 142
Neamine (See neomycin A), 123, 124,
    125, 127
Nebramycin, 122–123
Nebramycin Factor 1, 122
Nebramycin Factor 1', 122
Nebramycin Factor 2, 122, 123
Nebramycin Factor 3, 122, 123
Nebramycin Factor 4, 122, 123
Nebramycin Factor 5, 122, 123
Nebramycin Factor 6 (cf. tobramycin),
    122, 123
Negamycin, 123
Neocarzinostatin, 123
Neomycins (See also N-acetyl neomycins),
    123–128

Neomycin A (See neamine), 123, 124, 125, 127
Neomycin B, 124, 125, 126, 127, 128
Neomycin C, 124, 125, 126, 127, 128
Neopluramycin, 128
Neomycin methanesulfonate, 124
Netropsin, 30, 128
Neutramycin, 128
Niddamycin, 128–129
Nifimycin, 129
Nogalamycin, 129
Nogalarol, 130
Nogalarene, 130
Novobiocin, 130
Novobiocin acid, 130
Nystatin, 130–131

Ochramycin, 131
Oleandomycins, 131–133
Oleandomycin base, 132
Oleficin, 132–133
Oligomycin, 133
Olivomycin, 133
Oncastatin C, 23
Oospora virescens (Link) Vallr. antibiotic glycosides, 133
Oryzoxymycin, 133–134
Ossamycin, 134
Oudemansiella mucida antibiotic, 134
Oxacillin, 140, 142, 145
Oxychlortetracycline, reduction product of, 185
Oxypyrrolnitrin, 161
Oxytetracycline (See hydroxytetracycline; tetracycline; specific derivatives), 134, 181, 182, 183, 184, 187, 189
5-oxytetracycline, 190
Oxytocin, 134

Paecilomycerol, 134–135
Paromomycin, 135
Pathocidin, 135
Patulin, 135
Peliomycin, 135–136
Penicillanic acid, 145
Penicillins (See also benzylpenicillins; 6-amino penicillanic acid; penicillin G; specific penicillins), 136–146
Penicillin F, 137
Penicillin FH$_2$, 137

Penicillin G (cf. benzylpenicillin), 136, 137, 138, 139, 145
Penicillin K, 137
Penicillin V, 137, 139, 145
Penicillin X, 137, 139
Penicillin 1, 137
Penicillin 2, 137
Penicillin 3, 137
Penicillin 4, 137
Penicillin nucleus (cf. 6-Amino penicillanic acid)
Penicillins derived from:
    ε-Aminocaproic acid, 140
    DL-α-aminophenylacetamine, 140
    p-Aminophenylacetamide, 140
    m-Aminophenylacetic acid, 140
    p-Aminophenylacetic acid, 140
    D-α-aminophenylacetylglycine, 140
    γ-Amino-n-valeric acid, 140
    Benzoylglycine, 140
    Butylthioacetic acid, 140
    n-Butyric acid, 140
    Carboxylic acids, 140
    p-Chlorophenoxyacetic acid, 140
    3,4-Dichloro-α-methoxybenzyl side chain, 145
    3,4-Dichlorophenylacetic acid, 140
    3,4-Dihydroxyphenylacetic acid, 140
    Ethionine, 138
    S-Ethylcysteine, 138
    DL-α-Ethylphenylacetic acid, 140
    2-Furylmethylpenicillin methyl ester, 141
    Heptanamide, 140
    n-Heptanoic acid, 140
    Heptanoylglycine, 140
    Hexanamide, 140
    n-Hexanoic acid, 140
    3-Hexanoic acid, 140
    Hexanoylglycine, 140
    Homogentisic acid lactone, 140
    p-Hydroxy-α-hydroxyphenylacetic acid, 140
    α-Hydroxyisocaproic acid, 140
    DL-α-hydroxyphenylacetic acid, 140
    p-Hydroxphenylacetic acid, 140
    α-Ketophenylacetic acid, 140
    DL-α-hydroxyphenylacetylglycine, 140
    DL-mandelamide, 140
    Methionine, 138

DL-α-Methoxyphenylacetic acid, 140
p-Methoxyphenylacetic acid, 140
S-methylcysteine, 138
α-Methyl-α-hydroxyphenylacetic acid,
  140
1-Naphthylacetic acid, 140
2-Naphthylacetic acid, 140
n-Octanoic acid, 140
Octanoylglycine, 140
Phenoxyacetic acid, 140
Phenoxyacetylglycine, 140
Phenoxy methylpenicillin methyl
  ether, 138
DL-α-phenoxypropionamide, 140
DL-α-phenoxypropionylglycine, 140
Phenylacetic acid, 140
N-phenylacetyl-cyclic-DL-cysteinyl-D-
  valine, 141
Phenylacetylglycine, 140
N-phenylglycine, 140
Pimelic acid, 140
n-Propoxymethylpenicillin cyanomethyl
  ester, 141
2-Thienylacetic acid, 141
Valeramide, 141
n-Valeric acid, 141
Valerylglycine, 141
Perimycin, 146
Petrin, 146
Phenazines, 146–147
1,6-phenazinediol, 146
1,6-phenazinediol-5,10 dioside (Iodinin),
  146, 147
Phenethicillin, 139, 141, 142
D-Phenethicillin, 145
L-Phenethicillin, 145
Phenethicillin K, 142
Phenomycin, 147
Phenoxazinones, 146
α-phenoxyethylpenicillin side-chain, 145
Phenoxylethyl penicillin, 140
Phenoxymethylpenicillanic acid, 143
Phenoxymethyl penicillic acid, 143
Phenoxymethyl penicillin, 140, 141, 143,
  145
Phenoxymethyl penicillin K, 142
Phenoxymethyl penicilloic acid, 143
Phenoxymethyl penilloic acid, 143
7-phenylacetamido-cephalosporanic acid,
  49

N-phenylacetyl cephalosporin C, 47, 51
N-phenylacetyl cephalosporin C_C, 47, 51
Phleomycins, 147–148
Phleomycin C, 147, 148
Phleomycin D, 147
Phleomycin D_1, 147, 148
Phleomycin D_2, 147, 148
Phleomycin E, 147, 148
Phleomycin F, 147, 148
Phleomycin G, 147, 148
Phleomycin H, 147, 148
Phleomycin I, 147, 148
Phleomycin J, 147, 148
Phleomycin K, 147, 148
Phosphonomycin, 148–149
Picromycin, 149
Pilosomycins, 149
Pilosomycin A, 149
Pilosomycin B, 149
Pimaricin, 150
Piomycin, 150
Pleocidin complex, 176
Plicacetin, 151
Plurallin, 151
Polyangium cellulosum var. *fulvum*
  antibiotic, 151
Polyetherin A, 151–152
Polyfungins, 152
Polyketo acidomycin (PKAM), 152
Polymyxins, 152–155
Polymyxin A, 152, 153, 154
Polymyxin A_1, 153, 154
Polymyxin A_2, 153, 154
Polymyxin B, 125, 126, 152, 153, 154
Polymyxin B_1, 153, 154
Polymyxin B_2, 153, 154
Polymyxin D, 152, 154
Polymyxin E, 152, 153, 154
Polymyxin E-methane-sulfonate, 154
Polymyxin E_1, 153, 154
Polymyxin E_2, 153, 154
Polymyxin M, 154
Polyoxins, 155–156
Polyoxin A, 155, 156
Polyoxin B, 155, 156
Polyoxin D, 155, 156
Polyoxin E, 155, 156
Polyoxin F, 155, 156
Polyoxin G, 155, 156
Polyoxin H, 155, 156

Polyoxin I, 155, 156
Porfiromycin, 156
Prechromene A, 170
Primycin, 156
Proactinomycins, 156–157
Proactinomycin A, 157
Proactinomycin B, 157
Proactinomycin C, 157
Proceomycin, 157
Propionyl erythromycin, 71
Propionyl holothin, 90
Proticin, 157
Protomycin, 157
Prumycin, 157–158
Prunacetin, 158
Pseudomonas antifungal substance, 158
Psicofuranine, 158–159
Pyracrimycin A, 159
Pyridomycin, 159
Pyrrole antibiotic from Marine Bacterium,
  159–160
Pyrrolnitrin, 160–161

Quinomycins, 161–162
Quinomycin A, 161, 162
NX Quinomycin A, 162
QN Quinomycin A, 162
Quinomycin B, 161
Quinomycin B_0, 161
Quinomycin C, 161
Quinomycin D, 161
Quinomycin E, 161

Rabelomycin, 162
Racemomycin, 162
Racemomycin A, 162
Racemomycin B, 162
Racemomycin C, 162
Racemomycin D, 162
Ramnacin, 162
Relomycin, 162
Resistaphyllin, 162
Rhodomycins, 163
Rhodomycin A, 163
iso-Rhodomycin A, 163
Rhodomycin B, 163
iso-Rhodomycin B, 163
Rifampicin, 164
Rifamycins, 163–164
Rifamycin A, 163, 164

Rifamycin B, 163, 164
Rifamycin C, 163, 164
Rifamycin D, 163, 164
Rifamycin E, 163, 164
Rifamycin O, 163, 164
Rifamycin S, 163, 164
Rifamycin SV, 163, 164
Rimocidin, 165
Ristocetin, 165
Ristocetin A, 165
Ristocetin B, 165
Roridines, 166
Roridine A, 166
Roridine B, 166
Roridine C, 166
Roridine D, 166
Roridine E, 166
Rosamicin (See 67-694)
Roseothricin A, 176
Roseothricin B, 176
Roseothricin C, 176
Rubidin, 166
Rubiflavin, 166
Rubradirin, 166–167

Safynol, 167
Sarganin, 167
Sclerothricin, 167–168
Scopafungin, 168
Senfolomycins, 168
Senfolomycin A, 168
Senfolomycin B, 168
Shartresin, 168
Shincomycins, 169
Shincomycin A, 169
Shincomycin B, 169
Showdomycin, 169–170
Siccanin, 170
Siccanochromene A, 170
Siccanochromene B, 170
Siomycins, 170
Siomycin A, 170
Siomycin B, 170
Siomycin C, 170
Sisomicin, 171
Sparsogenin, 171
Sparsomycin, 171
Sphaeropsidin, 171
Spinamycin, 171–172
Sporangiomycin, 172

Sporocytophage cauliformis antibiotic, 172
Sporoviridinin, 172
Staphylomycin, 172–173
Steffisburgensimycin, 173
Streptimidone, 173
Streptolin, 173
Streptolin A, 173
Streptolin B, 173
Streptolydigin, 173
Streptomyces collinus, Lindenbein dipeptide antibiotic, 173–174
Streptomyces ramocissimus antibiotic, 174
Streptomyces viridochromogenes antibiotic, 174
Streptomycin, 174–175
Streptonigrin, 175
Streptonivicin, 175–176
Streptothricin; streptothricin-like antibiotics, 176
Streptothricin VI, 176
Streptovaricin, 176–177
Streptovaricin A, 176, 177
Streptovaricin B, 176, 177
Streptovaricin C, 176, 177
Streptovaricin D, 176, 177
Streptovaricin E, 176, 177
Streptovitacins, 177–178
Streptozotocin, 178
Subsporins, 178
Subsporin A, 178
Subsporin B, 178
Subsporin C, 178
Subtilin, 178
Succinimycin, 178–179
Sulfocidin, 179
Sulfomycins, 179
Sulfomycin I, 179
Sulfomycin II, 179
Sulfomycin III, 179

Taimycines, 180 (cf. Thaimycins)
Taimycine A, 180
Taimycine B, 180
Taimycine C, 180
Tbilimycin, 180
Tennecetin, 180
Tertiomycins, 180–181
Tertiomycin A, 180, 181

Tertiomycin B, 180
Tetracyclines (See: specific derivatives; chlortetracycline; demethylchlortetracycline; doxycycline; hydroxytetracycline; methacycline; oxytetracycline, tetracycline) 181–190
Tetracycline, 181, 182, 183, 184, 186, 187, 188, 189, 190
Tetracycline epimers, 184
Tetramycin, 190–191
Tetranactin, 191
Tetrangomycin, 191
Tetrin, 191
Thaimycins, 191–192 (cf. Taimycines)
2-Thienylmethylcephalosporin, 141
2-Thienylmethylcephalosporin pyridine, 141
(+)-1-Thiogriseofulvin, 86
Thiolutin, 192
Thiopeptins, 192
Thiopeptin A_1, 192
Thiopeptin A_2, 192
Thiopeptin A_3, 192
Thiopeptin A_4, 192
Thiopeptin B, 192
Thiostrepton, 192
Tilomycin, 193
Tobramycin (See: nebramycin factor 6)
Tolypomycin R, 193
Tolypomycin Y, 193
Tomaymycin, 193–194
Trehalosamine, 194
Triacetyloleandomycin, 132
Trichomycin, 194
Trienine, 194
4'-Trifluoromethyl-3'-dechloroaminopyrrolnitrin, 161
Triostin, 194–195
Triostin A, 195
Triostin B, 195
Triostin C, 195
6-Tritylamino-penicillanic acid, 145
Trypanomycin A_2, 195
Tsushimycin, 195
Tuberactinomycins, 196
Tuberactinomycin A, 196
Tuberactinomycin B^2, 196
Tuberactinomycin N, 196
Tuberactinomycin O, 196
Tumimycin, 196

Tylosin, 196–197
Tyrothricin, 197

Umbrinomycin, 197

Validamycins, 197–198
Validamycin A, 198
Validamycin B, 198
Validamycin C, 198
Validamycin D, 198
Validamycin E, 198
Validamycin F, 198
Vancomycin, 198–199
Variotin, 199
Venturicidins, 199
Venturicidin A, 199
Venturicidin B, 199
Venturicidin X, 199
Vermiculine, 199
Verrucarines, 199–200
Verrucarine A, 199
Verrucarine B, 199, 200
Verrucarine C, 199
Verrucarine D, 199
Verrucarine E, 199
Verrucarine F, 199
Verrucarine G, 199
Verrucarine H, 200
Verrucarine J, 200
Versicolin, 200
Viomycin, 200–201

Xanthocidin, 201
Xanthomycin A, 201

Yazumycin, 201
Yeminimycin, 201–202

Zorbamycin; zorbonomycins, 202
Zorbonamycin B, 202
Zorbonomycin C, 202
Zygomycins, 202
Zygomycin A, 202
Zygomycin B, 202
Zygosporins, 202–203
Zygosporin A, 203
Zygosporin D, 203
Zygosporin E, 203
Zygosporin F, 203
Zygosporin G, 203

VIIa, 176
IXa, 176
15 A, 203
15 B, 203
15 C, 203
15 D, 203
15 E, 203
15 F, 203
19 A, 203
136, 176
67-694 (rosamicin), 203
106-7, 204
136 A, 204
136 B, 204
136 C, 204
136 D, 204
136 E, 204
289 F, 204
289 FO, 204
Acetyl 289 F, 204
460, 204
1985/11, 204–205
2814 P, 205
3035/48, 205
3950, 205
4205 A, 205
4205 B, 205
4205 C, 205
6270, 205
16,511 R.P., 205, 206
16,511 A, 206
16,511 B, 206
16,511 C, 206
16,511 D, 206
17,967 RP, 206
18,051 RP, 206
18,631 RP, 206
19,402 RP, 206–207
24010, 207
A204, 207
A-396-I, 207
A/672, 208
A4993A, 208
A4993B, 208
A16884, 208–209
A16886B factor A, 209
A16886B factor B, 209
A16886-I, 209
A16886-II, 209
A-21101, 209–210

A22765, 210
AB-664α, 210
ABBOTT 29119, 210
AC-98 mixture, 210
AC-98 complex A, 210
AC-98 complex B, 210
AC541A, 210–211
AC541B, 210–211
AF 283α, 211
AF283β, 211
AO-341, 211
B4-81, 211
B-2847-R, 211–212
B-2847-Y, 211–212
B-15645, 212
BA-6903, 212
BD-12, 212–213
CP 21,635, 213
E-749-C, 213
G-253A, 214
G-253B, 214
G-253B$_1$, 214
G-253B$_2$, 214
G-253C, 214
G-253C$_1$, 214
K-288, 214
L.A. 5352, 214
L.A. 5937, 215
LA-7017, 133, 215
LL-21220, 215
LL-AB664, 215
LL-AC541, 215
LL-AO341A, 216
LL-AO341B, 216
LL-AV290, 216
LL-BL136 (cf. SF-701), 216
MSD-235S$_1$, 216
MSD-235S$_2$, 216
MSD-235S$_3$, 216
NSCA-649, 133, 216–217
O-2867α, 217
O-2867β, 217
PA-108, 217
PA-133A, 217
PA-133B, 217
PA-148, 217
R-468, 217–218

Ro 5-2667, 218
Ro 7-7730, 218
Ro 7-7731, 218
S-520, 218
DNP-S-520, 218
Acetyl-S-520, 218
S-583-A-II, 218
S-583-A-III, 218
S-583-B, 218
S-666, 218–219
SF-689, 219
SF-701, 219
SF-733, 219–220
SF-767-A, 220
SF-767-L, 220
n-Acetyl SF-767-A, 220
n-Acetyl SF-767-L, 220
SF-837, 220
SF-837-A$_2$, 220
SF-837-A$_3$, 220
SF-837-A$_4$, 220
T-2636, 220–221
T-2636 A, 221
T-2636B, 221
T-2636C, 221
T-2636D, 221
T-2636E, 221
T-2636-F, 221
T-2636M, 221
TA2407, 221
U-11,973, 108
U-12,898, 221–222
U-13,714, 222
U-13,933, 222
U-20,661, 222
U-21,699, 108
U-21,963, 223
U-22,324, 223
U-22,956, 223
VD 844, 223
YA 56-X, 223
YA 56-Y, 223
YC 73, 224
YL 704 A$_1$, 224
YL 704A$_2$, 224
YL 704B$_1$, 224
YL 704B$_2$, 224